Intraoperative Pathologic Diagnosis

FROZEN SECTION
AND OTHER TECHNIQUES

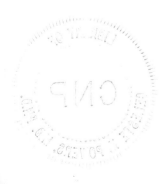

Intraoperative Pathologic Diagnosis

FROZEN SECTION AND OTHER TECHNIQUES

Elvio G. Silva, M.D.

Associate Professor
Department of Pathology
M. D. Anderson Hospital and Tumor Institute
Houston, Texas

B. Balfour Kraemer, M.D.

Department of Pathology
St. John's Mercy Medical Center
St. Louis, Missouri
Formerly
Faculty Associate
Department of Pathology
M. D. Anderson Hospital and Tumor Institute
Houston, Texas

With additional chapters by
John G. Batsakis, M.D.
Luis Guarda, M.D.
Bernd W. Scheithauer, M.D.

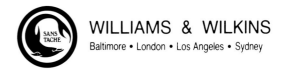

WILLIAMS & WILKINS
Baltimore • London • Los Angeles • Sydney

Editor: Timothy H. Grayson
Associate Editor: Carol Eckhart
Copy Editor: Kay Casteel
Design: JoAnne Janowiak
Illustration Planning: Wayne Hubbel
Production: Anne G. Seitz

Copyright © 1987
Williams & Wilkins
428 East Preston Street
Baltimore, MD 21202, U.S.A.

Accurate indications, adverse reactions, and dosage schedules for drugs are provided in this book, but it is possible that they may change. The reader is urged to review the package information data of the manufacturers of the medications mentioned.

Printed in the United States of America

Library of Congress Catologing-in-Publication Data

Intraoperative pathologic diagnosis.

    Includes index.
    1. Pathology, Surgical—Technique.   2. Frozen
tissue sections. I. Silva, Elvio G. [DNLM: 1. Microtomy
—methods. WO 142 I61]
RD57.I67 1987   616.07'583   86-13321
ISBN 0-683-07711-2

87 88 89 90 91   10 9 8 7 6 5 4 3 2

To my wife, Betty, and children, Natalia and Nicholas,
for their love, patience, and support.

ELVIO G. SILVA

To my husband, Bruce,
for his encouragement, support, forbearance,
and sustaining love.

B. BALFOUR KRAEMER

Preface

Over the years, the traditional practice of surgical pathology has been expanded by the application of electron microscopy, immunocytochemistry, and flow cytometry. New techniques, such as DNA hybridization, and an increasing reliance upon computers will undoubtedly further expand our diagnostic abilities in the future. Amidst such technologic advances, the frozen section has remained a valid and indispensable tool by which important therapeutic decisions are made. Since the impact of a given frozen section diagnosis is often great, the diagnostic process can create stressful moments in the life of the pathologist. Surprisingly, no source of information has heretofore been compiled to assist the pathologist with intraoperative diagnostic difficulties, or to help delineate the implications of a particular frozen section interpretation.

This text is designed for use at the time of frozen section. Both pathologists and surgeons should find it a helpful reference. The fact that it is arranged according to organ systems should make for convenient access to a desired topic. On occasion, the reader will find some overlap; the same topic may be discussed in two different sections. Here, two different authors have provided commentary on their respective approaches to a given problem. In addition, there is a separate chapter devoted exclusively to neuroendocrine neoplasms. The overall emphasis placed on neoplastic proliferations reflects the nature of accessions examined at a large referral center (M. D. Anderson Hospital and Tumor Institute). Experience provided by a high volume of frozen sections has allowed us to develop what we believe is a comprehensive analysis of the problems and situations most likely to be encountered at the time of frozen section.

Our book represents a unique offering. By sharing our combined experience with frozen section diagnosis, we hope to benefit those like ourselves who are fated to struggle with the frozen section and, of necessity, must not be confounded by it.

E.G.S.
B.B.K.

Acknowledgments

We wish to express our thanks to the supervisor of our frozen section laboratory, Mrs. Betty McKinney, and to our laboratory technicians, Mrs. Patricia Wilson and Mrs. Imogene Petitt, for their excellent assistance. We express our deep gratitude to the M. D. Anderson Pathology staff for their support, collaboration, and expert advice. We are indebted to the following surgeons at M. D. Anderson Hospital and Tumor Institute who offered their valuable suggestions and constructive criticism: Drs. Richard Martin, Helmuth Goepfert, Felix Rutledge, David Swanson, Robert McKenna, and Douglas Johnson. We extend our appreciation to Dr. Scott Martin, Director, Surgical Pathology, St. John's Mercy Medical Center, St. Louis, Missouri for his helpful advice and useful comments. We also thank Mrs. Brenda Clayton, Mrs. Elsa Ramos, Mrs. Kathy Shanks, and Mr. Mannie Steglich for their assistance in the preparation of this book.

Contributors

John G. Batsakis, M.D.
Professor and Chairman, Department of Pathology
M. D. Anderson Hospital and Tumor Institute
Houson, Texas

Luis Guarda, M.D.
Department of Pathology
Florida Hospital
Orlando, Florida
formerly
Assistant Professor, Department of Pathology
M. D. Anderson Hospital and Tumor Institute
Houston, Texas

Bernd W. Scheithauer, M.D.
Associate Professor, Department of Pathology
Mayo Graduate School of Medicine
Rochester, Minnesota

Contents

1

Preparing and Evaluating Frozen Tissue Sections: Techniques and Cytology

Elvio G. Silva, M.D.

The methods to be used in diagnosing frozen tissue sections will vary with the number of frozen sections needed, the staff working in the frozen section laboratory, the technicians' familiarity with a given method, and the pathologists' preferences. These are probably the reasons that no method for frozen section diagnosis has been universally accepted.

The method selected for tissue freezing is usually related to the laboratory's work load. In our department, in which an average of 75 frozen sections is performed daily and there are five full time technicians at work, we prefer to use the dry-ice box technique, a method of tissue freezing that allows us to freeze 40 blocks of tissue in two separate boxes at any given time with a high degree of safety and efficiency. In a frozen section laboratory with an average of five frozen sections a day and fewer technical personnel, an entirely different situation is presented. Under these conditions, a device that uses Freon, isopentane, or liquid nitrogen may be more efficient.

Methods of fixation, dehydration, staining, and hydration of the frozen tissue sections also depend on the technicians' and pathologists' preferences. Some centers use cytologic preparations, which in some cases might obviate the need for frozen section.

In this chapter, different methods of preparing frozen sections are discussed, and the most common problems in frozen section technique and evaluation are outlined.

INDICATIONS FOR FROZEN SECTION

The primary reasons for preparing and evaluating a frozen tissue section are as follows: *a*) to obtain a diagnosis from which a therapeutic decision may be made, such as checking the margins of resection, determining the extent of disease and type of operation needed, and identifying the tissue in question; *b*) to ascertain the adequacy of the biopsy material; and *c*) to provide tissue for ancillary studies.

Margins of Resection

Tissue sections are not usually taken to confirm resection margins when the tumor and margin of the specimen are separated by 3 (or more) cm of uninvolved tissue. When the margins must be examined microscopically, the first step is to study a representative tumor section. This will help the pathologist to better search out areas of tumor in the resection margins if he is acquainted with the features of the primary. The second step is to section the margin and avoid contaminating it with tumor cells during the procedure. To achieve this, blades are changed after the tumor is sectioned. If tumor is intentionally sectioned in continuity with a respective margin, the section should be made such that the area containing tumor is sectioned last.

An acceptable pathology report on the margins of resection includes information on the margin itself and the distance from tumor to margin; the latter is often important in differentiating between a margin and a safe margin. In endocrine carcinoma of the skin (Merkel cell carcinoma), for example, a safe margin means that a tumor is more than 2.0 mm from the margin (1). The report of a negative margin for this tumor could be meaningless if the tumor was 0.5 mm from the margin. There is no ideal method for checking margins of resection. A section perpendicular to the margin for the purposes of determining distance from tumor to margin is often performed, but such a section will usually not sample the entire margin of resection. A tissue section parallel to the margin, on the other hand, will not be informative about the distance from tumor to margin. We believe that, in most cases, sections perpendicular to the margin and from the area closest to the tumor should be taken to verify a safe margin.

In 1974, a new technique was proposed as an "exacting method for the surgical removal of cutaneous tumors" (2). This technique, a modification of Mohs chemosurgery (3), was called microscopic-controlled excision. Using this method, the surgeon removes the tumor, examines the margins of excision, and submits for microscopic examination, by means of frozen section, tissue from the convex parts of the specimen or, with a second excision, tissue from the surgical defect (4, 5). Sections are always taken parallel to the scalp blade. This technique does not provide information about the distance from tumor to margin (see also Other Indications for Frozen Section, this chapter).

Other Indications for Frozen Section

During surgical operations, frozen section is commonly used to determine the extent of the patient's disease. The information will determine the resectability of the lesion and the extent of the operative procedure. Often this indication for frozen section overlaps with checking the margins of resection.

Probably the most common situation in which frozen section is performed for tissue identification is during exploration of the neck and anterior mediastinum to search for parathyroids. Diagnostic differentiation between parathyroid adenoma and hyperplasia is often based on identification of all the parathyroid glands to determine whether the process involves one or more glands. Since it may be difficult to distinguish parathyroid glands from lymph node and thyroid outgrowths, frozen sections help to make this distinction.

When frozen section is used to confirm the presence of the lesion in question in the biopsy material, the procedure will avoid a delay in diagnosis and a second operation. This is so for patients who have tumors with extensive fibrosis, ulceration, and necrosis and for patients whose lesions cannot be biopsied without general anesthesia or who have lesions in difficult to visualize areas, such as the nasopharynx.

Frozen sections are used also for ancillary studies of tissues, such as tissue markers in lymphomas.

Contraindications

In our experience, the only contraindication for freezing tissue is a situation in which the sample submitted for examination is so small that it is impossible to process enough tissue for permanent section. Our arbitrary minimum is 3 mm for the tissue's largest dimension, a sample size that is difficult to bisect without creating crush artifacts. Most of the time there is not enough residual tissue to make a diagnosis on the basis of the permanent section. The situation obviously varies in each case and applies with regularity only in cases without a previous definite diagnosis.

TISSUE FREEZING

The specimen received for frozen section examination should be fresh and free of excess moisture, but not entirely dry. Wrapping the specimen in gauze with saline solution may produce severe artifacts and create holes in the tissue.

During the freezing of tissue, water molecules aggregate into ice crystals, and once the nuclei of the crystals are formed, they expand and destroy all organelles around them. When the frozen section is picked up with a warm slide, the thawing ice crystals will leave holes in the tissue. The number of crystals in tissue is inverse to the speed of tissue freezing (6, 7). Thus, slow-freezing methods should be avoided.

Use of a specimen holder (tissue chuck) is a good technique for freezing tissue because the metal has high thermal conductivity. A supporting medium is needed in this situation to make the tissue adhere to the specimen holder. A few years ago, the medium of choice was saline; but now the one in widest use is optimal cutting temperature solution (OCT). This polysaccharide, a mixture of glycols and resins, is water-soluble and will rinse away during fixation and staining. Different types of OCT solidify at different temperatures: $-10°$ to $-20°C$, $-20°$ to $-35°C$, and $-35°$ to $-50°C$. We use the middle one. OCT is applied to the corrugated surface of the specimen holder (the surface promotes OCT adhesion), then the specimen is deposited on the OCT and frozen on the holder.

We use the slide method in setting the tissue on top of the specimen holder, selecting the face from which the frozen section is cut and placing this slide downward on a glass slide. The slide is then inverted on top of the specimen holder containing OCT, and the tissue is placed on it. We prefer slides to forceps in setting tissue on top of the holder, because with this method we can be certain that the desired surface will be cut. In addition, after the tissue is set on the OCT, exerting minor pressure with the glass slide helps to create a flat surface for cutting, which will substantially reduce the need for specimen trimming. For small specimens, a cork disc can be placed between the holder and the specimen.

Rapid freezing of the tissue depends on the size of the specimen, the temperature of the cooling agent, and the rate at which heat is removed from the specimen (the three basic characteristics of heat transfer). Specimen size is very important, because all freezing techniques dissipate the heat present on the tissue surface; thinner specimens will, of course, freeze faster. The ideal thickness is probably 1 to 2 mm; and tissue to be frozen should never be thicker than 3 mm.

Tables 1.1 and 1.2 list some coolant characteristics. The ideal coolant is liquid, with a boiling point above room temperature, a freezing point as low as possible, low viscosity near the freezing point, and high thermal conductivity (8). By these criteria, isopentane is the best coolant, followed by Freon; but many laboratory workers prefer Freon because isopentane is highly flammable (ignition temperature, 420°C). In addition, near the freezing point, Freon is less viscous than isopentane.

The thermal conductivity of nitrogen, isopentane, and Freon differs significantly. Liquid nitrogen forms a "film coat," an insulated layer of vapor, around the specimen, which interferes with heat transfer. Isopentane and Freon have high thermal conductivity, because they do not form such coats.

Among these three biochemical components, liquid nitrogen is the only one that does not require a special cooling method; as long as it is maintained in a liquid state, its temperature will be between $-209°$ and

Table 1.1.
Most Commonly Used Coolants and Different Methods of Tissue Freezing

Coolant	Temperature Obtained, °C	Freezing Time, s	Disadvantages
Liquid nitrogen	−196	10	Produces a film coat that interferes with heat transfer Frostbite Requires constant supply In nonventilated areas, N_2 may consume O_2
Isopentane	−40 to −60	25	Explosive Requires constant supply
Freon	−40 to −60	25	Requires constant supply
Dry-ice box	−60	30	Requires constant supply
CO_2 quick-freeze	−40 to −70	15	Cumbersome Requires constant supply
Quick-freeze	−30	110	
Rapid-freeze attachment or heat extractor box	−35	90	Number of specimens that may be frozen depends on brand of cryostat

Table 1.2.
Some Characteristics of Biochemical Coolants[a]

Coolant	Freezing[b] Point, °C	Boiling[c] Point, °C
Liquid nitrogen	−209	−195
Isopentane (2-methyl butane)	−160	27.9
Freon (chlorofluorocarbon)	−160	−29

[a]Indicates temperature limit between solid and liquid phases.
[b]Below this temperature the biochemical component will become solid.
[c]Indicates temperature at which a liquid will transform into a gas.

−195°C. Isopentane and Freon are maintained at −40° and −60°C by surrounding their containment vessel with a second container filled with dry ice or liquid nitrogen or by use of an electronic device that creates a cold bath with magnetic stirring. These devices reach −60°C in 30 min.

FREEZING DEVICES

To freeze tissue in the different coolants, the tissue block is immersed in the coolant container by means of special forceps. Since this could be a problem when 10 or more specimens must be frozen at the same time, we use a dry-ice box. This is a styrofoam-insulated, stainless steel box in which are located four metal bars containing five holes each, such that 20 tissue blocks per box can be frozen simultaneously (Fig. 1.1). The holes are filled

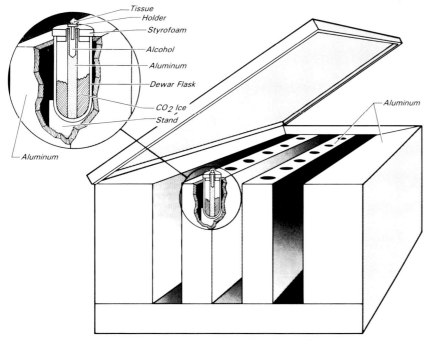

Figure 1.1. Diagram of the dry-ice box.

with 95% ethyl alcohol, which acts as a heat transfer bond (9). To freeze a tissue block, the specimen holder is set in a hole, and a small amount of OCT is laid on the holder's surface. When the OCT begins to solidify, the specimen is placed on it. A layer of OCT between the holder and the bottom part of the specimen prevents the knife from hitting the tissue holder when deeper tissue sections are needed. Placing a cork disc between holder and specimen will also eliminate this problem.

The CO_2 quick-freeze attachment is a device that connects to a cylinder of CO_2. The specimen holder is placed into the device, and the tissue is frozen immediately on contact with the CO_2. The primary difficulty with the CO_2 procedure is that the specimen must be held with forceps, because the flow of CO_2 may displace it from the holder. Some CO_2 quick-freeze attachments include a metal box designed to minimize movement. Cryostats are sometimes equipped with a quick-freeze system powered by the main processor and connected to a lateral bar inside the chamber. Freezing specimens with this system takes more than 1 min, and therefore additional artifacts will be induced.

The quick-freeze attachment, also called a heat extractor block, consists of one or two metal discs applied on top of the specimen to be frozen. The principle of high thermal conductivity is again applied in this device. Since the discs are solid metal, their temperature is probably 10° or 15°C below the temperature in the chamber; they will rapidly transmit this lower temperature to the specimen and extract the heat.

Freon aerosol spray, which is commonly used, is stored in small containers and discharged through a 5-in. flexible nozzle. Freon spray is effective when the surface to be cut in a frozen block has not hardened. In this situation the block is frozen, but, because of manipulation or friction, only a superficial part of the block is not at optimal temperature. However, freezing an entire fresh tissue block with Freon spray is difficult, expensive, and requires more than 1 min of freezing time.

Most tissues are cut well at −10° to −20°C. Extremely soft tissue, such as brain, spleen, adrenal gland, or lymph node, is best cut at −7° to −10°C. A very low temperature of −20° to −40°C is needed for fat. The temperature of the frozen tissue block is usually lower than the optimal temperature at which tissue should be cut, but it will rise from the time the block is taken from the freezing device to the moment it is cut in the cryostat. When the tissue block temperature is too high, the tissue sections will become compressed, forming a mass that adheres to the knife. In this situation, the block may be refrozen by the previously used method or with Freon spray. When the tissue block temperature is too low, the tissue will fragment. In this case, the optimal temperature may be obtained by removing the block from the cryostat or applying the thumb to the top of the block.

Cryostats

Pieter de Riemer, a 19th century anatomist, was probably the first man to freeze tissue by immersing it in a freezing mixture (10). He was trying to discover a method for increasing tissue's consistency in order to obtain sections thin enough to be examined with a microscope. In 1891, Welch was one of the first pathologists to prepare and evaluate a diagnostic frozen section (11). He used CO_2 to freeze tissue taken by Halsted (a biopsy of the breast). Wilson in 1905 and MacCarty in 1929, both working at the Mayo Clinic, gave great impetus to the CO_2 method of freezing tissue (12, 13).

Next in the development of sectioning frozen tissue was the design of a closed cabinet in which the microtome and knife could be maintained at low temperature. Linderstrom-Lang and Mogensen first attempted this in 1938 by placing dry ice inside a cabinet and using a fan to blow the cool air to the front where the microtome was located (14). When a refrigerated system was attached to the cabinet, the unit was designated a cryostat. Russel, Chang, Ibanez, and Speece at The University of Texas M. D. Anderson Hospital and Tumor Institute at Houston in 1955 were the first pathologists to use a closed-chamber cryostat in diagnostic pathology (9, 15, 16). These physicians modified the cryostat Linderstrom-Lang and Mogensen had designed for histochemical research, and they published their results in 1960 (15, 16). At the same time, Klionsky and Nunnally reported their experience with cryostats in surgical pathology (17, 18).

Two types of cryostats are used for freeze sectioning.

The Closed Unit. Tissue blocks are placed in the closed cryostat through a small door, and slides with sections are taken out, although the door remains closed most of the time. All necessary movements in the cryostat are performed with hands covered by special, insulated cryogloves, and the process is observed through at 7 × 7-in. window. The closed cryostat has some disadvantage, because the large cryogloves are clumsy, and operators need experience to operate the instrument.

The Open Top. The open-top cryostat unit has a large sliding top window through which the specimen is introduced, the microtome and knife adjusted, the section made, and the slides taken out.

A microtome that uses CO_2 is not a cryostat, because it is not a cooled chamber containing a microtome. In these CO_2 microtomes, sections tend to adhere to the knife, because it is at room temperature. The major limitations of the CO_2 microtome are the special skills necessary to obtain satisfactory sections (sections are usually thinner than 12 μm and are difficult to obtain). By use of closed or open cryostats it is not difficult to cut sections as thin as 5 μm.

The temperature at which a cryostat should be maintained depends on its use. For surgical pathology, a cryostat should be maintained at −20°C, because this is the best temperature for cutting tissue. Cryostats that reach −40° or −50°C are suitable, therefore, for diagnoses based on surgical frozen sections. If histochemical studies are to be performed on the tissue, the cryostat should be able to reach a temperature of −80°C. In laboratories in which only a small number of frozen sections are done, the cryostat cannot be permanently maintained at −20°C. In this situation, it is advisable to work with a cryostat equipped with a quick-freeze system that can drop the temperature from −10° to −30°C in 5 min or less.

Cryostat Maintenance

One problem with the cryostat, primarily with the open-top unit, is the difficulty of maintaining a uniform temperature throughout the chamber.

Some cryostats are equipped with fans inside the chamber to circulate the cold air, but these fans may also blow small tissue particles around. During sectioning, the knife produces a dynamic energy that is dissipated as heat, so it is important to obtain a temperature reading at the level of the blade. Some cryostats are designed to maintain a specific temperature in the specimen holder that is independent of the temperature in the chamber. When the temperature in the block rises, cryostats equipped with this system save considerable time, because it is unnecessary to cool the entire cabinet to lower the temperature in the tissue block. A main compressor cools the entire cabinet while a second compressor cools the specimen holder area. A small thermostat is located in the area of the specimen holder. Since the temperature of the knife is of paramount importance in preparing frozen sections, the knife blade should always be kept inside the cryostat.

The difference in temperature between the inside of a cryostat and the ambient temperature of the room produces a fog on the cryostat window. Windows heated by electric wires passing through them and by other means have been designed to correct this problem.

When the cold chamber of a cryostat is open to ambience it produces water molecules, which transform into ice crystals in different parts of the cabinet, primarily on the inner walls. In this situation, it is necessary to defrost the cabinet. In our laboratory, cryostats are defrosted every 3 months. Some cryostats have a defrost system connected only to areas in which ice accumulates most frequently. Since ice crystals are rarely seen on the knife, this selective defrost system protects the knife from changes in temperature. Rarely is a microtome out of operation because of the formation of ice crystals; crystals can be dissolved with drops of absolute alcohol, but the previously stiffened parts should then be dried and oiled. Proper maintenance of a microtome will avoid frosting of its parts. In our laboratory, the microtomes are completely cleaned of debris at the end of each day. They are then lubricated with a special low-temperature cryostat oil that protects moving parts and prevents frosting. Some of the adjustment wheels on the microtome are coated with nylon to protect the operator from frostbite.

Cutting Techniques

The technique of cutting tissue in a cryostat is similar to that used for permanent sectioning of tissue embedded in paraffin. The best knife angle for cutting frozen section is 30°. A vertical position of the knife should be avoided to prevent sections from falling to the bottom of the cabinet. Section thickness varies according to the type of tissue, sharpness of microtome knives, and skill of the operator. We try to obtain sections no thicker than 4 to 5 μm. In open-top cryostats, the sections tend to roll over on the surface of the knife, probably because of temperature differences in tissue, knife, and room, a problem that does not usually occur in closed cryostats. To avoid this situation, most open-top cryostats have a transparent plastic antiroll plate. This plate must be positioned immediately over the knife edge and be parallel to and approximately 1/64th of an inch from the knife facet.

The microtome knife may be cleaned with various solutions to lessen compression and eliminate static electricity. Teflon spray, antistatic spray, or solutions containing copper sulfate, stannous chloride, sodium thiosulfate, and sodium chromate may be used to diminish compression and friction. The most common causes of compression, however, are a dull knife, an improper knife angle, and too warm a temperature.

After the sections are cut, they may be picked up from the knife with glass slides, or transferred to a Petri dish containing water and then recovered with a glass slide. The thickness of the sections can be observed in the Petri dish. Sections that float rigidly are too thick, whereas those that fold and unfold freely are of the proper thickness. Tissue sections tend to fold over and often appear wrinkled on the glass slide. A camel hair brush or one of softer, more expensive, sable hair (our preference) is used to unfold and correct the position of the tissue sections.

Slides for use in picking up sections may be outside the cryostat at room temperature or inside the cabinet at $-15°$ to $20°C$. The difference between the cold tissue section and the warmer glass slide is an important factor in the adherence of tissue to slide. We prefer to maintain glass slides inside the cryostat because sections adhere weakly to cold surfaces, allowing for easy correction of folds and wrinkles. When the tissue has flattened on the slide, it is taken out of the cryostat, and the warmer outside temperature helps the tissue adhere to the slide. This can be accelerated by holding the slide face without tissue in one's hand.

Most important in the adherence of tissue to slide is the presence of proteins in the tissue sections. Since fixation denatures proteins, frozen sections cut from fixed tissue will not adhere to slides. To correct for this, slides may be dipped in a solution of gelatin, albumin, chrome alum, and distilled water; the tissue on the slide should be air dried or placed inside a drying oven for several minutes before staining.

FIXATION AND STAINING

We stain frozen sections with hematoxylin and eosin because it preserves them indefinitely and it is a familiar technique. Our fixation and staining procedure has five basic steps (see PROCEDURES AND SOLUTIONS, this chapter; and Fig. 1.2).

1. Fixation

Time required is 30 to 50 s. We prefer to use equal parts of ether and methanol, but formaldehyde solution, 95% alcohol, or a mixture of both (one part formaldehyde at 40% plus nine parts of alcohol), or 100% acetone may also be used. The fastest fixative is methanol (20 to 30 s). For fatty tissue avoid alcoholic fixatives. Fixation will be faster if the fixative is at room temperature. To minimize artifacts, it is preferable to pick up sections with a cold glass slide and to fix the tissue in a solution containing osmium tetroxide, acetone and alcohol at a temperature below $0°C$. This technique is similar to the one used for fixation of tissue by freeze substitution, in which the ice in the tissue is not melted but slowly dissolved (substituted) in a fluid solvent. The principle of this method is that ice is soluble in some solvents at temperatures far below the melting point of ice (19). This method, however, presents some problems when frozen sections are used for diagnosis. It is difficult to maintain the adhesion of a section on a cold slide when it is fixed in a cold fixative, without allowing the temperature of the tissue or slide to increase. Moreover, the use of a cold fixative will prolong the time necessary to obtain a frozen section.

2. Hydration

Time required is 3 to 6 s. This step is necessary to prepare the tissue for staining. We dip the slide in tap water for 3 s, or we add two passages through absolute alcohol and 95% alcohol before a dip in tap water. In our frozen section laboratory, slides are dipped in tetrahydrofuran (THF) before absolute alcohol (Fig. 1.2); the passage through THF helps to clear the tissue.

3. Hematoxylin

Time required is from 45 s to 2 min. After hematoxylin is added (we use Harris's hematoxylin) the slides are rinsed in tap water and passed through 1% aqueous hydrochloric acid to remove excess hematoxylin. An additional step is to use ammonia water (2 drops of ammonia in 50 ml of distilled water), which will enhance the blue color of the hematoxylin.

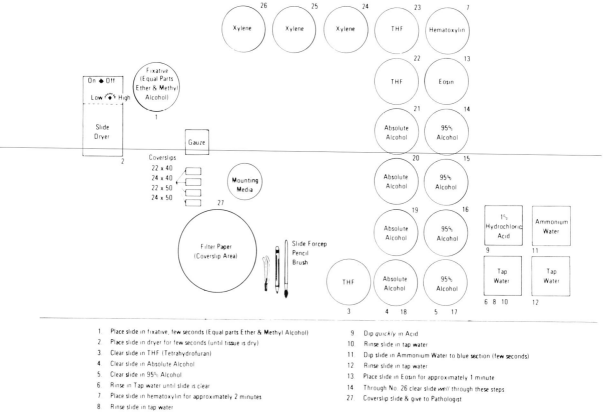

1. Place slide in fixative, few seconds (Equal parts Ether & Methyl Alcohol)
2. Place slide in dryer for few seconds (until tissue is dry)
3. Clear slide in THF (Tetrahydrofuran)
4. Clear slide in Absolute Alcohol
5. Clear slide in 95% Alcohol
6. Rinse in Tap water until slide is clear
7. Place slide in hematoxylin for approximately 2 minutes
8. Rinse slide in tap water
9. Dip *quickly* in Acid
10. Rinse slide in tap water
11. Dip slide in Ammonium Water to blue section (few seconds)
12. Rinse slide in tap water
13. Place slide in Eosin for approximately 1 minute
14. Through No. 26 clear slide *well* through these steps
27. Coverslip slide & give to Pathologist

Figure 1.2. Diagram of the different steps used at M. D. Anderson Hospital for fixation and staining of frozen sections.

4. Eosin

Time required is 20 s to 1 min.

5. Dehydration

Time required is 6 to 30 s. The minimal dehydration necessary can probably be obtained with passages through three steps in alcohol—one in 95% alcohol and two in absolute alcohol. We use four passages through 95% alcohol and four through absolute alcohol. We add two passages through THF to clarify the slide, and three passages through xylene to clear it and facilitate the distribution of the mounting medium over the section.

With toluidine blue and polychrome stains, slides can be stained in less than 2 min and coverslipped with water. The primary disadvantage of this technique is that the color will eventually fade.

Technique for Toluidine Blue or Polychrome Staining

Procedure

1. Fix slide in 100% methanol 0.5 to 2.0 min.
2. Dip slide in toluidine blue or polychrome for 6 to 10 s.
3. Dip in distilled water twice, after which sections may be mounted from water.
4. Dip slide in acetone, two changes, three dips each, then place slide on a warming table at 60°C for 30 to 60 s.
5. Dip slide in xylene, two changes, three dips each.
6. Affix coverslip.

Some polychrome stains are *a*) 1% methylene, blue, 0.5% thionin in 20% alcohol, 1% toluidine blue and 20% alcohol, and *b*) paragon multiple stain: toluidine blue, 0.365 g, basic fuchsin 0.136 g, and ethyl alcohol, 30%, 50 ml.

With these techniques, the nuclei are deep purple to black, and the color of the cytoplasm will vary according to the type of cells. Epithelial cells are pale blue-purple, smooth muscle cells are pale blue, elastic tissue is green-blue, and mast cells are red-purple. When toluidine blue or polychrome stains are used, collagen and cartilage may show only a pale color or they may remain totally unstained, which is the reason why these stains should not be used for lesions containing cartilage.

INTRAOPERATIVE CYTOLOGY

Cytologic preparations of specimens submitted for frozen tissue section evaluation, now widely used, are a valuable adjunct to frozen sections, and they are sometimes essential to diagnosis. The application of cytology to intraoperative diagnoses was introduced by Dudgeon and Patrick in 1927 (20, 21).

Technique

Three types of cytologic preparation are most commonly used for frozen section specimens; smears prepared by scraping the tissue, touch imprints, and the "squash" type of preparation.

Smears prepared by scraping the tissue with a scalpel or glass slide are probably best for cytologic preparations, with the most optimally prepared cells usually found in the middle portion of the smear. Often these smears are too thick and difficult to see at one end, and too thin, showing drying artifacts, at the other end.

Touch imprints are probably the only method for obtaining cytologic preparations when the material submitted for frozen section evaluation is very small, extremely soft, or multi-fragmented.

In the squash preparation, which is especially useful for evaluating brain tumors, a small fragment of tissue is set between two glass slides and the tissue squeezed between the slides with a rotary movement.

Fixation. Cytologic preparations can be air dried or fixed in 95% alcohol. Air-dried slides are usually stained with Romanovsky's solution. Drying the specimen at room temperature will produce only partial denaturation of proteins; the cells will not be entirely fixed. Complete fixation will be obtained by immersing in alcohol (22). If the slide is to be fixed in 95% alcohol, it should be immersed in alcohol immediately, because thin smears or imprints will dry out within seconds. This is particularly important when touch imprints are used. If fixation is delayed to obtain several imprints on one slide, the first imprints will have dried.

Staining. As for frozen sections, hematoxylin and eosin, (see PROCEDURES AND SOLUTIONS, this chapter), Romanovsky's polychrome, and Papanicolaou's stains may be used for routine slides. These cytologic preparations are also useful as special stains for micro-organisms and for immunocytochemistry.

Indications

Cytologic preparations might be useful in many different situations during the evaluations of frozen tissue sections, but the following are instances in which cytologic study is essential for diagnosis.

Epithelial Tumor Versus Lymphoma. Classic examples of this problem of differential diagnosis are thymoma and nasopharyngeal carcinoma versus lymphoma.

Undifferentiated Carcinoma and Some Sarcomas Versus Hodgkin's Disease.

Carcinoma Versus Neuroendocrine Tumors. An example is pancreatic carcinoma versus islet cell tumor.

Pituitary Tumor Versus Normal Pituitary Tissue. We prefer to stain such slides with Papanicolaou's stain because this makes it easier to recognize different cell types in normal pituitary tissue. A cytologic preparation from normal pituitary shows fewer cells than one from pituitary adenoma.

Tumors Characterized by Uniform Cells Difficult to Recognize in Frozen Section. Because of freezing artifacts, oligodendroglioma, for example, may easily be confused with metastatic carcinoma, and the clear cell cytoplasm in renal cell carcinoma may not be appreciated.

In all of these differential diagnoses, the therapeutic approach to patients differs so significantly that every available diagnostic method should be used to achieve accuracy. In these cases, cell characteristics are more important than pattern, and since freezing will affect these characteristics, smears or imprints are vital for diagnosis.

The study of cytologic preparations may be indispensable when evaluating frozen sections, under other conditions, including the following: *a*) frozen sections of a tissue contain bone—for example, the margin of resection or a calcified nodule from a patient with a history of bone tumor—it is advisable to scrape the soft tissue from around the calcification to prepare smears; *b*) when an infectious process is suspected, cytologic study may avoid contamination of cryostats; *c*) in the case of very small biopsies, a diagnosis may be based on cytology while the rest of the tissue is saved for permanent sections; *d*) in the case of necrotic tumor.

The use of cytologic preparations in frozen section evaluation has some other advantages. Since preparing frozen sections takes twice as long as preparing cytologic slides, the pathologist can evaluate the cytology until the tissue sections are ready. Moreover, tissue samples from different areas may be placed on one slide. We sometimes use cytologic instead of frozen section evaluation for patients whose diagnosis seems clear and needs only to be confirmed, as in the case of a cancer patient undergoing lymph node resection. If gross examination suggests carcinoma in the lymph node, cytologic examination will suffice to confirm the diagnosis and will save considerable time.

Finally, our experience includes some rare situations in which cytologic examination is not helpful or may complicate interpretation of the lesion submitted for frozen section evaluation. Some examples are: *a*) tumors, such as nodular lymphomas, in which the pattern is very important, and *b*) extremely soft tumors containing round cells, which, because of technical artifacts of the smear, appear as spindle cells.

TECHNICAL PROBLEMS

Many technical problems may occur during the preparation of tissue sections for study. Some of these are:

Tissue Section Fragmentation

This problem may be caused by a damaged knife or low temperature in the tissue block.

Tissue Section Adherence to the Knife Edge

Possible causes of tissue adherence to the knife are high block temperature and an incorrectly positioned antiroll plate.

Tissue Section Floating During Staining

This problem occurs frequently during staining of small cauterized specimens, necrotic tissue, and cartilage. When we see that a tissue section tends to float (by folding of the margins), we skip steps 9 and 11 (Fig. 1.2; hydrochloric acid and ammonia water in staining); if a tissue tends to float, it will probably do so during these steps.

Precautions to be taken if a section has already floated and a new section is cut include *a*) using a slide dryer after fixation, and *b*) avoiding hydrochloric acid and ammonia water after hematoxylin and water. If tissue sections continue to float, the problem may be corrected by *a*) picking up the section with an albuminated slide; *b*) drying the slide thoroughly before and after fixation; *c*) skipping hydration of tissue and going from fixative to hematoxylin; *d*) using only two changes, 95% alcohol and absolute alcohol, during final dehydration of the slide; and *e*) rinsing carefully. These changes will, however, reduce the final quality of the slide and produce some artifacts.

Tissue Containing Abundant Fat

Fatty tissue tends to fall off the slide. To avoid this problem the following procedures are recommended: *a*) do not use alcohol fixative; *b*) cut the tissue as soon as possible because the lower temperature in the tissue block will facilitate cutting fat; *c*) cut sections thicker; and *d*) wash the tissues carefully.

Adherence Problem of Formaldehyde-Fixed Tissue

Tissue adherence to the slide is difficult to attain after tissue has been fixed, because the proteins have been denatured. Sometimes the sections can be maintained on the slide by dipping it in albumin, 3.0 g of gelatin plus distilled water and 0.5 g of chrome alum, or by letting the tissue dry on the slide before staining.

Frozen sections of formaldehyde-fixed tissue also display large ice crystals, because formaldehyde freezes at $-3°C$ (23). These tissues should be washed before freezing.

Presence of Fungi

If fungi are present over and around the tissue section, but not actually within the tissue itself, this is an indication that contamination occurred during some step in the frozen section procedure, and most probably is from the OCT medium.

ARTIFACTS AND SPECIAL PROBLEMS

Tissue Quality

One of the important elements in frozen section based diagnosis is ensuring that the quality of the frozen tissue will allow accurate evaluation. We have seen *serious* mistakes in frozen section diagnoses that have resulted from overinterpretation of suboptimally prepared sections. For example, the crush artifact commonly seen in permanent tissue sections of small undifferentiated (oat) cell carcinoma, was used to support the frozen section based diagnosis of oat cell carcinoma in a lung lesion. This is a very dangerous situation, because, for a given neoplasm, diagnostic artifacts present on permanent tissue section may not necessarily be present in the frozen section. The pathologist should observe viable cells without artifacts before making a definite diagnosis.

Irradiation Change

One great difficulty in frozen section based diagnosis is the evaluation of tissues that have been irradiated. This is probably the most frequently encountered diagnostic pitfall in frozen section evaluation of soft tissue neoplasms. Epithelial structures may also be affected. In our experience, the most reliable histologic indicator of irradiation change is the presence of atypical cells scattered in an isolated, random fashion. Uniformly atypical cells or atypical cells forming solid areas argue for a neoplastic rather than a reactive process (see also chapter 14, **Bone, Radiation-Injured Tissue, Skin, and Soft Tissue**).

Section Thickness

The invasion depth of a given tumor can be rendered in frozen section, but the pathologist should remember that in frozen sections tumors are 0.1 to 0.2 mm thicker than in permanent sections (EG Silva, unpublished observations). This is probably because the tissue retracts after fixation.

Mitotic Rate

We have seen cases in which a diagnosis of an aggressive tumor was rendered on the basis of the mitotic rate, but in which permanent tissue sections showed a lower mitotic count than that observed in the frozen sections. This phenomenon caused us to study a group of rat tumors, and we were able to confirm previous studies that had shown the number of mitoses to vary according to fixation time (24–26). After 12 h, specimens left unfixed have 20 to 50% fewer mitoses compared with those of promptly fixed specimens, a difference that occurs even if the specimens are refrigerated. For specimens left unfixed for fewer than 12 h, the mitotic rate is lower also, but more variable.

Tumor Cells in Vessels

The report of a positive or negative margin in a frozen tissue section is usually clear and does not create a problem of interpretation. When the only tumor cells present at the margin are within vessels, however, the next step in surgical treatment depends on the pathologist's interpretation. In such a situation, we try to determine whether the tumor cells are within blood or lymphatic vessels. If the tumor cells are in blood vessels, it is important to determine whether they are within or attached to an intramural thrombus. If so, new tissue should be taken at the margin. On the other hand, if few tumor cells are floating freely in the lumen of the vessel, the pathologist cannot be sure whether the cells are an artifact or a tumor embolus. In either case, it is not necessary to resect new tissue at the margin. When tumor cells are identified within lymphatics, and if resection of regional lymph nodes was not planned as part of the original operation, a sampling of the regional lymph nodes is advisable.

Marking the Margins

We routinely mark the lateral and deep margins of lesions with india ink. It is important that small amounts of ink be used, since india ink is indelible and may diffuse within the tissue, thus interfering with the diagnosis. This is important when special stains are needed, especially stains for melanin and silver stains for fungi. We presently use regular tattoo ink, because it is dense and does not smear within the tissue. In addition, the various colors of tattoo ink allow the pathologist to delineate the different margins of a specimen.

SPECIAL STAINS FOR FROZEN SECTIONS

Signet-ring Cell Carcinoma

Identifying signet-ring cell carcinoma on frozen tissue section may be a problem, because the membranes of these cells are difficult to evaluate after they have been subjected to rapid freezing. That is why in questionable cases in which the therapeutic approach depends on the diagnosis of the frozen section, we perform a rapid stain for mucin. We use a rapid alcian blue stain (1% alcian blue, pH 2.5, for 1 min; Ref. 27). Stromal mucin and the cytoplasm of mast cells also stain with this technique. We also use alcian blue stain when the suspicious cells are in the epithelium—for example, when checking margins in Paget's disease, but not when evaluating suspected cells in connective tissue. In the latter situation, when necessary, we perform a rapid mucicarmine stain procedure (see PROCEDURES AND SOLUTIONS, this chapter). The primary differences between rapid and regular mucicarmine stains are that, in the rapid stain, the picric acid passage is skipped, Weighert hematoxylin (requiring 10 min) is replaced by Harris's hematoxylin (1 min), tap water (1 min) by ammonia water (3 s), and mucicarmine with water by pure mucicarmine (5 min).

The problem of visualizing the signet-ring appearance of the cells in the frozen section may be related to the mucinous component or type of mucin present in the cytoplasm of these cells. The signet-ring cells of myxoid liposarcoma are, in comparison, easy to see.

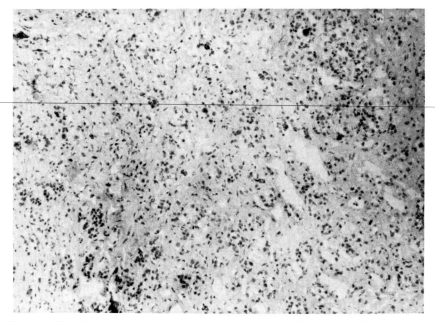

Figure 1.3. Pituitary adenoma, frozen section stained with hematoxylin and eosin. With this technique it is often impossible to differentiate normal pituitary from adenoma.

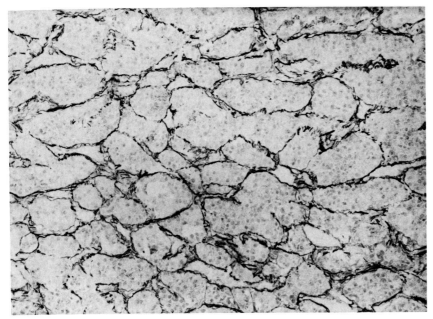

Figure 1.4. Normal pituitary. Reticulin stain shows abundant reticulum fibers demarcating nests of cells.

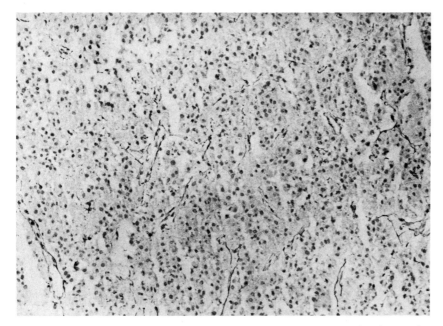

Figure 1.5. Pituitary adenoma. Reticulin stain shows scanty, isolated reticulum fibers.

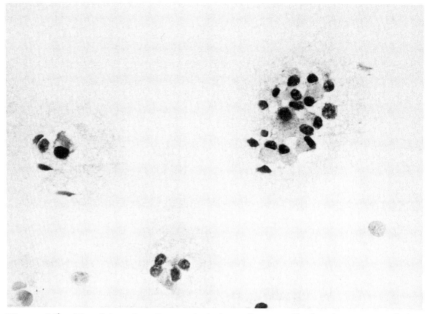

Figure 1.6. Touch imprint of normal pituitary. Sparse cells showing some variation in size and shape.

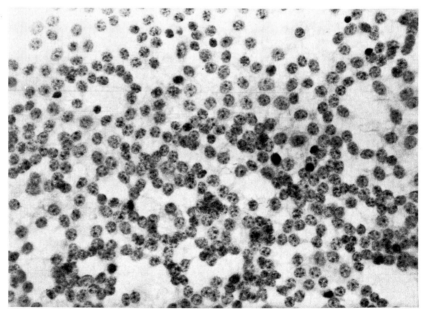

Figure 1.7. Touch imprints of pituitary adenoma. Numerous cells having similar size and shape.

Stereotactic Biopsies

Occasionally, stereotactic biopsies create problems in frozen section diagnosis, particularly those done to evaluate a possible pituitary adenoma (Fig. 1.3). In this situation, the neurosurgeon must know whether the pituitary adenoma has been resected and whether normal pituitary is present in the resected tissue. In this case, the operative procedure is terminated. If the tissue sample is large enough, we perform a rapid reticulin stain (see PROCEDURES AND SOLUTIONS, this chapter), which can be done in 10 min. In the normal pituitary, reticulin fibers form well-defined nests (Fig. 1.4). In an adenoma, a few reticulin fibers are seen; but no obvious nesting pattern or organoid cellular arrangement appears (Fig. 1.5; Ref. 28). If the tissue sample is very small, the cytologic interpretation with imprints will be more useful. The combination of scanty cells and a mixture of cell types is characteristic of normal pituitary (Fig. 1.6). Large numbers of cells of one histologic type are indicative of adenoma (Fig. 1.7). We have found these touch imprints from pituitary tissue easier to interpret if the slides are stained with rapid Papanicolaou's stain.

Frozen tissue sections may also be stained for bacteria or fungi. Monheit et al. reported the use of calcofluor white and fluorescence microscopy to detect fungi in frozen sections in 1 min (29).

PROCEDURES AND SOLUTIONS

Rapid Alcian Blue (4 to 6 min)

Procedure

1. Use frozen sections fixed in either/methanol (50/50) solution.
2. Postfix in 10% formaldehyde for 1 min (10 ml of 37–40% formaldehyde in 90 ml of tap water).
3. Rinse in tap water three times.
4. Dry slide by blotting or wiping off excess water with gauze, then hold slide in the exhaust airflow from the fume guard.
5. Stain in 2% alcian blue 8GX made up in 3% acetic acid, pH 2.5, for 3 min, or in 1% alcian blue, pH 2.5, for 1 min (27).
6. Rinse in tap water three times.
7. Counterstain in 0.2% nuclear fast red, made up in 5% aluminum sulfate, for 1 min.
8. Rinse twice in distilled water.
9. Dehydrate, clear, and apply coverslip.

Solutions

10% Formaldehyde. Distilled water, 90 ml; formaldehyde solution of 37–40%, 10 ml.

Alcian Blues. *1*) 0.2% alcian blue 8GX, 2 g; 3% acetic acid, 100 ml; adjust pH to 2.5+ with concentrated acetic acid.

2) −1% alcian blue 8GX, 1.0 g; 3% acetic acid, 100 ml; adjust pH to 2.5 ± 0.2 with concentrated acetic acid.

Nuclear Fast Red. Kernechtrot nuclear fast red, 0.2 g; 5% aluminum sulfate, 100 ml. Dissolve 5 g of aluminum sulfate in 100 ml of distilled water; heat and stir. Add nuclear fast red, continue stirring while bringing solution to a boil. Boil for 3 min, keeping solution covered to avoid evaporation. Nuclear fast red requires boiling to dissolve. Remove from heat, add a grain of thymol; cool and store. Filter before using.

Ammonia Water. Tap water, 450 ml; concentrated ammonium hydroxide, 2 ml.

Hydrochloric Acid. Tap water, 99 ml; concentrated hydrochloric acid, 1 ml.

Eosin. Eosin Y (CI 48380; 100% dye content, 10 g or 90% dye content, 11.11 g); orange G (CI 16230), 0.5 g; absolute alcohol, 1, 800 ml; distilled water, 200 ml; concentrated acetic acid, 2 ml; phloxine B (CI 45410), 0.2 ml. Dissolve the three dyes in a small amount of the distilled water. Add remaining water, alcohol, and acid; mix well. Ready for use.

Rapid Mucicarmine (7 to 8 min)

Procedure

1. Fix frozen sections for several seconds in ether/methanol (50/50) solution.
2. Hydrate fixed frozen sections. This is an important step and should not be eliminated.
3. Stain in Harris's hematoxylin for 20 to 30 s.
4. Rinse in tap water.
5. Dip in acid alcohol.
6. Rinse in tap water.
7. Dip in ammonia water.
8. Rinse in tap water.
9. Stain for 5 min in full-strength, unfiltered, mucicarmine solution.
10. Rinse in distilled water.
11. Stain for 1 min in metanil yellow.
12. Rinse in distilled water.
13. Dehydrate through 95% and 100% ethyl alcohol and THF, and clear in xylene.
14. Mount with a commercial synthetic mounting medium, such as Pro-Texx or Permount.

Solutions

Harris's Hematoxylin.

Southgate's Mucicarmine. Carmine (CI 75470, 1.0 g; aluminum hydroxide, 1.0 g; 50% ethyl alcohol, 100 ml; anhydrous aluminum chloride, 1.0 g. Mix carmine and aluminum hydroxide as dry compounds with a magnetic stirrer in a 500-ml flask. While stirring, add alcohol and aluminum chloride. Bring dye solution to boil by placing flask into boiling water bath; this may take 10 to 20 min. Allow solution to boil for at least 5 min while watching for color change from bright red to dark red. Color change is more important than time; boiling longer will not harm the solution. Cool solution quickly with cold water; it will be somewhat thick and syruplike. Filter and refrigerate.

Metanil Yellow.   Metanil yellow (CI 13065), 0.25 g; distilled water, 100 ml; acetic acid, 0.25 ml.

Results

Mucin will be pink to red, nuclei will show as blue, and other tissue elements will be yellow.

Papanicolaou Quick-Staining Technique

Procedure

1. Fix frozen section in ether/methanol (50/50) solution.
2. Hydrate in tap water, 10 dips.
3. Stain in Harris's hematoxylin, 3 to 5 s.
4. Rinse in tap water, 10 dips.
5. Dip in 95% ethyl alcohol 10 times.
6. Stain with orange G-6 for 1 min.
7. Dip in 95% ethyl alcohol 10 times.
8. Stain with EA-modified solution for 2 min.
9. Dip in 95% ethyl alcohol 10 times.
10. Dip in 100% ethyl alcohol 10 times.
11. Rinse in xylene, 10 dips, or until cleared.

Solutions

Orange G Counterstain.   The orange G-6 (OG-6) staining solution is 0.5% (wt/vol) orange G in 95% ethyl alcohol. Since the crystalline dye is not readily soluble in 95% alcohol, the following procedure should be followed: *a*) prepare a 10% aqueous solution of orange G (CI on 16230, certified) using distilled water; allow it to stand for several days; *b*) prepare the OG-6 staining solution (0.5%) by combining 50 ml of 10% orange G in aqueous solution with 950 ml of 95% ethyl alcohol and 0.15 g of phosphotungstic acid. Store in a well-stoppered, dark bottle, and filter well before using.

EA-Modified.   To prepare a working modified EA staining solution, combine these ingredients: 95% ethyl alcohol, 700 ml; absolute methanol, 250 ml; glacial acetic acid, 20 ml; light green (3% TDC) aqueous solution, 10 ml; eosin (20% TDC) aqueous solution, 20 ml; phosphotungstic acid, 2 g.

Snook Reticulin

Procedure

1. Fix frozen sections in ether/methanol (50/50) solution.
2. Hydrate in distilled water.
3. Oxidize in 0.25% potassium permanganate (5 min regular; 3 min rapid).
4. Rinse in tap water.
5. Clear by agitating in 50% oxalic acid.

6. Rinse well in tap water.
7. Place in distilled water. From here to step 10, process each slide individually.
8. Mordant in 1% uranium nitrate by agitating for 10 to 12 s.
9. Rinse in distilled water.
10. Place in ammoniacal silver solution (8 min regular; 5 min rapid).
11. Carry the slides quickly through two changes of distilled water.
12. Agitate in 1% formaldehyde for a few seconds, until color changes to yellowish-brown.
13. Rinse in distilled water.
14. Agitate in 1% gold chloride until color changes to gray.
15. Rinse in distilled water.
16. Place slides in 5% sodium thiosulfate for 1 min.
17. Rinse in distilled water.
18. Place in 0.2% nuclear fast red (5 min regular; 1 min rapid).
19. Rinse twice in distilled water.
20. Dehydrate, clear, and mount.

Solutions

Potassium Permanganate (0.25%). Potassium permanganate, 0.25 g; and distilled water, 100 ml.

Oxalic Acid (5%). Oxalic acid, 5 g; and distilled water, 100 ml.

Uranium nitrate (1%). Uranium nitrate (uranyl nitrate), 1 g; and distilled water, 100 ml.

Formaldehyde Solution (1%). Formaldehyde solution (40%), 1 ml; and distilled water, 100 ml.

Gold Chloride (1%). Gold chloride, 1 g; and distilled water, 100 ml.

Sodium Thiosulfate (5%). Sodium thiosulfate, 5 g; and distilled water, 100 ml.

Nuclear Fast Red. Nuclear fast red (Kernechtrot) 0.20 g; and 5% aluminum sulfate, 100 ml.

Silver Nitrate (5%). Silver nitrate, 5 g; and distilled water, 100 ml. Store in chemically clear, dark bottle.

Sodium Hydroxide (10%). Sodium hydroxide, 1.5 g; and distilled water, 25 ml.

Ammoniacal Silver Solution. To 15 ml of 5% silver nitrate, add 15 drops of 10% sodium hydroxide in a chemically clean, graduated, stoppered cylinder. Use plastic disposable or chemically clean droppers. Add concentrated ammonium hydroxide to this solution, drop by drop, until only a few granules remain in the solution. Be sure to insert the stopper and shake the cylinder after each drop. Add distilled water to the clear (or almost clear) solution to the 45-ml level. This solution must be kept covered and can be used all day.

REFERENCES

1. Silva EG, Mackay B, Goepfert H, Burgess MA, Fields RS: Endocrine carcinoma of the skin (Merkel cell carcinoma). *Pathol Annu* 19:1–30, 1984.
2. Tromovitch TA, Stegman SJ: Microscopically-controlled excision of skin tumors: Chemosurgery (Mohs)—fresh tissue technique. *Arch Dermatol* 110:231–232, 1974.

3. Mohs FE: Chemosurgery: A microscopically controlled method of excision. *Arch Surg* 48:478–481, 1944.

4. Swanson NA, Grekin RC, Baker SR: Mohs surgery: Techniques, indications, and applications in head and neck surgery. *Head Neck Surg* 6:683–692, 1983.

5. Davidson TM, Nahum AM, Haghight P, Astarita RW, Saltzstein SL, Seagren S: The biology of head and neck cancer. *Head Neck Cancer* 110:193–196, 1984.

6. Terracio L, Schwabe KG: Freezing and drying of biological tissues for electron microscopy. *J Histochem Cytochem* 29:1021–1028, 1981.

7. Pearse DC (ed): Fixation: Rapid freezing. In *Histological Techniques for Electron Microscopy.* New York, Academic, 1964, p 67.

8. Bullivant S: Present status of freezing techniques. In Parsons DF (ed): *Some Biological Techniques in Electron Microscopy.* New York, Academic, 1970, p 101.

9. Russell WO, Ibanez ML, Chang JP, Speece AJ: Improved diagnosis of cancer with cold chamber frozen sections. *Acta Union Int Contre Cancer* 26:351–357, 1960.

10. Long ER (ed): Pathological histology and the last third of the nineteenth century. In *A History of Pathology.* New York, Dover, 1965, p 127.

11. Jennings ER, Landers JW: The use of frozen section in cancer diagnosis. *Surg Gynecol Obstet* 104:60–62, 1957.

12. Wilson LB: A method for the rapid preparation of fresh tissues for the microscope. *JAMA* 45:1737, 1905.

13. MacCarty WC: The diagnostic reliability of frozen sections. *Am J Pathol* 5:377–380, 1929.

14. Linderstrom-Lang K, Mogensen KR: Studies on enzymatic histochemistry. XXXI. Histological control of histochemical investigations. *Compt-rend Lab Carlsberg Ser Chim* 23:27–35, 1938.

15. Ibanez ML, Russell WO, Chang JP, Speece AJ: Cold chamber frozen sections for operating room diagnosis and routine surgical pathology. *Lab Invest* 9:98–109. 1960.

16. Chang JP, Russell WO, Moore EB, Sinclair WK: A new cryostat for frozen section technic. *Am J Clin Pathol* 35:14–19, 1961.

17. Klionsky B, Smith OD: Application of the refrigerated microtome in surgical pathology. *Am J Clin Pathol* 33:144–151, 1960.

18. Nunnally RM, Abbott JP: Use of the microtome cryostat for rapid frozen sections. *Am J Clin Pathol* 35:20–25, 1961.

19. Feder N, Sidman RL: Methods and principles of fixation by freeze-substitution. *Biophys Biochem Cytol* 4:593–600, 1958.

20. Dudgeon LS, Patrick CV: A new method for the rapid microscopical diagnosis of tumors: With an account of 200 cases so examined. *Br J Surg* 15:250–261, 1927.

21. Dudgeon LS, Barrett NR: The examination of fresh tissues by the wet-film method. *Br J Surg* 22:4–22, 1934.

22. Petersen H: Fixation. In Blackith RE, Kovoor A (eds): *Histological Techniques.* Paris, Masson, 1976, p 30.

23. Rosen Y, Ahuja SC: Ice crystal distortion of formalin-fixed tissues following freezing. *Am J Surg Pathol* 1: 179–181, 1977.

24. Graem N, Helweg-Larson K: Mitotic activity and delay in fixation of tumour tissue. *Path Microbiol Scand* 87:375–378, 1979.

25. Edwards JL, Donalson JT: The time of fixation and the mitotic index. *Am J Clin Pathol* 41:158–162, 1964.

26. Franzini DA, Silva EG, Maizel A: Variability of mitotic count dependent on fixation time. *Lab Invest* 44:20A–21A, 1981.

27. Rosai J (ed): Gastrointestinal tract/stomach. In *Ackerman's Surgical Pathology.* St. Louis, C. V. Mosby Company, 1981, p 417.

28. Velasco ME, Sindley SD, Roessmann U: Reticulin stain for frozen section diagnosis of pituitary adenomas. *J Neurosurg* 46:548–550, 1977.

29. Monheit JE, Cowan DF, Moore DG: Rapid detection of fungi in tissues using calcofluor white and fluorescence microscopy. *Arch Pathol Lab Med* 108:616–618, 1984.

2

Breast

Elvio G. Silva, M.D.

Twenty to thirty-five percent of all frozen sections are from the breast. In our experience, and judging by data in the literature, the percentage of false positive frozen section diagnoses of breast lesions varies from 0.03% to 0.1%, and false negative diagnoses varies from 0.5% to 1%. Frozen section diagnosis is deferred in 0.5 to 3% of all breast biopsies (1, 2).

INDICATIONS FOR FROZEN SECTION

Diagnosis of Breast Lesion to Reach a Therapeutic Decision. Deciding on treatment was and, in some institutions, still is the most important indication for frozen section diagnosis of breast tissue. This type of biopsy, however, is increasingly being replaced by the fine-needle aspiration (FNA) biopsy. In our hospital, diagnoses based on frozen sections from breast are only performed for patients whose FNA results were equivocal.

Tumor Near Margins of Resection. For a small carcinoma of the breast, which is commonly treated with wide excision instead of mastectomy, the success of the treatment depends largely on the absence of tumor at the margin or resection. When we receive wide excisions of breast for frozen section, we slice the tissue thinly to examine the relationship of tumor to the margins of resection. If gross examination shows the tumor to be close to the resection margin, we perform frozen sections of that specific margin. If all the margins appear to be clear of tumor, we discuss with the surgeon the need for random frozen sections of the margins for each individual case. The presence of in situ carcinoma, at the margin of resection, is associated with a high local recurrence rate (3).

Tissue for Ancillary Studies. To determine the appropriateness of tissue for further studies, we perform frozen section in situations in which *a*) because of a low index of suspicion, scant availability of tissue, or human error, tumor tissue was not separated during the biopsy for ancillary studies and *b*) when, because of previous biopsy, subsequent mastectomy, or wide excision, areas in the breast show fibrosis or fat necrosis that could be difficult to differentiate from carcinoma.

TYPES OF SPECIMENS

At our institution, breast biopsy material submitted for frozen section is usually obtained by needle biopsy with a Vim Silverman or "Tru cut" needle. When there is a palpable breast mass, this biopsy is a fast procedure that provides a sterile specimen. It can be done with local anesthesia or as the first step in the operating room after general anesthesia before the operative field is prepared. When the result of the needle biopsy is negative, the surgeon performs an incisional or excisional biopsy according to the size of the mass and submits this second biopsy for frozen section diagnosis.

SPECIAL TECHNIQUES: SPECIMEN RADIOGRAPHY OF EXCISED BREAST TISSUE

Specimen radiography is indicated when the results of mammography raise suspicion of a tumor although there is no palpable mass. A needle localization may be performed at the time of the biopsy, in which case the laboratory receives the tissue with a needle embedded in it. Alternatively, the radiologist may inject a drop of contrast medium mixed with Evan's blue dye, to mark the suspected area (4). We prefer to remove the needle from the specimen before radiographic examination because the metal interferes with the identification of the calcifications. The specimen is immediately examined with a small x-ray unit, the Faxitron (for convenience we have a Faxitron in our frozen section laboratory). We use 3 mA for 1 min, 30 kV (peak), and expose film at 25.5 cm. At our institution, the surgeon personally delivers mammograms and biopsy specimens to the frozen section suite and reviews the mammographic findings with the pathologist. If the initial specimen radiograph shows the areas that aroused suspicion in the mammogram, the biopsy material is sliced into pieces no thicker than 1 cm, and then the pieces are x-rayed together again. The radiograph of these thin slices clearly locates microcalcifications or any area of increased density, indicating the area that should be submitted for microscopic examination. When the specimen radiography fails to show the suspected area present in the mammogram, more breast tissue must be resected. Once either the areas of calcification or the suspected area is shown in specimen radiographs, the question of submitting tissue for frozen section examination arises. Our policy is to perform frozen section study only on biopsy specimens in which the area suspected of malignancy is *grossly* identified, provided that enough lesional tissue is available for permanent sections.

Table 2.1.
Microcalcifications[a]

	Associated with Benign Conditions	Associated with Malignant Neoplasms
Amount	Scanty	Numerous to uncountable
Distribution	Wide	Confined to measurable area
Density	Uniformly dense	Faint to dense
Location	Intraductal, regular	Scattered in one area

[a]Based on Snyder RE: Specimen radiography and preoperative localization of nonpalpable breast cancer. *Cancer* 46:950–956, 1980; and Egan RL: *Technologist's Guide to Mammography.* Baltimore, Williams & Wilkins, 1968, p 93.

The characteristics of calcifications in benign and malignant breast lesions are shown in Table 2.1. In addition to these, one must note that calcifications associated with a mass usually indicate a malignant neoplasm, especially if the mass is poorly demarcated. Calcifications characteristic of such benign conditions as sclerosing adenosis and papillomatosis may be useful for detecting lobular carcinoma in situ in the vicinity of the benign lesion(s).

FROZEN SECTION DIAGNOSIS

A simple approach to the different lesions encountered in frozen sections is to determine whether the lesions are ductal or lobular, or whether they originate in the stroma. The main features of breast lesions, with emphasis on those particularly important to differential diagnosis, are discussed in Proliferation of Ductal Epithelial Cells (this chapter). The diagnosis of any borderline lesion should, however, be deferred from frozen section until the permanent sections have been examined.

Proliferation of Ductal Epithelial Cells

Benign Versus Malignant Conditions

This category includes cases in which the differential diagnosis is between epitheliosis or papillomatosis and in situ carcinoma.

Except in the case of solitary papillomas, the macroscopic appearance of these lesions does not help to differentiate between benign and malignant ones. Carcinoma in situ is the only exception to the rule in that the microscopic diagnosis should always be in harmony with the lesion's gross appearance. In cases of carcinoma in situ, the macroscopic findings could be completely negative for malignancy. Focal areas of white, dense tissue, with or without small cysts with yellow or brown contents, are the only macroscopic findings in these ductal epithelial proliferations.

Table 2.2 lists the main histologic features useful in differentiating benign (Fig. 2.1) and malignant proliferations of ductal epithelium (Fig. 2.2 and 2.3).

In the differential diagnosis between benign and malignant ductal epithelial proliferations, the cytologic characteristics are the most reliable indicators, but unfortunately, during examination of frozen sections it is difficult to determine what proportion of cellular atypia is the result of freezing artifact. In this situation, it is important to compare cells from the area in question with those areas that are obviously benign; this comparison indicates how much atypia was caused by freezing artifact. Atypia produced by a neoplastic process is, however, clear in cytologic preparations.

In Situ Versus Infiltrating Carcinoma

Identifying a breast carcinoma as infiltrating is usually not difficult. The main histologic feature of invasion is the totally disorganized arrangement of the neoplastic cells. Even in cases of tubular carcinoma, which might be confused with adenosis, well-formed glands infiltrate the stroma, whereas hyperplastic lesions maintain the normal breast architecture of central ducts with small lobular units at the periphery. Other unequivocal indicators of

Table 2.2.
Histological Differentiation of Benign and Malignant Proliferations of Ductal Epithelium

Feature	Epitheliosis (papillomatosis)	Ductal Carcinoma
Pattern	Solid or forming glandular spaces of irregular shape	Solid, comedo, or forming glandular spaces that are round and similar in size and shape (cribriform)
Necrosis and/or hemorrhage	Rare	May be present
Cytologic characteristics	Usually a mixture of spindle and polygonal cells	Uniform population of cuboidal cells
Cellular atypia	Rare	Present
Individual cell necrosis	Rare	Frequent
Enlarged nucleolus	Rare	Frequent
Suggested therapeutic approach	Excisional biopsy	For focal involvement of few ducts, wide excision or extended simple mastectomy
		If present in several ducts or multifocal, modified radical mastectomy

infiltrating carcinoma are single cells (sometimes forming a single-file, Indian-file pattern) isolated in the stroma, a tendency for cells to form small groups, clear vacuoles in the cytoplasm (giving a signet-ring appearance), invasion of fat, desmoplastic reaction around tumor cells, and vascular invasion. Comedocarcinoma is one form of breast carcinoma often difficult to distinguish with certainty as to whether it is in situ or invasive. Carcinoma of the breast with a comedo pattern may infiltrate the stroma in a fashion similar to that of other breast carcinomas and pose no diagnostic problem; or it may infiltrate the stroma to form comedones that resemble the intraductal comedones. In the latter situation, the reaction of the stroma around the tumor may make the tissue look like the wall of a duct, so that the diagnosis of stromal invasion may be difficult, if not impossible. The presence of comedones in the metastases proves that this pattern can be maintained in the tumor's invasive portion.

For practical purposes, the differentiation of in situ and invasive carcinoma is significant only in patients who have a small focus of in situ disease. Extensive in situ carcinoma and invasive carcinoma should be treated in the same way, that is, with modified radical mastectomy. Patients with a small focus of in situ carcinoma are treated in our hospital with wide excision or extended simple mastectomy, because the possibility of metastases to the lymph nodes is very slight in this situation.

Primary Versus Metastatic Carcinoma

After a diagnosis of carcinoma, the next step is to determine whether the tumor is primary or metastatic. The diagnosis of primary carcinoma in

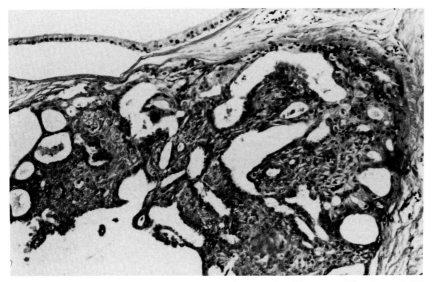

Figure 2.1. Benign epithelial hyperplasia characterized by a proliferation of different cell types, irregular glandular spaces, and absence of atypia and necrosis.

the breast is based on two histologic features, the microscopic evidence of tumor tissue and the presence of an in situ component, both of which are usually present in conjunction. Some breast carcinomas do not, however, show an in situ component; in these cases, the diagnosis must be based on histologic appearance alone. In typical medullary carcinoma of breast, for example, the intraductal component is absent (5), and diagnosis is based on the well-circumscribed appearance, syncytial growth pattern, mononu-

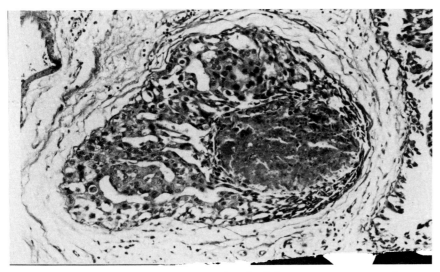

Figure 2.2. Intraductal carcinoma. Irregular glandular spaces are present, however, the uniform cell population, the cytologic atypia, and necrosis present are diagnostic of carcinoma.

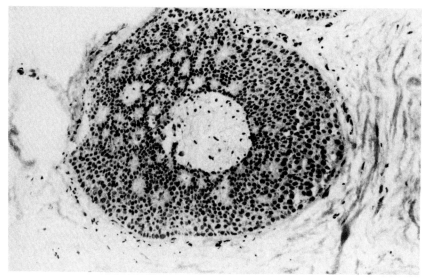

Figure 2.3. Intraductal carcinoma. Uniform proliferation of atypical cells with cribriform pattern.

clear inflammatory infiltrate, marked nuclear pleomorphism, and absence of glands. Another carcinoma of breast in which the in situ component may be absent is tubular carcinoma. Reported rates of an in situ component with tubular carcinoma of breast have varied in the literature from 0 (6) to almost 70% (7). Open glands of irregular shape, including several angulated forms distributed haphazardly, are characteristic of tubular carcinoma. The stroma may be elastotic or demosplastic, and the glandular epithelium may show intraluminal bridging and apocrine snouts. The main characteristic of

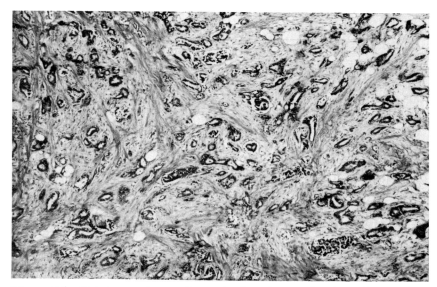

Figure 2.4. Tubular carcinoma. Open glands with irregular shape showing haphazard arrangement, infiltrating fat.

Table 2.3.
Differential Diagnosis Between Lobular Hyperplasia and Lobular Carcinoma in Situ

Characteristics	Lobular Hyperplasia	Lobular Carcinoma *in situ*
Lobular size	Similar to other units or minor distention	Marked distention
Residual lumina between cells	Present	Absent; compact groups of tumor cells
Cells	Could show some variation in size and shape	Uniform size and shape (polygonal)
Suggested therapeutic approach	Excisional biopsy	Controversial[a]

[a]At our hospital, lobular carcinoma *in situ* is treated with extended simple mastectomy, and management of the opposite breast is discussed with the patient. Several other treatment modalities for the opposite breast have been proposed for lobular carcinoma *in situ*, ranging from excisional biopsy only, with close follow-up, to bilateral mastectomy (35, 36).

this neoplasm is its invasive component at the periphery. This neoplasm has an infiltrative margin, and it often infiltrates fat (Fig. 2.4).

The designation of these two types of breast carcinoma, medullary and tubular, as primary in the breast should be made only after it is certain that no other primary carcinoma could have originated a breast metastasis. Medullary carcinoma can be confused with an undifferentiated carcinoma.

Proliferation of Lobular Epithelial Cells

Lobular carcinoma in situ is rarely identified at the time of frozen section. This form of breast carcinoma is almost always an incidental finding in a biopsy performed for conditions that appear benign on radiographic examination, so that frozen section is not requested. Table 2.3 outlines the differences between lobular hyperplasia and lobular carcinoma in situ.

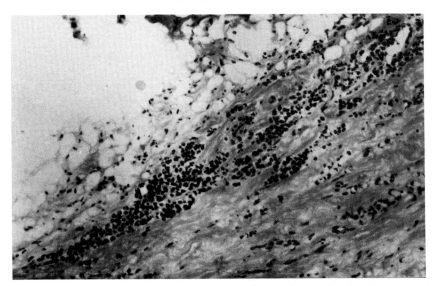

Figure 2.5. Frozen section of infiltrating lobular carcinoma. Small cells arranged in single lines or forming small groups infiltrate the stroma.

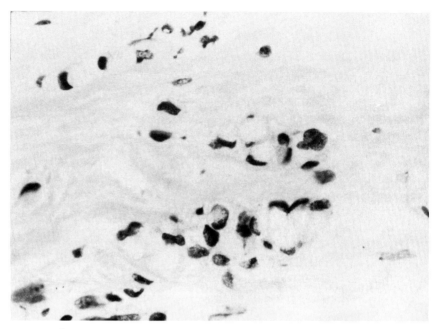

Figure 2.6. Frozen section of infiltrating lobular carcinoma showing clear vacuoles in the cytoplasm of the tumor cells.

The presence of necrosis of individual cells favors a diagnosis of lobular carcinoma in situ, but such necrosis is not a frequent finding. Mitoses are rare in benign lobular proliferations.

The differentiation of lobular carcinoma in situ from invasion of lobules by ductal carcinoma does not need to be made in frozen section. This

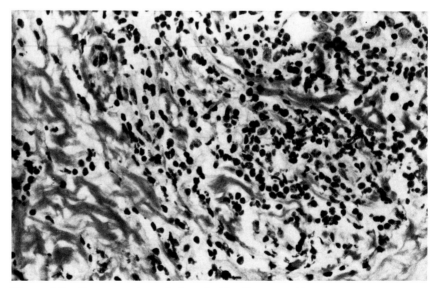

Figure 2.7. Frozen section of a lymphoid infiltration of breast. Conspicuous lack of cohesion between lymphoid cells.

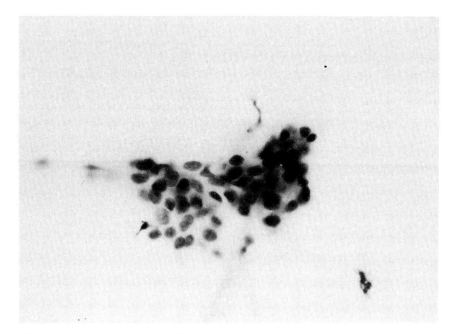

Figure 2.8. Touch imprint of breast carcinoma. Irregular groups of tumor cells.

differential diagnosis is very important for determining treatment for the opposite breast, but not for immediate management of the ipsilateral breast.

The in situ component may be absent in invasive lobular carcinoma of the breast, for which diagnosis is based on the infiltration of the stroma by small cells arranged in an Indian-file pattern, or on formations of small cell groups (Fig. 2.5). On occasion, clear vacuoles with eosinophilic material

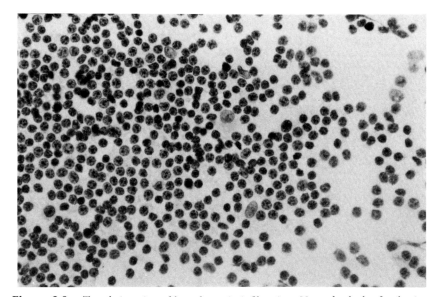

Figure 2.9. Touch imprint of lymphocytic infiltration. Note the lack of cohesion between cells.

may be observed in the tumor cell cytoplasm (Fig. 2.6).

A lymphoid infiltrate is characterized by the lack of cell cohesion and the disorganized arrangement of the cells (Fig. 2.7). It cannot be overemphasized that the difficulties in the differential diagnosis between any type of epithelial cell and lymphoid cell in tissue sections can be easily avoided by examining the cytologic preparations. The tendency to form small groups (Fig. 2.8) is a characteristic of epithelial cells, and is not seen with lymphoid cells (Fig. 2.9). Moreover, skeletal muscle atrophy may be confused with an inflammatory disorder or even infiltrating carcinoma. The location of the skeletal muscle nuclei, at the periphery of the degenerating muscle fiber, is diagnostic of muscle atrophy and should not be confused with the other processes described above (Figs. 2.10 and 2.11).

Unusual Variants of Breast Carcinoma

Squamous Carcinoma of Breast

We believe there are different types of squamous carcinoma of breast. Squamous metaplasia in a typical carcinoma of breast and squamous carcinoma (usually with a spindle cell component) are two easily diagnosed neoplasms (8) that should be treated with modified radical mastectomy. We have seen some carcinomas characterized by irregular islands of squamous cells within a diffuse proliferation of spindle cells. Mitotic figures and atypia are rarely seen in both the squamous and spindle cells. We believe that this neoplasm is a low-grade squamous carcinoma that may be adequately treated by extended simple mastectomy, but unfortunately our data are insufficient to give a more definitive statement on this entity (EG Silva, unpublished observations).

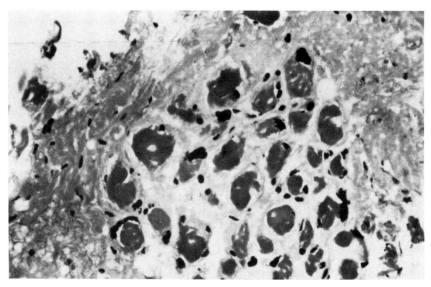

Figure 2.10. Frozen section of atrophic muscle showing groups of nuclei at the periphery of the fibers.

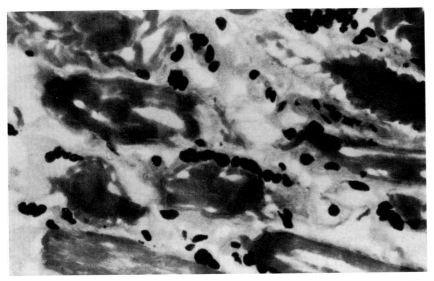

Figure 2.11. Frozen section of atrophic muscle. Residual skeletal muscle nuclei are arranged in single rows.

Adenoid Cystic Carcinoma

In our recent review of adenoid cystic carcinoma of breast (9), we found that the grading of this tumor with a system similar to the one applied to these tumors in salivary glands may be an important factor in surgical management. The grading system is based on the tumor's solid component. Adenoid cystic carcinoma without a solid component is designated grade I; if solid component is present but makes up less than 30% of the tumor, the designation is grade II; and tumor with more than 30% solid component is grade III. In our experience, one case of grade III adenoid cystic carcinoma metastasized to axillary lymph nodes. We believe that simple or extended simple mastectomy is the optimal treatment for well-differentiated and moderately differentiated adenoid cystic carcinoma, but that the poorly differentiated type should be treated with modified radical mastectomy.

Other Lesions Often Confused with Breast Carcinoma

The lesions most often confused with breast carcinoma are sclerosing papillomatosis, radial scar, and sclerosing adenosis. It may be also difficult to differentiate breast carcinoma from breast adenoma, microglandular adenosis, and epithelioid hemangioendothelioma.

Sclerosing Papillomatosis

In this lesion, characterized by areas of sclerosis in a papilloma, the sclerosis may be present at the base, in one lateral border, or, more often, at the center of the papilloma. The distortion that the sclerosis causes in

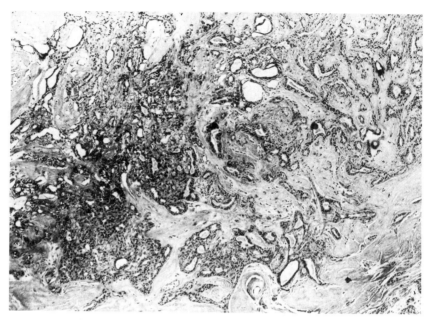

Figure 2.12. Sclerosing papilloma. The distortion produced by the sclerosis simulates an infiltrating carcinoma.

the glands creates an appearance of tubular carcinoma; however, at the periphery of the lesion there are usually dilated residual lumina (Figs. 2.12–2.15). In cases in which the sclerosis completely effaces the papilloma, the benign nature of the lesion is indicated by the absence of infiltrative margins. The problems of differentiating sclerosing papillomatosis from car-

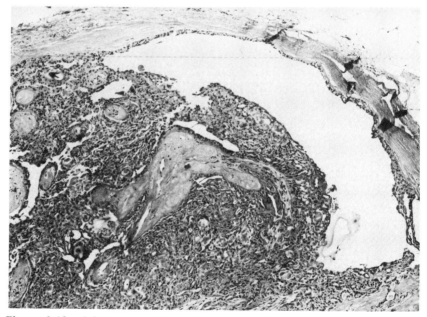

Figure 2.13. Sclerosing papilloma. Same case as Fig 2.12. At the periphery, the lesion is well circumscribed and contains a dilated space.

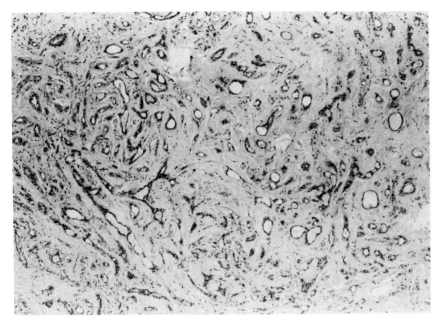

Figure 2.14. Sclerosing papilloma. Central portion of the lesion showing small ducts, many of them with open irregular lumina.

cinoma may be amplified by small biopsy specimens that include only sclerotic areas. The pathologist should concentrate on the microscopic features at the periphery, rather than on those in the center of the lesion. The glands at the center of the lesion or in areas of sclerosis are indistinguishable from those affected by tubular carcinoma.

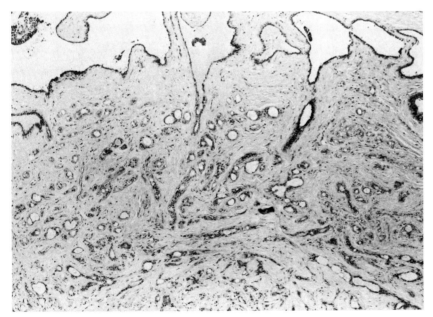

Figure 2.15. Sclerosing papilloma. Same case as Fig 2.14. Periphery of the papilloma showing cystic spaces.

Radial Scar

This lesion is characterized by a central focus of sclerosis with several ducts radiating to the periphery in a disorganized fashion (Fig. 2.16). These ducts are usually distorted by papillomatosis or epitheliosis. Radial scars are most often microscopic lesions that do not infiltrate the peripheral fat.

Although some publications (10–12) use the two terms, "sclerosing papillomatosis" and "radial scar," for the same process, in our opinion the two entities are distinct. Both are basically sclerosing processes. Sclerosing papilloma, however, does not resemble tubular carcinoma except in the situation where very small biopsy specimens include only sclerotic material at the center of the lesion, or when the process is very advanced and the periphery of the papilloma is obliterated by sclerosis. In this latter situation, one of sclerosing papilloma's most important typical features, the well circumscribed border, is not recognizable. Radial scar has an infiltrative border and therefore is more easily confused with tubular carcinoma. The main clue for the differential diagnosis is that in tubular carcinoma the glands are small, without epitheliosis or papillomatosis, and in radial scar the majority of the ducts are large and show papillomatosis. Some researchers believe, however, that tubular carcinoma originates in radial scars (11).

Sclerosing Adenosis

The breast lesion of sclerosing adenosis is well circumscribed and characterized by glands that have closed lumina and two cell types, epithelial and myoepithelial (Fig. 2.17). Glands in perineural spaces may be seen in instances of sclerosing adenosis. Table 2.4 shows the differences between sclerosing lesions and tubular carcinoma.

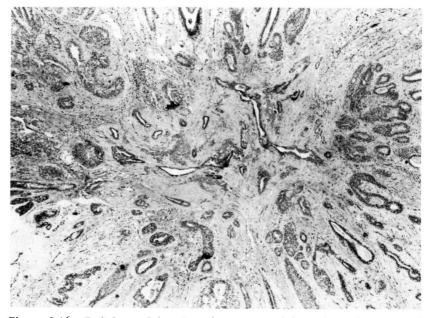

Figure 2.16. Radial scar. Sclerosis at the center with large ducts showing papillomatosis radiating to the periphery.

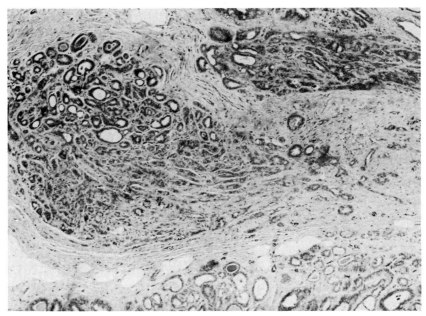

Figure 2.17. Sclerosing adenosis. The sclerosis present distorts this mammary lobule, however the lesion is still well circumscribed. In addition, most of the lumina of the glands are closed.

Table 2.4.
Differential Diagnosis Between Tubular Carcinoma and Sclerosing Breast Lesions

Characteristics	Tubular Carcinoma	Sclerosing Adenosis	Sclerosing Papilloma	Radial Scar
Gland distribution	Haphazard	Nodular or lobular	Nodular	Haphazard
Margin	Infiltrative	Well circumscribed	Well circumscribed	Infiltrative
Collagen	Evenly distributed	More abundant at periphery	Predominant in focal areas	Evenly distributed
Glands	Small, all open, angulated	Small, the majority closed	Small, angulated	Large ducts with epitheliosis or papillomatosis
Miscellaneous	Glands have one cell layer	Glands have two cell layers, epithelial and myoepithelial	In areas without sclerosis, papillary projections and dilated spaces are prominent	
Associated *in situ* carcinoma	Present in 50% to 70% of patients	No association	No association	No association

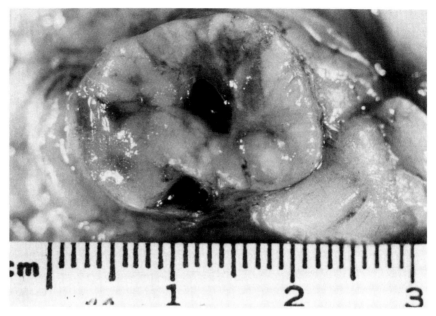

Figure 2.18. Adenoma of breast. A well circumscribed homogeneous appearing lesion.

Adenoma of Breast

Tubular adenoma (13) of breast could be confused with carcinoma of breast; however, the complete circumscription of the lesion, the presence of two cell layers (epithelial and myoepithelial), and the absence of atypia are basic features that distinguish adenoma from carcinoma (Figs. 2.18–2.22).

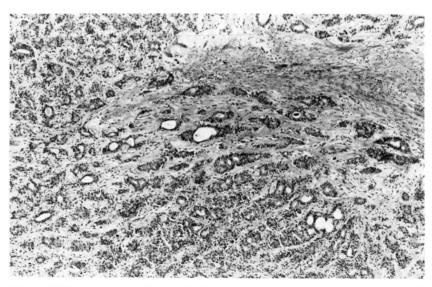

Figure 2.19. Adenoma of breast. In this area, the adenoma is distorted by sclerosis, however the regular, uniform proliferation of similarly sized glands is still preserved.

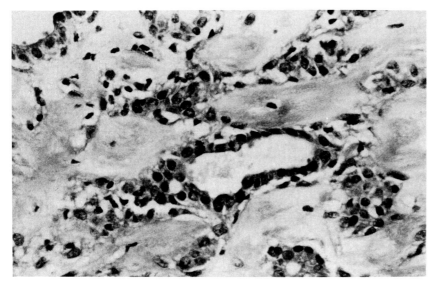

Figure 2.20. Adenoma of breast. Glands lined by epithelial and myoepithelial cells, the latter showing clear cytoplasm.

Microglandular Adenosis

The peculiar breast lesion of microglandular adenosis is characterized by a proliferation of small, round glands lined by one layer of cuboidal cells with clear cytoplasm without atypia or mitoses. Eosinophilic dense material is present in the lumina of the glands. Instead of being confined to lobular areas, this lesion infiltrates the breast stroma in a diffuse form (Fig. 2.23). In most publications, microglandular adenosis (14–17) is described as a benign condition, but the consistent absence of myoepithelial cells, the infiltrative pattern, and the association with carcinoma (15, 18) has raised some doubts about its benign behavior. Until the prognosis of microglandular adenosis is clearly determined, the lesion should be treated with wide excision and regular clinical follow-up. In frozen section, the clear cytoplasm of the cells lining the lumina in microglandular adenosis is not seen. On occasion it is difficult to see the cytoplasmic border, and the glands are characterized by round spaces with a layer of naked nuclei at the periphery of the space. The diagnosis of microglandular adenosis in these cases should be based on the characteristic pattern, round glands, absence of atypia and mitoses, and dense eosinophilic material in the lumina (Fig. 2.24).

Epithelioid Hemangioendothelioma

Yet another lesion, epithelioid hemangioendothelioma (19), has been confused with breast carcinoma. We have seen cases of two patients with epithelioid hemangioendothelioma that were misinterpreted as infiltrating carcinoma of breast. In these cases, the lesion was in soft tissue overlying breast. In this situation, the location and characteristics of the lesion must be identified. Invasive carcinoma of breast (other than medullary) and nearly

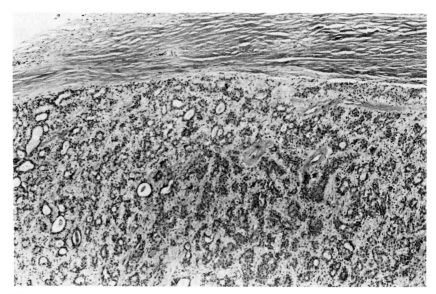

Figure 2.21. Adenoma of breast. Well circumscribed margin. Orderly proliferation of glands having similar size.

a third of tubular carcinomas are accompanied by intraductal or intralobular neoplasia. Carcinomas also form glands, and cellular atypia is present. Epithelioid hemangioendothelioma may be located in the soft tissue around the breast, and associated in situ neoplasm and cellular atypia will be absent.

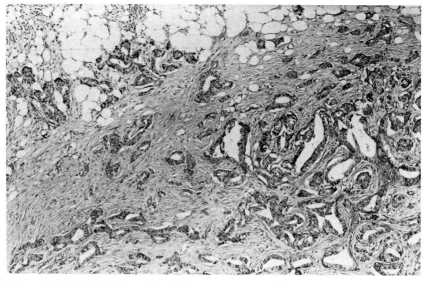

Figure 2.22. Well differentiated adenocarcinoma of breast. Compare with Figure 2.21. Disorderly proliferation of glands show significant variation in size and shape. In addition, this lesion has an infiltrating margin.

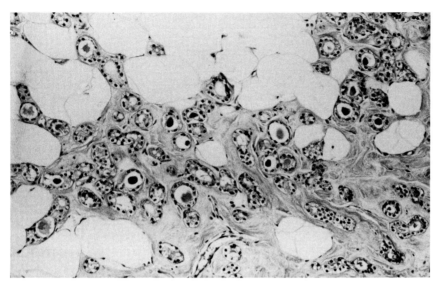

Figure 2.23. Microglandular adenosis. Small, round glands, lined by cuboidal cells with clear cytoplasm having dense eosinophillic material in the lumina.

Overdiagnosis

The most common overdiagnoses of breast carcinoma occur *a*) in mammography, when the lesion is chronic abscess; *b*) in macroscopic examination, when the correct diagnosis is granular cell tumor and fat necrosis; and *c*) in microscopic examination, in cases of adenoma and

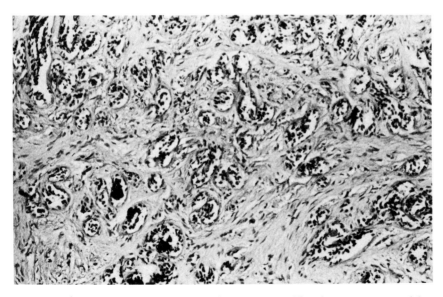

Figure 2.24. Microglandular adenosis, frozen section. The clear appearance of the cells can not be appreciated in the frozen section. Diagnosis must be based on the uniform, regular appearance of small glands containing dense material in the lumina.

the sclerosing lesions (radial scar, sclerosing adenosis, and sclerosing papillomatosis).

SURGICAL MANAGEMENT OF BREAST CARCINOMA

The standard treatment for patients with carcinoma of the breast is modified radical mastectomy. In most institutions, extended simple mastectomy is done for patients who have small foci of intraductal carcinoma and lobular carcinoma in situ, pure tubular carcinoma smaller than 2 cm in diameter, and well- or moderately differentiated adenoid cystic carcinoma. There is, however, an increasing tendency to treat small carcinomas of breast with wide local excision and partial resection of the axillary nodes.

Mixed Stromal And Epithelial Proliferations

The three most common fibroepithelial proliferations of breast (Figs. 2.25–2.28) are fibroadenoma, benign phyllodes tumor, and malignant phyllodes tumor. Table 2.5 shows the main differences between these three fibroepithelial lesions (20, 21). Grossly, phyllodes tumor is a gelatinous neoplasm that sometimes shows cystic areas with broad papillary projections. Size should not be used to separate fibroadenoma from phyllodes tumor. A fibroepithelial lesion in the breast having moderate cellularity in the stroma, atypical cells, and two to three mitoses per 10 high power fields (HPF) should be classified as a phyllodes tumor, regardless of its size.

Some authors (22) have divided phyllodes tumors into three groups:

Table 2.5.
Differential Diagnosis of Fibroepithelial Lesions

	Benign		Malignant
	Fibroadenoma	Phyllodes Tumor	Phyllodes Tumor
Mean age of patients	25	44	44
Tumor border	Sharply demarcated	Well circumscribed	Focally infiltrating
Stromal cellularity	Hypocellular	Intermediate	Hypercellular
Atypia	Absent	Mild to moderate	Moderate to severe
Mitoses	Rare	Less than 4/10 HPF[a]	More than 5/10 HPF
Stromal overgrowth[b]	Absent	Absent	Present
Miscellaneous			Heterologous component may be present
Suggested therapeutic approach	Excision	Wide excision	Simple mastectomy

[a]HPF, high-power field
[b]Stromal overgrowth refers to an entire low-power field without epithelial elements. Ward RM, and Evans HL:Cystosareoma phyllodes: A Clinicopathologic Study of 26 cases. _Cancer_ 58:2282–2289, 1986.

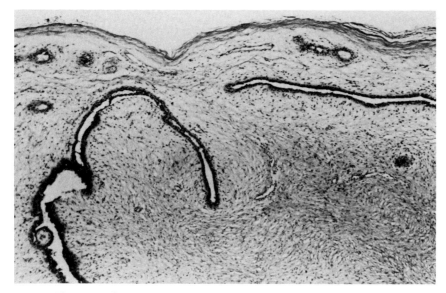

Figure 2.25. Fibroadenoma showing well circumscribed margins.

benign, borderline, and malignant. Tumors are designated as borderline if they have pushing or infiltrating margins, five to nine mitoses per 10 HPF, and moderate atypia.

It is not unusual to see proliferation of the epithelial cells of ducts within phyllodes tumors. Most often this process represents simple hyperplasia, but ductal carcinoma, whether in situ or invasive, may be associated with phyllodes tumor (23). Patients with this type of tumor should be treated like those who have conventional breast carcinoma.

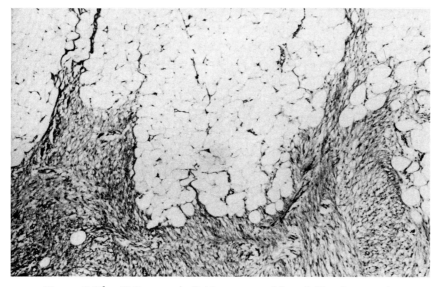

Figure 2.26. Malignant phylloides tumor with an infiltrating margin.

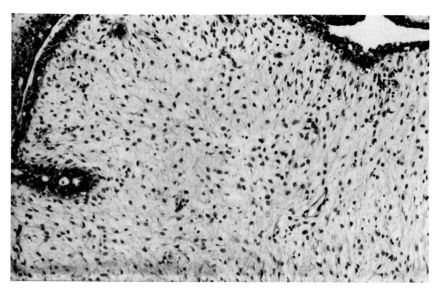

Figure 2.27. Fibroadenoma exhibiting mild to moderate cellularity in the stroma.

DEFERRED DIAGNOSIS

Proliferations of Epithelial Cells

Breast Papillomas. Whether breast papillomas are solitary or multiple, they should not be diagnosed by means of frozen section analysis. The differential diagnosis between papilloma and papillary carcinoma rests mainly on cytologic characteristics that are often distorted by freezing artifact.

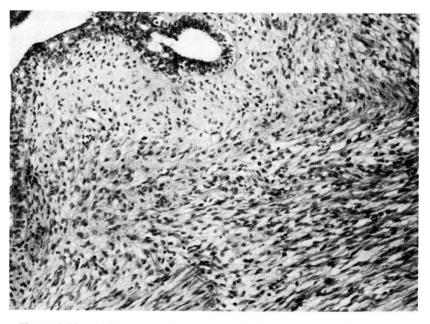

Figure 2.28. Malignant phylloides tumor displaying a hypercellular stroma.

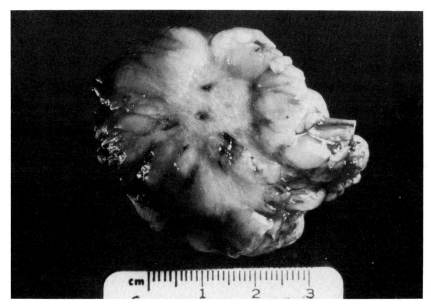

Figure 2.29. Carcinoma of breast with irregular, stellate scarlike area.

If the papillary nature of the lesion is discovered during macroscopic examination, a frozen section should not be performed.

Epithelial Proliferations in Young Patients. Diagnosis of epithelial proliferations in young patients should always be deferred until the permanent sections have been examined, because even severe atypia may be

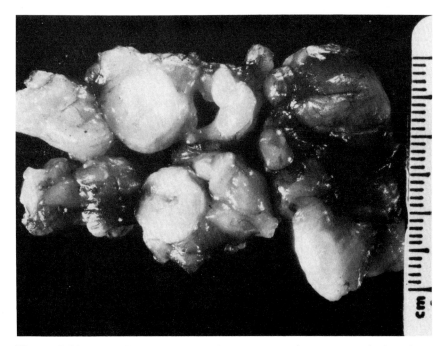

Figure 2.30. Medullary carcinoma of breast. Note the circumscribed uniform, homogeneous mass.

present in lesions that are not yet considered to be carcinomas (24). The age range of patients studied by Rosen et al. was 10 to 44 yrs, with an average age of 19.

Uncommon Carcinomas. We defer the diagnosis of all uncommon types of breast carcinoma. Included in this category are secretory carcinoma (25, 26), lipid-rich carcinoma (27), and glycogen-rich carcinoma (28).

Stromal Lesions

Vascular Proliferations. The microscopic diagnosis of grossly identifiable vascular tumor (29, 30) should be deferred until permanent section examination has been done. It is difficult in frozen section to evaluate some microscopic features that are crucial for the diagnosis of vascular tumors (e.g., endothelial tuftings and intercommunicating channels). Another important motive for deferring diagnosis is that variations in the sampled area often make it difficult to identify and categorize the neoplasm. Biopsy specimens from the peripheral portions, for example, often show low grade areas in otherwise higher grade tumor (29).

Fibromatosis. Diagnosis should be deferred in cases of fibromatosis (31) because it is often difficult to separate this disease from a reactive process and from sarcomas. To avoid causing under- or overtreatment, it is advisable to wait for the permanent sections.

Pure Sarcomas. To rule out the possibility of sarcomatoid (metaplastic) breast carcinoma, a thorough examination of multiple tumor sections is necessary when a pure sarcoma (32, 33) is suspected. Some surgeons may treat sarcomatoid carcinoma with radical mastectomy, in contrast to simple mastectomy which is prescribed for pure sarcomas. Obviously, such different treatments cannot be decided on the basis of examination of one or a few frozen sections.

MACROSCOPIC CHARACTERISTICS

Table 2.6 contains a summary of the most common breast lesions according to their macroscopic appearance (Figs. 2.29 and 2.30). There is always an absolute correlation between macroscopic appearance and microscopic features, except for those in situ lesions that can be differentiated only on the basis of microscopic examination.

TISSUE FOR ESTROGEN RECEPTORS

Tissue for examination of estrogen receptors is needed from all carcinomas of breast. Most laboratories require 0.25 to 0.50 g of tumor to perform this examination. Immunoperoxidase may also be used to determine estrogen receptors in tissue sections (34), but this method does not provide information about number of receptors.

REFERENCES

1. Nakazawa H, Rosen P, Lane N, Lattes R: Frozen section experience in 3000 cases: Accuracy, limitations, and value in Residency Training. *Am J Clin Pathol* 49:41–51, 1968.

Table 2.6.
Classification of Most Common Breast Lesions According to
Macroscopic Appearance

Breast showing area of scar
  Benign
    Fat necrosis
    Radial scar
    Granular cell tumor
  Malignant
    Carcinoma[a]
Well-circumscribed lesion in breast (most are also soft)
  Primary in breast
    Benign
      Fibroadenoma[a]
      Adenoma
    Malignant
      Medullary carcinoma
      Sarcomatoid carcinoma
      Sarcoma
  Metastasis (including lymphoma)
Cystic lesions in breast
  Benign
    Fibrocystic disease[a]
  Malignant
    Cystic carcinoma
    Phyllodes tumor

[a]Indicates that diagnosis is the most common entity in each group.

2. Holaday WJ, Assor D: Ten thousand consecutive frozen sections: A retrospective study focusing on accuracy and quality control. *Am J Clin Pathol* 61:769–777, 1974.

3. Lagios MD, Richards VE, Rose MR, Yee E: Segmental mastectomy without radiotherapy: Short-term follow-up. *Cancer* 52:2173–2179, 1983.

4. Snyder RE: Specimen radiography and preoperative localization of nonpalpable breast cancer. *Cancer* 46:950–956, 1980.

5. Ridolfi RL, Rosen PP, Port A, Kinne D, Mike V: Medullary carcinoma of the breast: A clinicopathologic study with 10 year follow-up. *Cancer* 40:1365–1385, 1977.

6. van Bogaert L-J: Clinicopathologic hallmarks of mammary tubular carcinoma. *Hum Pathol* 13:558–562, 1982.

7. Deos PH, Norris HJ: Well-differentiated (tubular) carcinoma of the breast: A clinicopathologic study of 145 pure and mixed cases. *Am J Clin Pathol* 78:1–7, 1982.

8. Eggers JW, Chesney TM: Squamous cell carcinoma of the breast: A clinicopathologic analysis of eight cases and review of the literature. *Hum Pathol* 15:526–531, 1984.

9. Ro J, Silva EG, Gallager HS: Adenoid cystic carcinoma of breast. (submitted for publication).

10. Fenoglio C, Lattes R: Sclerosing papillary proliferations in the female breast: A benign lesion often mistaken for carcinoma. *Cancer* 33:691–700, 1974.

11. Linell F, Ljungberg O, Andersson I: *Breast Carcinoma: Aspects of Early Stages, Progression, and Related Problems.* Acta Pathol Microbiol Scan, 1980, p 14.

12. Wellings SR, Alpers CE: Subgross pathologic features and incidence of radial scars in the breast. *Hum Pathol* 15:475–479, 1984.

13. Hertel BF, Zaloudek C, Kempson RL: Breast adenomas. *Cancer* 37:2891–2905, 1976.

14. McDivitt RW, Stewart FW, Berg JW: *Atlas of Tumor Pathology of Armed Forces Institute of Pathology, Tumors of the Breast,* ed 2. Bethesda, 1968, p 91.

15. Rosen PL: Microglandular adenosis. *Am J Surg Pathol* 7:137–144, 1983.

16. Tavassoli F, Norris HJ: Microglandular adenosis of the breast. *Am J Surg Pathol* 7:731–737, 1983.

17. Clement PB, Azzopardi JG: Microglandular adenosis of the breast: A lesion simulating tubular carcinoma. *Histopathology* 7:169–180, 1983.

18. Rosenblum MK, Purrazzella R, Rosen PP: Is microglandular adenosis a precancerous disease: A study of carcinoma arising in microglandular adenosis. *Lab Invest* 52:57A, 1985.

19. Weiss SW, Enzinger FM: Epithelioid hemangioendothelioma: A vascular tumor often mistaken for a carcinoma. *Cancer* 50:970–981, 1982.

20. Norris HJ, Taylor HB: Relationship of histologic features to behavior of cystosarcoma phyllodes: Analysis of ninety-four cases. *Cancer* 20:2090–2099, 1967.

21. Hart WR, Bauer RC, Oberman HA: Cystosarcoma phyllodes: A clinicopathologic study of twenty-six hypercellular periductal stromal tumors of the breast. *Am J Clin Pathol* 70:211–216, 1978.

22. Pietruszka M, Barnes L: Cystosarcoma phyllodes: A clinicopathologic analysis of 42 cases. *Cancer* 41:1974–1983, 1978.

23. Rosen PP, Urban JA: Coexistent mammary carcinoma and cystosarcoma phyllodes. *Breast* 1:9–15, 1975.

24. Rosen PP, Cantrell B, Mullen DL, DePalo A: Juvenile papillomatosis (Swiss cheese disease) of the breast. *Am J Surg Pathol* 4:3–12, 1980.

25. Oberman HA: Secretory carcinoma of the breast in adults. *Am J Surg Pathol* 4:465–470, 1980.

26. Akhtar M, Robinson C, Ali MA, Godwin JT: Secretory carcinoma of the breast in adults: Light and electron microscopic study of three cases with review of the literature. *Cancer* 51:2245–2254, 1983.

27. Azzopardi JG: *Problems in Breast Pathology,* ed 2. Philadelphia, W. B. Saunders, 1979, p 301.

28. Hull MT, Priest JB, Broadie TA, Ransburg RC, McCarthy LJ: Glycogen-rich clear cell carcinoma of the breast: A light and electron microscopic study. *Cancer* 48:2003–2009, 1981.

29. Donnell RM, Rosen PP, Lieberman PH, Kaufman RJ, Kay S, Braun DW Jr, Kinne DW: Angiosarcoma and other vascular tumors of the breast: Pathologic analysis as a guide to prognosis. *Am J Surg Pathol* 5:629–642, 1981.

30. Merino MJ, Carter D, Berman M: Angiosarcoma of the breast. *Am J Surg Pathol* 7:53–60, 1983.

31. Hanna WM, Jambrosic J, Fish E: Aggressive fibromatosis of the breast. *Arch Pathol Lab Med* 109:260–262, 1985.

32. Norris HJ, Taylor HB: Sarcomas and related mesenchymal tumors of the breast. *Cancer* 22:21–28, 1968.

33. Barnes L, Pietruszka M: Sarcomas of the breast: A clinicopathologic analysis of ten cases. *Cancer* 40:1577–1585, 1977.

34. Pertschuk LP, Eisenberg KB, Carter AC, Feldman JG: Immunohistologic localization of estrogen receptors in breast cancer with monoclonal antibodies: Correlation with biochemistry and clinical endocrine response. *Cancer* 55:1513–1518, 1985.

35. Haagensen CD: *Diseases of the Breast,* ed 2. Philadelphia, W. B. Saunders, 1971, p 503.

36. Andersen JA, Fechner RE, Lattes R, Rosen PP, Toker C: *Pathology Annual,* ed 1. New York, Appleton-Century Crofts, 1980, p 193.

3

Thyroid

B. Balfour Kraemer, M.D.

Thyroid and thyroid-related specimens account for 12–15% of all diagnostic frozen sections. Accurate frozen section diagnosis approaches 98% in the author's experience, provided that an adequate sample is initially obtained. Diagnostic errors are explained either by sampling error or inaccurate tissue identification. In the case of sampling errors, false-negative diagnoses are the most common. Such is the case with a follicular lesion where frozen section may not display invasion, but on permanent sections one or more areas of invasion are demonstrated. Inaccurate tissue identification is the other situation in which frozen section misdiagnosis occurs. Thyroid carcinoma metastatic in a lymph node can be easily confused with lymphocytic thyroiditis. Distinction of thyroid from parathyroid can be difficult, especially if one is given only a small biopsy to evaluate (see Chapter 11 (**Parathyroid**).

INDICATIONS FOR FROZEN SECTION OF THE THYROID

During the course of thyroidectomy, the surgeon will almost always request a frozen section of the thyroid in order to evaluate a suspicious nodule or other palpable or radiologically demonstrated abnormality. The frozen section diagnosis directs the surgeon's hand in performing either a more radical procedure or terminating the operation. Indications for frozen section at the time of thyroid surgery include the following:

1. A hypofunctioning or nonfunctioning solid nodule with physical findings suggestive of malignancy (i.e., fixation or vocal cord paralysis).
2. A hyperfunctioning nodule that has failed suppression therapy.
3. Dominant cold nodule(s) in a multinodular gland.
4. A cystic nodule *a*) greater than 4 cm in diameter; *b*) having positive or indeterminate cytology; *c*) with serosanguinous contents; or *d*) recurrent or persistent after aspiration.
5. A rapidly enlarging thyroid or thyroid nodule.
6. A thyroid in a patient with a diagnosis or family history of MEN II with an elevated plasma calcitonin level.

7. A palpable nodule or an abnormal radionuclide scan in a patient who has received prior irradiation to the head and neck.

8. Any thyroid nodule in a child or adolescent.

The surgical treatment of thyroid carcinoma remains controversial and is often individualized. Many factors influence the initial surgical approach and include: *a*) the presumed clinical extent of disease; *b*) the prognosis based on age and sex; *c*) the histologic type of malignancy (if known); *d*) a history of prior irradiation to the head and neck; *e*) the expected rate of complications; and *f*) the mode of patient follow-up.

TYPES OF SPECIMENS RECEIVED FOR FROZEN SECTION DIAGNOSIS

Needle Biopsy

In recent years, the utilization of fine-needle aspiration biopsy (FNAB) and tissue core needle biopsy has gained popularity as a cost-effective screening procedure in the initial evaluation of patients with suspicious thyroid nodules (1–4). Both of these procedures are subject to sampling errors, failure to obtain an adequate or representative specimen, and interpretative errors.

Our cumulative experience with frozen section interpretation of tissue core needle biopsies of thyroid nodules is limited, since the majority of surgeons prefer to rely upon either FNAB, or to proceed with definitive thyroid surgery. Tissue core needle biopsy for frozen section diagnosis may be submitted when the patient is considered a poor surgical candidate, or when there is acute tracheal compression secondary to a rapidly enlarging thyroid mass. A rapid tissue diagnosis will establish the histologic type of neoplasm and thus determine whether external irradiation would be beneficial in reducing the size of the mass.

Lobectomy, Subtotal and Total Thyroidectomy

The type of resection of a given thyroid nodule may vary depending on its size and location. The initial surgical specimen delivered for frozen section evaluation is usually a lobectomy specimen (5,6). If the nodule is located within the isthmus, the entire isthmus and medial third of each thyroid lobe are resected in continuity. At the time of lobectomy, if the clinical suspicion of carcinoma is high, usually no attempt is made to identify or preserve the ipsilateral parathyroids. If the parathyroids are to be preserved, the surgeon may submit small biopsies of parathyroid tissue for tissue identification (see Chapter 11, **Parathyroid**).

If a definitive frozen section diagnosis of benign thyroid disease is made, the procedure is terminated. If a definitive diagnosis of carcinoma cannot be made, the surgeon may either terminate the procedure and wait for the permanent sections, or perform a subtotal thyroidectomy. The latter approach is justified on the basis that re-exploration is avoided should the diagnosis of carcinoma be confirmed in the permanent sections (6,7). A compartmental dissection may be included as part of the subtotal thyroidectomy (7). Such a dissection includes lymph nodes in the tracheo-esophageal groove, along the recurrent laryngeal nerve, and in the anterosuperior mediastinum. Occasionally, the compartmental dissection will also include lymph nodes medial to the jugular vein, from the carotid bifurcation caudally. The contralateral parathyroids are identified and preserved, and a small rim of posterolateral thyroid tissue lying immediately adjacent to the preserved parathyroids is left in situ (intracapsular lobectomy). From this procedure, approximately 80–85% of the thyroid and at least two parathyroids have been surgically excised.

Although the need for total thyroidectomy in thyroid carcinoma remains controversial, it is generally accepted that there are specific patient groups that benefit from this procedure. Total thyroidectomy allows for a more complete regional lymph node dissection than does subtotal thyroidectomy, and it is routinely performed for medullary carcinoma, follicular carcinoma with extrathyroidal invasion and/or distant metastases, papillary carcinomas in patients with a history of irradiation and grossly bilateral disease, and thyroid carcinomas in patients in the high risk category (males over 50). As in subtotal thyroidectomy, the parathyroids are identified, preserved if possible, and autotransplanted if necessary (8) (see Chapter 11, **Parathyroid**).

Thyroid-Related Specimens

Parathyroid Glands

These are discussed in Chapter 11, **Parathyroid.**

Cervical Lymph Nodes

Neck lymph nodes are submitted for frozen section diagnosis because the surgeon wants a diagnostic confirmation of metastatic disease in order to proceed with a neck dissection. Often, the lymph nodes submitted for frozen section are clinically positive. When neck lymph nodes are clinically negative, a midjugular lymph node may be submitted for frozen section. If positive, a lateral cervial lymph node dissection will follow (6).

To make a definitive diagnosis of metastatic thyroid carcinoma in a lymph node, the pathologist must first ascertain that the submitted tissue is actually a lymph node. This requires identification of a true subcapsular sinus. Such as task may be impossible when metastases are present, since the sinuses will often be obliterated or secondarily compressed by tumor. Furthermore, it is not uncommon for the lymph node to be replaced entirely by carcinoma, precluding accurate tissue identification.

Frozen section evaluation of lymph node metastases from papillary thyroid carcinoma can pose special problems. Lymph node metastases from papillary carcinoma tend to undergo cystic degeneration. These cystic metastases may have a minimal neoplastic epithelial component in the frozen section. Psammoma bodies may or may not be present. The frozen section differential diagnosis includes thyroglossal duct cyst (see Thyroid Ectopias, this chapter). The clinical history and lateral location may help to make the distinction.

Another common problem encountered with papillary carcinoma is the situation in which both the primary tumor and metastasis are submitted for frozen section evaluation, and the histology of the metastasis appears different from the primary. This situation may be encountered in papillary carcinoma, follicular variant, in which the primary is by definition, entirely follicular (9). The corresponding metastasis may be purely papillary, or mixed papillary-follicular.

The differential diagnostic problem presented in distinguishing lymph node metastasis from lymphocytic thyroiditis is fully discussed later in this chapter.

Occasionally, metastases from an occult primary thyroid carcinoma are identified in cervical lymph nodes removed for other reasons (10) (see Chapter 12, **Lymph Nodes**). If the thyroid appears grossly abnormal, the surgeon may elect to perform a lobectomy on the side from which the positive lymph nodes were identified. If, on the other hand, the thyroid lobe appears normal, the surgeon may elect not to disturb the thyroid bed. Since the overwhelming majority of occult thyroid carcinomas are small sclerosing papillary carcinomas, the prognosis for the patient who has such a malignancy will not be influenced by either decision, provided there is no clinical evidence of distant metastasis.

If ever in doubt about the frozen section diagnosis, the pathologist should request information about the patient's clinical history and gross appearance of the thyroid. If needed, additional tissue should be submitted for frozen section evaluation.

Thyroid Ectopias

Thyroid parenchyma dissociated from the thyroid gland may be found in a variety of anatomic locations in the neck and mediastinum:

<u>Midline</u>
lingual
sublingual
perihyoid
intratracheal
substernal (intrathoracic goiter)
anomalous pyramidal lobe
<u>Midline or lateral</u>
suture-associated implants
sequestered nodular goiter
thyroiditis

Midline

Midline thyroid ectopias are usually associated with thyroglossal duct remnants and are most commonly found around the hyoid bone (11,12). When lingual in location, the thyroid tissue is often functional. It is estimated that approximately 75% of patients who have aberrant lingual thyroid tissue have no other functional thyroid. If a lingual thyroid is identified on frozen section, the pathologist should remind the surgeon that complete excision could possibly render the patient permanently hypothyroid. In the exceedingly rare event that a lingual thyroid carcinoma is identified (13), total resection is warranted, since these carcinomas may behave aggressively.

Thyroglossal Cysts

A thyroglossal cyst typically presents as an anterior midline fluctuant cystic mass, most often located at the level of the hyoid bone. These cysts may develop secondary sinus and/or fistula formation. A sudden increase in the relative size of the cyst arouses clinical suspicion of abscess or carcinoma, and prompts surgical exploration. Frozen section of the cyst may be requested. Ideally, in such resections, the cyst should be delivered intact for pathologic examination. When carcinoma arises in a thyroglossal cyst, a grossly visible mass is often identifiable within the cyst wall. Histologically, the majority of thyroglossal cyst carcinomas are well differentiated papillary carcinomas (14–18). Accurate frozen section interpretation is especially important in this situation because if a carcinoma is identified, the surgeon can carefully inspect the thyroid gland and regional neck lymph nodes to exclude the possibility of metastatic disease. Although most thyroglossal cyst carcinomas are believed to arise de novo from thyroid tissue rests within the cyst wall, metastasis from an occult thyroid primary must be considered in the differential diagnosis (15,18). To complicate the problem further, cystic lymph node metastases from papillary carcinoma may closely resemble thyroglossal duct cysts. The features of a thyroglossal cyst that distinguish it from other entities are *a*) a benign epithelial lining composed of embryonic ciliated, cuboidal, or squamous epithelium, and *b*) the presence of histologically unremarkable thyroid tissue in the cyst wall. The treatment of choice for thyroglossal cysts (with or without carcinoma) is complete en bloc excision of the entire duct, including the central portion of the hyoid bone to remove all epithelial remnants (Sistrunk procedure) (12,19). Some surgeons may also submit a frozen section of the thyroid if it appears clinically suspicious, or they may proceed with a thyroidectomy.

Midline or Lateral Thyroid Ectopia

So-called "lateral aberrant thyroid" refers to the presence of thyroid tissue lateral to the jugular veins. Some authors have used this term in conjunction with thyroid tissue found within cervical lymph nodes (20,21). Patients who have undergone previous neck surgery and who have had the thyroid manipulated during the procedure will rarely develop suture-associated thyroid implants. These implants histologically resemble normal thyroid and often reside around unabsorbed suture material (22,23) or within the perimysium of neck muscles (Fig. 3.1). A history of prior neck surgery is helpful when evaluating such tissue by frozen section. If the patient has a history of follicular carcinoma, the differential diagnosis becomes more complicated. In this situation, the presence of vascular invasion or tissue destruction is helpful in making the distinction.

Invasive fibrous (Reidel's) thyroiditis is a ligneous fibrosing process that may invade tracheal soft tissues and compromise the airway. To relieve respiratory distress, the isthmus and adjacent tissues are resected, if possible. Tissue may be submitted for frozen section to confirm that there is no malignant process. Histologically, thyroid follicles may become secondarily entrapped at the periphery of the fibrosis, superficially resembling follicular

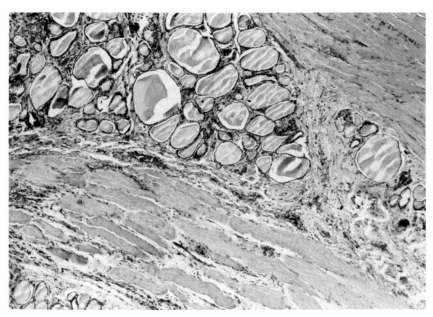

Figure 3.1. Suture-associated thyroid implant in skeletal muscle. Histologically normal thyroid resides in perimysium.

carcinoma. One feature which helps to identify Reidel's thyroiditis is the presence of an accompanying vasculitis, usually an occlusive phlebitis (24).

Thyroid affected by nodular goiter may become mechanically disconnected from the rest of the thyroid, presumably due to the continuous movement of the overlying neck muscles (25) (Fig. 3.2). The histologic appearance of these detached nodules is identical to that of the goitrous thyroid. They reside in the same fascial plane and receive a vascular supply from the same arterial bed which furnishes blood to the thyroid.

Hashimoto's thyroiditis, fibrous variant (26), may pose special problems at the time of frozen section. In a process similar to sequestered nodular goiter (vide supra), progressive interlobular fibrosis can lead to peripheral sequestration of thyroid tissues (Fig. 3.3). Small islands or lobules of thyroid can become entirely surrounded by broad fibrous bands and may eventually become separated from the rest of the thyroid. These nodules may remain attached by only a thin fibrous band, or they may become totally dissociated. This process of sequestration is particularly common in the area of the pyramidal lobe.

As the surgeon initially explores the thyroid, one of the first lymph node compartments visualized is the juxtavisceral group of anterior cervical lymph nodes. In Hashimoto's thyroiditis, fibrous variant, small sequestered nodules of thyroid tissue may be indistinguishable from cervical lymph nodes to the surgeon. He may biopsy one such thyroid nodule and submit it for frozen section, designating it as "lymph node."

One of the classic pitfalls in frozen section diagnosis of thyroid is to mistake Hashimoto's thyroiditis, particularly the fibrous variant, for metastatic thyroid carcinoma involving a neck lymph node. Why is this mistake made? First, the progressive fibrosis of Hashimoto's thyroiditis grossly dis-

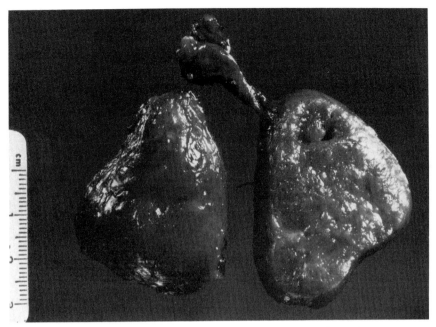

Figure 3.2. Sequestered nodular goiter. A small amount of thyroid remains connected to the rest of the gland by a fibrous band.

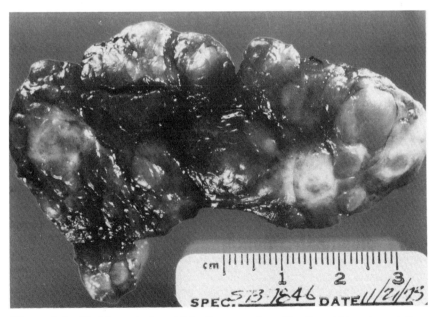

Figure 3.3. Hashimoto's thyroiditis, fibrous variant. The thyroid is enlarged, firm, and nodular. A lobule at the periphery remains partially attached to the gland.

torts the thyroid compartment, making surgical anatomic landmarks difficult to evaluate. The thyroid involved by Hashimoto's thyroiditis is usually enlarged, firm, and multinodular (Figs. 3.3 and 3.4). To the surgeon, firm nodules around the thyroid most likely represent clinically positive lymph nodes. Second, the pathologist is often biased by the surgeon, who designates the tissue as "lymph node." The pathologist presumes that the surgeon has actually biopsied a lymph node, and views the frozen section with this bias.

In addition to the misleading clinical circumstances, there are four main histologic features which create diagnostic confusion at the time of frozen section. Hashimoto's thyroiditis, fibrous variant, has:

1. A lymphocytic infiltrate, complete with germinal centers, resembling a lymph node.
2. Follicular thyroid epithelium intimately intermingled with the lymphocytic proliferation, resembling lymph node metastasis.
3. Follicles with oxyphilic and squamous metaplasia, often with marked cytologic atypia.
4. Broad fibrous bands, resembling desmoplasia.

The low-power appearance of the frozen section in Hashimoto's thyroiditis is extremely helpful and probably the most reliable feature in arriving at an accurate frozen section diagnosis. The broad fibrous bands are exaggerations of the interlobular septae, which separate the thyroid tissue into fairly well compartmentalized lobules of degenerating thyroid parenchyma. On high-power magnification, plasma cells are often numerous. The cytologic atypia of the degenerating follicular epithelial cells along with the oxyphilic and squamous metaplasia can be alarming when combined with

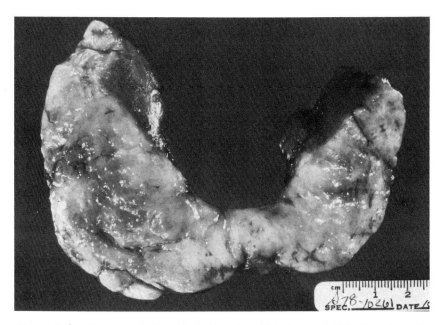

Figure 3.4. Hashimoto's thyroiditis. The thyroid is firm and diffusely enlarged.

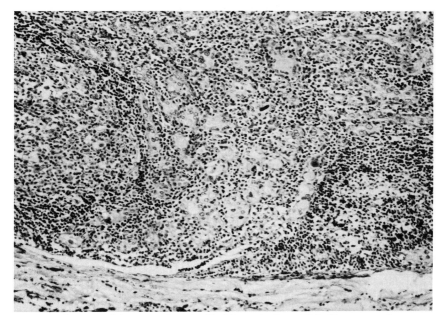

Figure 3.5. Oxyphilic metaplasia in Hashimoto's thyroiditis. Frozen section.

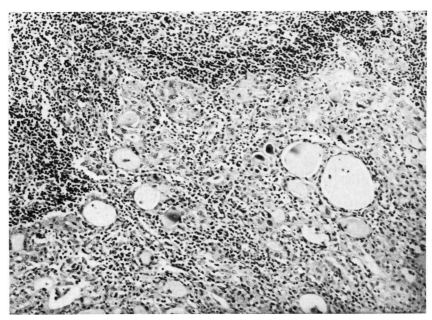

Figure 3.6. Oxyphilic metaplasia of the follicular epithelium in Hashimoto's thyroiditis. Note cytologic atypia and degenerative features of the follicular epithelium. Frozen section.

frozen section artifact (Figs. 3.5 and 3.6). This combination of atypia and peculiar metaplasia should not lure the pathologist into an erroneous diagnosis of malignancy.

FROZEN SECTION DIAGNOSIS OF THYROID NEOPLASMS

Papillary Carcinoma

The gross appearance of papillary carcinoma is variable. It often presents as a small, firm, nondescript nodule that appears vaguely sclerotic. It may also diffusely infiltrate the thyroid, be partially calcified, or almost entirely cystic. Papillary excrescences may or may not be found within the cystic component. The overall appearance may resemble a benign follicular adenoma.

One of the most reliable light microscopic features of papillary carcinoma is the presence of "optically clear" or ground glass nuclei (27) (Fig. 3.7). This feature is reported to be a formaldehyde fixation artifact and is usually not present in tissue that has been frozen. Even after the frozen section is thawed and routinely processed, ground glass nuclei are absent. Hematoxylin and eosin or Papanicolaou touch preparations may rarely display optically clear nuclei, but this is not a striking cytologic feature. Nuclear pseudoinclusions (Fig. 3.8), reported to be a reliable cytologic feature of papillary carcinoma (28) are best seen in hematoxylin and eosin or Papanicolaou touch preparations.

After recognizing the above inherent disadvantage in evaluating a papillary lesion of the thyroid, other features must be relied upon in the frozen section to make the diagnosis of papillary carcinoma. The most important features include the presence of true papillae having fibrovascular cores

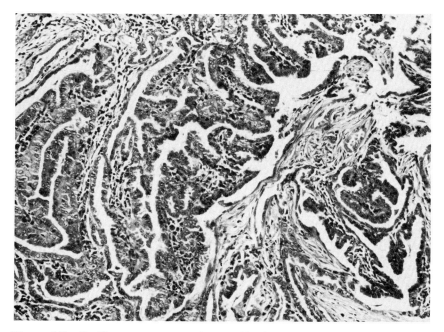

Figure 3.7. Papillary carcinoma with optically clear nuclei.

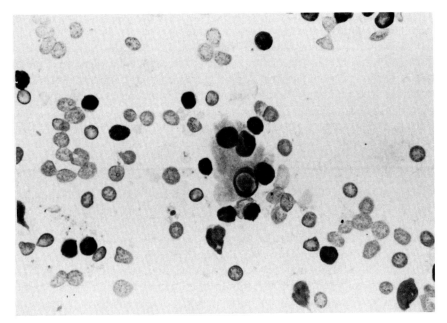

Figure 3.8. Nuclear pseudoinclusion in papillary carcinoma. Touch preparation, Papanicolaou stain.

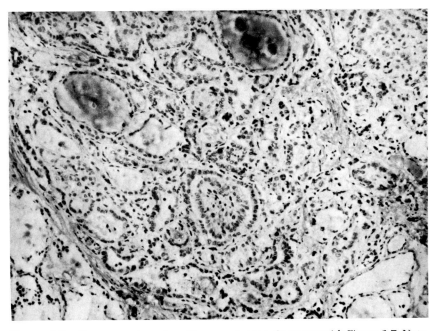

Figure 3.9. Frozen section of papillary carcinoma. Compare with Figure 3.7. Note papillary projection in the center.

(Fig. 3.9), an infiltrative complex arrangement of papillae, and a mixture of papillary, follicular, and solid areas. Squamous metaplasia can be found in 40% of papillary carcinomas, and when present is helpful, especially if it is located within the papillary component of the carcinoma. Squamous metaplasia without accompanying carcinoma can also be seen in a variety of other disorders and should not be confused with squamous carcinoma (29). Another helpful feature commonly present in papillary carcinoma is an abrupt transition from carcinoma to normal thyroid, best appreciated by low-power examination. Psammoma bodies are often present within or immediately adjacent to a papillary carcinoma, and their presence in histologically normal thyroid should prompt a search for a nearby carcinoma. Deeper levels of the frozen section block often resolve the problem. Very rarely, psammoma bodies are associated with reactive or benign thyroid disease such as diffuse toxic or adenomatous goiter (30). Untreated diffuse toxic goiter may display marked papillary hyperplasia and may very rarely have psammoma bodies. However, the papillary hyperplasia represents papillary infoldings of follicular epithelium rather than true papillae with fibrovascular cores. In addition, the lobular architecture of the thyroid is preserved, and there is usually an associated thyroiditis. Papillary hyperplasia in adenomatous goiter is often a focal microscopic finding, surrounded by changes characteristic of adenomatous goiter.

The special problem of papillary carcinoma, follicular, variant, is discussed in Follicular Lesions, this chapter.

Follicular Lesions

There continues to be controversy regarding the histologic criteria for follicular carcinoma (31,32). Traditional criteria include: *a*) destructive invasion of the neoplasm's capsule, *b*) capsular angioinvasion, *c*) thyroid parenchymal destruction, and *d*) extrathyroidal extension and/or metastasis. The gross appearance of follicular adenoma and follicular carcinoma is of little aid in frozen section evaluation, unless there is gross extension of tumor beyond the thyroid capsule into perithyroidal soft tissues. Likewise, the cytologic evaluation of follicular lesions is of little assistance, since follicular adenomas may display marked cytologic atypia, and follicular carcinomas may be histologically bland.

The differential diagnosis for follicular lesions is listed in Table 3.1.

The most common thyroid lesions clinically confused with follicular carcinoma are adenomatous goiter and follicular adenoma. Grossly, an adenomatous nodule is one of several nodules in the thyroid, whereas follicular adenoma or carcinoma tends to be unifocal. In addition, the luminal diameter of follicles in adenomatous goiter is variable, and often larger relative to that of normal thyroid follicles. In contrast, the diameter of neoplastic follicles in follicular carcinoma tends to be smaller relative to that of the normal thyroid (so-called "microfollicular pattern") (31) (Fig. 3.10), although this is not a consistently reliable finding.

In evaluating a follicular lesion at the time of frozen section, the following guideline for handling such lesions is recommended: for any encapsulated mass within the thyroid, one section containing the mass-capsule-

Table 3.1.
Frozen Section Differential Diagnosis of Follicular Lesions of the Thyroid

Lesion	Gross	Histology
Goiter	One or more nodules; thin capsule or nonencapsulated	Micro/macrofollicular; focal papillary hyperplasia; colloid usually abundant
Adenoma	Nodule(s); thin or thick capsule	Microfollicular; trabeculated; atypical follicles with mitoses; colloid sparse
Follicular carcinoma	Encapsulated nodule; often invading capsule or perithyroid tissues	Microfollicular; cystic pattern; atypical follicles with mitoses
Papillary carcinoma, follicular variant	Partially or nonencapsulated nodule	Follicular with abundant colloid; psammoma bodies

thyroid interface should be submitted for frozen section. If the frozen section displays a follicular lesion with no obvious invasive capsular destruction or capsular vascular invasion, and if the mass is at least 1.5 cm in diameter, three additional sections representing the same interface are taken from remaining quadrants and submitted for frozen section. If no invasion is identified in these additional sections, the frozen section diagnosis is reported as "follicular lesion, most consistent with adenoma," and the rest of the mass is submitted for permanent section (Fig. 3.11).

For follicular carcinomas with proven metastases and/or obvious ex-

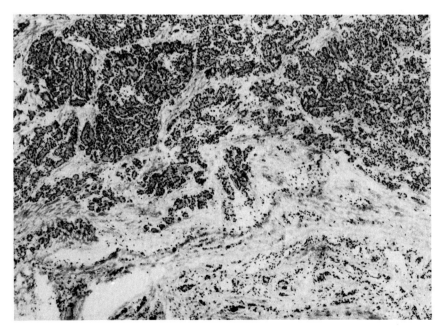

Figure 3.10. Frozen section of follicular carcinoma, with microfollicular pattern. Obvious invasion is absent. This patient had distant metastases.

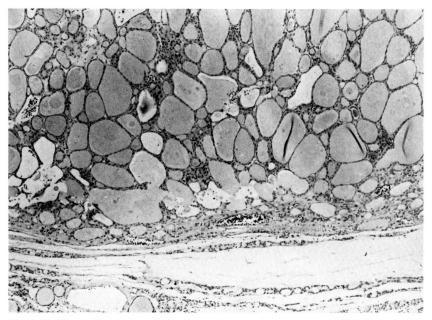

Figure 3.11. Follicular lesion, most consistent with follicular adenoma.

trathyroidal vascular invasion, total thyroidectomy is the treatment of choice. For follicular carcinomas with "minimal invasion" (microscopic invasion of the neoplasm's capsule or vessels), the surgical management is controversial. Some surgeons will perform a simple lobectomy, whereas others will pursue a more aggressive approach, removing most or all of the thyroid. Since the

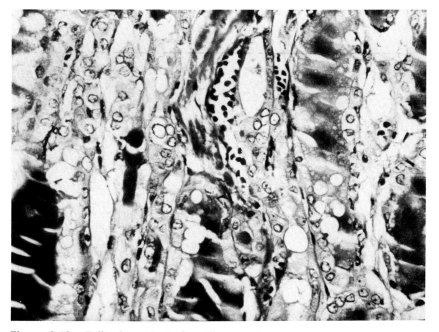

Figure 3.12. Follicular variant of papillary carcinoma.

incidence of lymph node metastases in follicular carcinoma is low, en bloc lymph node resections are usually not performed.

The follicular variant of papillary carcinoma should always be included in the differential diagnosis of follicular lesions. Frozen section diagnosis relies on the presence of psammoma bodies, and, if metastases are examined, the presence of a papillary component. By definition, a papillary carcinoma, follicular variant, is entirely follicular. Optically clear nuclei can usually be appreciated only on permanent section (Fig. 3.12). Metastases often show a mixed papillary and follicular pattern.

Hürthle Cell Lesions

Hürthle cells may be found in a variety of disorders affecting the thyroid:

1. Aging (especially women)
2. Goiter
3. Thyroiditis
     Lymphocytic
     Hashimoto's
     Idiopathic myxedema
4. Therapy-related
     Excess iodide
     Lithium
     Chemotherapy
     Radiation
5. Neoplastic
     Pure Hürthle cell
     Hürthle cell with follicular features
     Hürthle cell with papillary features

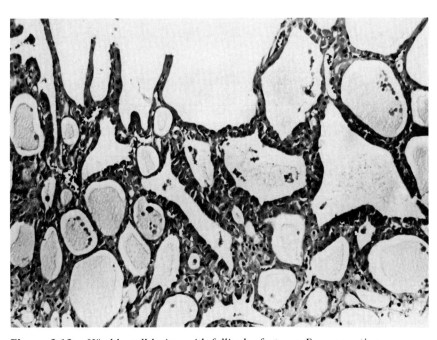

Figure 3.13. Hürthle cell lesion with follicular features. Frozen section.

The gross appearance of a Hürthle cell neoplasm is variable. It may have the gross features of a papillary or follicular carcinoma, or it may closely resemble a follicular adenoma. The frozen section diagnosis of "Hurthle cell neoplasm" provokes controversy among surgeons as to the appropriate management. The prevailing opinion is that Hurthle cell neoplasms, regardless of histology, are potentially malignant, especially if they are 2 cm or greater in diameter, and should therefore be treated with subtotal or total thyroidectomy (7,33,34).

Generally, a Hürthle cell neoplasm that is 2 cm or greater in diameter, displays a multicentric pattern, invades its surrounding capsule, or extends through the thyroid capsule is a biologically aggressive lesion that will behave in a malignant manner. Follicular or papillary differentiation may be present and may aid in more accurately predicting the behavior of the neoplasm (35) (Fig. 3.13). The pathologist examining a frozen section of any Hürthle cell neoplasm should evaluate the above characteristics and report these to the surgeon. If the lesion appears aggressive, regional lymph nodes may be biopsied.

Medullary Carcinoma

The majority of medullary carcinomas are diagnosed preoperatively from MEN II screening procedures and plasma calcitonin assays (36). The frozen section evaluation of such carcinomas is usually straightforward. Grossly, medullary carcinomas are located along the lateral aspect of the upper two-thirds of the thyroid and may be unifocal or multicentric. Microscopically, these carcinomas assume either an organoid (Fig. 3.14) or spindle cell pattern, or they may have an admixture of the two. When the spindle cell pattern predominates, confusion with fibrosarcoma or anaplastic

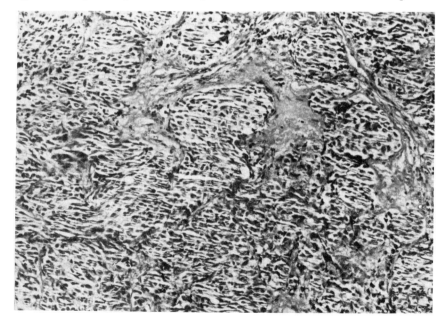

Figure 3.14. Medullary carcinoma. Note predominantly organoid arrangement. Frozen section.

carcinoma may arise. The deposition of amyloid is variable and may be difficult to assess on frozen section. Calcification may also be present, admixed with the amyloid.

Medullary carcinoma may display a microfollicular pattern, creating diagnostic confusion with follicular carcinoma (37). True thyroid follicles may be entrapped in the carcinoma, but they are usually confined to the periphery of the lesion when present. Medullary carcinomas that have large polygonal cells may be confused with Hürthle cell neoplasms. To make this important distinction, a touch imprint can be useful. Cells of medullary carcinoma contain cytoplasmic granules, which by use of immunoperoxidase have been proven to be calcitonin (38). On Giemsa or Papanicolaou preparations, these granules are punctate eosinophilic granules, which are often numerous (38,39). The other frozen section differential diagnoses include parathyroid carcinoma and metastatic adenocarcinoma. The problem of parathyroid carcinoma is discussed in Chapter 11, **Parathyroid.** If a metastatic adenocarcinoma is strongly suspected, the diagnosis should be deferred, especially in the absence of a supporting clinical history.

In patients with MEN syndromes (40), parathyroid chief cell hyperplasia or adenomas may be removed in continuity with a medullary carcinoma. During the course of thyroidectomy, a subtotal parathyroidectomy may also be performed.

Undifferentiated (Anaplastic) Carcinoma

Most anaplastic carcinomas occur in elderly patients and are typically rapidly growing masses that extensively infiltrate extrathyroidal tissues, making surgical resection difficult or impossible. Tissue core needle biopsy may be submitted for frozen section in order to establish a definitive diagnosis so that palliative therapy may be instituted.

Histologically, the main patterns exist as spindle and giant cell types. The spindle cell pattern may resemble fibrosarcoma and may be admixed with a giant cell component. A pure spindle cell neoplastic proliferation may represent a medullary carcinoma (41). Since anaplastic variants of medullary carcinoma have been reported (42), this morphologic variant must be considered in the differential diagnosis. The definitive diagnosis rests upon immunocytochemical and ultrastructural findings (42).

DEFERRED DIAGNOSIS

There are three main situations in which the frozen section diagnosis of a thyroid lesion should be deferred:

1.) Possible malignant lymphoma arising in the thyroid. The pathologist should inform the surgeon that the frozen section displays a lymphoproliferative process. An adequate volume of representative tissue should be obtained, and a portion of it should be processed in a manner similar to that for lymph nodes suspicious for malignant lymphoma (see Chapter 12, **Lymph Nodes**). The pathologist should also request that the surgeon perform an atraumatic excisional biopsy of one or more enlarged regional lymph nodes, taking care not to disrupt the capsule. The majority of malignant small cell proliferations involving the thyroid are malignant lymphomas (43,44). If a convincing thyroid epithelial neoplastic component cannot be recognized at the time of frozen section, the diagnosis should be deferred, and representative tissue should be processed as described above.

2.) Follicular lesions with no obvious invasion (see Follicular Lesions, this chapter).

3.) Suspected metastasis to the thyroid. Rarely, metastatic disease is discovered in the thyroid before the primary becomes clinically evident. The most common metastases to the thyroid include breast, lung, kidney, and malignant melanoma (45,46), and are the result of hematogenous or lymphatic spread. When the histology of the frozen section appears peculiar and incompatible with a thyroid primary, the diagnosis should be deferred. Depending on the size and location of the mass, the surgeon will most likely perform at least a simple lobectomy. Ultrastructural examination is valuable in this situation, and tissue should routinely be procured for electron microscopy where the histology of the thyroid lesion is unusual.

REFERENCES

1. Lowhagen T, Willems JS, Lundell G, Sundblad R, Granberg PO: Aspiration biopsy cytology in diagnosis of thyroid cancer. *World J Surg* 5:61–73, 1981.
2. Lowhagen T, Granberg PO, Lundell G: Aspiration biopsy cytology (ABC) in nodules of the thyroid gland suspected to be malignant. *Surg Clin N Am* 59:3–18, 1979.
3. Wallfish PG, Hazani E, Strawbridge HTG, Miskin M, Rosen IB: A prospective study of combined ultrasonography and needle aspiration biopsy in the assessment of the hypofunctioning thyroid nodule. *Surgery* 82:474–482, 1977.
4. Hamaker RC, Singer MI, DeRossi RV, Shockley W: Role of needle biopsy in thyroid nodules. *Arch Otolaryngol* 109:225–228, 1983.
5. Thompson NW: The resection therapy of carcinoma of the thyroid. *Surgical Rounds* (Jan):100–114, 1984.
6. Block MA: Management of carcinoma of the thyroid. *Ann Surg* 185:133–144, 1977.
7. Guillamondegui O, Goepfert H: Primary treatment of thyroid carcinoma. In Gates GA (ed): *Current Therapy in Otolaryngology, Head and Neck Surgery 1984–1985.* Philadelphia, BC Becker, 1985, p 270–275.
8. Paloyan E, Lawrence AM, Paloyan D: Successful autotransplantation of the parathyroid glands during total thyroidectomy. *Surg Gynecol Obstet* 145:364–368, 1977.
9. Chen KTK, Rosai J: Follicular variant of thyroid papillary carcinoma: A clinicopathologic study of six cases. *Am J Surg Pathol* 1:123–130, 1977.
10. Butler JJ, Tulinius H, Ibanez ML, Ballantyne AJ, Clark RL: Significance of thyroid tissue in lymph nodes associated with carcinoma of the head, neck, or lung. *Cancer* 20:103–112, 1967.
11. Baughman RA: Lingual thyroid and lingual thyroglossal duct remnants. *Oral Surg* 34:781–786, 1972.
12. Allard RHB: The thyroglossal cyst. *Head Neck Surg* 5:134–146, 1982.
13. Potdar GG, Desai PB: Carcinomas of the lingual thyroid. *Laryngoscope* 81:427–429, 1971.
14. Jacques DA, Chambers RG, Oertel, JE: Thyroglossal tract carcinoma: Review of the literature and addition of eighteen cases. *Am J Surg* 120:439–446, 1970.
15. Joseph TJ, Kamorowski RA: Thyroglossal duct carcinoma. *Hum Pathol* 6:717–729, 1975.
16. LiVolsi VA, Perzin KH, Savetsky L: Carcinoma arising in median ectopic thyroid (including thyroglossal duct tissue). *Cancer* 34:1303–1315, 1974.
17. Smithers DW: Carcinoma associated with thyroglossal duct anomalies. In Smithers DW (ed): *Tumors of the Thyroid Gland.* Edinburgh, Livingstone, 1970, p 155.
18. Weber AO: Carcinoma of the thyroglossal duct, primary or metastatic from the thyroid. *Calif Med J* 108:127–129, 1968.
19. Sistrunk WE: The surgical treatment of cysts of the thyroglossal tract. *Ann Surg* 111:950–957, 1940.

20. Gerard-Marchant R: Thyroid follicle inclusions in cervical lymph nodes. *Arch Pathol* 77:633–637, 1964.

21. Gricouroff G: Epithelial inclusions in the lymph nodes. Diagnostic, histogenetic, and prognostic problems. *Diagn Gyn Obstet* 4:285–294, 1982.

22. Moses DC, Thompson NW, Nishiyama RH, Sisson JC: Ectopic thyroid tissue in the neck. Benign or malignant? *Cancer* 38:361–365, 1976.

23. Block MA, Wylie JH, Patton RB, Miller HM: Does benign thyroid tissue occur in the lateral part of the neck? *Am J Surg* 112:476–482, 1966.

24. Harach HR, Williams ED: Fibrous thyroiditis-An immunopathological study. *Histopathology* 7:739–751, 1983.

25. Sisson JC, Schmidt RW, Beienvaltes WH: Sequestered nodular goiter. *N Engl J Med* 270:927–932, 1964.

26. Katz SM, Vickery AL: The fibrous variant of Hashimoto's thyroiditis. *Hum Pathol* 5:161–170, 1974.

27. Hapke M, Dehner LP: The optically clear nucleus. A reliable sign of papillary carcinoma of the thyroid? *Am J Surg Pathol* 3:31–38, 1979.

28. Soderstrom N, Biorklund A: Intranuclear cytoplasmic inclusions in some types of thyroid cancer. *Acta Cytol* 17:191–197, 1973.

29. LiVolsi VA, Merino MJ: Squamous cells in the human thyroid. *Am J Surg Pathol* 2:133–140, 1978.

30. Patchefsky AS, Hoch WS: Psammoma bodies in diffuse toxic goiter. *Am J Clin Pathol* 57:551–556, 1972.

31. Meissner WA: Follicular carcinoma of the thyroid. *Am J Surg Pathol* 1:171–173, 1977.

32. Evans HL: Follicular neoplasms of the thyroid. A study of 44 cases followed for a minimum of 10 years, with emphasis on differential diagnosis. *Cancer* 54:535–540, 1984.

33. Gundry SR, Burney RE, Thompson NW, Lloyd R: Total thyroidectomy for Hürthle cell neoplasm of the thyroid. *Arch Surg* 118:529–532, 1983.

34. Miller RH, Estrada R, Sneed WF, Mace ML: Hürthle cell tumors of the thyroid gland. *Laryngoscope* 93:884–888, 1983.

35. LiVolsi VA: Pathology of the Thyroid. In Greenfield LD (ed): *Thyroid Cancer.* West Palm Beach, CRC, 1978, p 108.

36. Jackson EC, Tashjian AH, Block MA: Detection of medullary thyroid cancer by calcitonin assay in families. *Ann Intern Med* 78:845–852, 1973.

37. Harach HR, Williams ED: Glandular (tubular and follicular) variants of medullary carcinoma of the thyroid. *Histopathology* 7:83–97, 1983.

38. Geddie WR, Bedard YC, Strawbridge E: Medullary carcinoma of the thyroid in fine needle aspiration biopsies. *Am J Clin Pathol* 82:552–557, 1984.

39. Soderstrom N, Telenius-Berg M, Akerman M: Diagnosis of medullary carcinoma of the thyroid by fine needle aspiration biopsy. *Acta Med Scand* 197:71–76, 1975.

40. Keisser HR, Bearen MA, Doppmann J, Wells S, Buja LM: Sipples's syndrome: Medullary carcinoma, pheochromocytoma, and parathyroid disease. *Ann Intern Med* 78:561–579, 1973.

41. Norman T, Johannessen JV, Gautvik KM, Olsen BR, Brennhord IO: Medullary carcinoma of the thyroid. *Cancer* 38:366–377, 1976.

42. Mendehlsohn G, Bigner SH, Eggleston JC, Baylin SB, Wells SA: Anaplastic variants of medullary thyroid carcinoma. A light microscopic and immunohistochemical study. *Am J Surg Pathol* 4:333–341, 1980.

43. Cameron RG, Seemayer TA, Wang NS, Ahmed MN, Tabath EJ: Small cell malignant tumors of the thyroid. *Hum Pathol* 6:731–740, 1975.

44. Walt AJ, Woolner LB, Black BM: Small cell malignant lesions of the thyroid gland. *J Clin Endocrinol Med* 17:45–60, 1957.

45. Silverberg SG, Vidone RA: Metastatic tumors in the thyroid. *Pac Med Surg* 74:175–179, 1966.

46. Elliott RHE, Frantz VK: Metastatic carcinoma masquerading as a primary thyroid carcinoma. *Ann Surg* 151:551–561, 1960.

4

Head and Neck

John G. Batsakis, M.D.

The use of frozen section consultations in surgery of the head and neck appears to equal the extent of use in general surgery, albeit frozen sections for clearance of surgical margins have a much greater use in head and neck surgery than in any other surgical discipline. The accuracy rate (frozen section compared with final surgical-pathologic impression) for head and neck specimens is also comparable to those from other sites. Dehner and Rosai report an accuracy rate of 96% on 1187 individual (nondeferred) frozen sections taken from all sites (1). This level of achievement is nearly identical to that given by others dealing only with lesions in the head and neck (Table 4.1) (2–8). Both of these values are less than those reported for frozen section accuracy in salivary gland lesions—preponderantly of the parotid glands (Table 4.2) (7, 9–11).

SPECIAL TECHNIQUES—PARALLEL SECTIONS IN FROZEN SECTION

The expression "microscopic-controlled excision", used in the routine practice of surgical pathologists and head and neck surgeons, has been appropriated as a contemporary term for what used to be the frozen section part of Mohs zinc chloride fixative chemosurgery (12, 13).

There are two modifications of the traditional method of frozen section, long employed by pathologists. The first is technical; if the conventional orientation of a section is perpendicular, the "new" method utilizes parallel histologic sections (microscopic sections that parallel the surgical margin). The second difference is that, in many instances, a pathologist is excluded from the therapeutic team. This is particularly true for so-called dermato-surgeons who excise and control their own frozen sections of basal cell and squamous cell carcinomas of the skin. To exclude the surgical pathologist from the interpretation does not serve the patient. Certainly the non-cutaneous lesions of the head and neck require a degree of expertise for interpretation not found in the training or background of a dermatologist.

Proponents of this form of microscopic-controlled surgery make two claims in support of parallel sections; a) "all head and neck surgical margins

Table 4.1.
Accuracy of Frozen Section Diagnoses in Head and Neck Lesions

Authors	No. Specimens	Accuracy, %
Pitts et al.[2]	274	96
Winship and Rosvoll[3]	418	96
Ackerman and Ramirez[4]	263	98
French and Lafler[5]	858	97
Nakazawa et al.[6]	628	99
Remsen et al.[7]	1146	96
Bauer[8]	296	96

are random sampling and . . . may examine as little as 1/1,000 of the actual margin," and *b*) "parallel histologic sections theoretically look at 100% of the margin" (12).

Such pejorative statements are further fueled by advocates of parallel sectioning, who claim that 75% of a series of mucosal carcinomas in the head and neck would have had positive surgical margins if parallel sections had not been examined (12).

The parallel section technique for frozen sections of mucosal lesions has the following limitations: *a*) it is labor intensive and requires multiple sections (Table 4.3); *b*) it requires an even more demanding collaboration with the surgeon for purposes of mapping and orienting the specimens; *c*) the possibility of overlooking discontinuous extension of carcinoma in parallel sections is no less than with perpendicular sections taken appropriately at margins; *d*) even with the time consuming parallel section technique, 100% of the margins will not be included.

Knowledge of the biologic behavior of mucosal carcinomas, that margins should include mucosa, submucosa, and muscle or soft tissue, and surgical judgment are effective rejoinders to the technical novelty of parallel sections (14).

INDICATIONS FOR FROZEN SECTION DIAGNOSIS

The indications for frozen section diagnosis in the anatomic region of the head and neck do not differ substantially from those espoused for other organ systems or regions. These are *a*) margins of excision, *b*) diagnosis, *c*) validation of appropriate tissues for additional study or the applications of other techniques (e.g., electron microscopy, immunocytochemistry, and flow cytometry), and *d*) to determine the resectability of a neoplasm.

Table 4.2.
Accuracy of Frozen Section Diagnoses of Parotid Lesions

Authors	No. Patients	Accuracy, %
Miller et al.[9]	132	90
Hillel and Fee[10]	108	91
Dindzans and van Nostrand[11]	110	94
Remsen et al.[7]	88	95

Table 4.3.
Parallel Frozen Section "Levels"[b] Found to be Necessary to Secure a Negative Margin in Carcinomas of the Head and Neck[a]

	Level I	Level II	Level III or more
Oral cavity	8	12	5
Sinonasal tract	1	2	1
Hypopharynx	1	1	2
Oropharynx	1	12	4
Larynx	6	7	5
	17(25%)	34(50%)	17(25%)

[a]Modified from data presented by Davidson TM, Naum AM, Haghighi P, Astarita RW, Saltzstein SL, Seagren S: The biology of head and neck cancer. Detection and control by parallel histologic sections. *Arch Otolaryngol* 110:193–196, 1984.
[b]"Levels" refers to what the authors call a "new round of frozen sectioning."

Margins

This request should be honored without question. Two types of margins apply: *a*) those taken by the surgical pathologist from a presumed extirpated lesion, or *b*) those taken by the surgeon for in situ/in vivo margins after removal of the neoplasm. Both are microscopically controlled resections. Randomly selected margins are never acceptable. All dimensions require evaluation and should always include the deep margin. If the pathologist is not in the operating room, he must be advised of the specific margins of importance in the resected specimen; he must also have information that indicates the orientation of the specimen so that marginal demographics may be accurately defined.

Definition of Positive and Negative Margin

That which constitutes positive or negative surgical margins lacks standardization and certainly precision. Irrefutable microscopic evidence is the presence or absence of invasive carcinoma at the resection line. Carcinoma in situ at the margins has also been considered as "positive" (Fig. 4.1). "Closeness" to a margin and severe dysplasia at the margin have not been systematically evaluated. Indeed, both of these are not easy to assess. Severe dysplasia remains a highly subjective pathologic impression and as such can be either over or under diagnosed. The grading of dysplasia by frozen section as espoused by some gynecologic pathologists is fallacious (15).

Measurement of margin clearance is more objective, but its reliability varies with the conditions of measurement (16). Postremoval and postfixative shrinkage render these measurements inferior to an estimation of distance based on a carcinoma in an in situ sample that has been frozen section monitored.

Given optimum surgical and pathological conditions, what are the prognostic implications of using frozen section to determine the "adequate" amount of squamous carcinoma to remove from the oral cavity and pharynx? Histologic grade is definitely secondary to size or T-stage of a squamous cell carcinoma as a prognostic indicator. The size of the tumor bears heavily

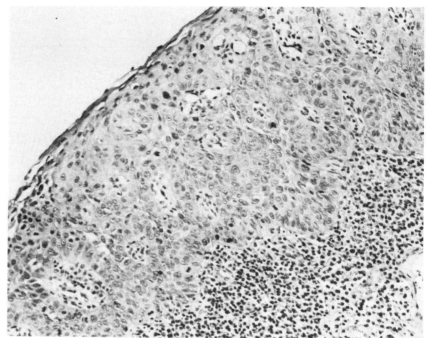

Figure 4.1. Severe dysplasia at mucosal margin of excision of a hypopharyngeal squamous cell carcinoma.

on the rate of local recurrences and more so on 2- and 5-yr survivals, even when there are surgically free margins. It is also important to note that a rather constant number of carcinomas (5 to 10%) will resist the surgical goal of clear margins, regardless of apparent T-stage.

On the basis of available information, there are indications that lesional tissue within 0.5 cm of a surgical margin, whether of severe dysplasia, in situ carcinoma, or invasive carcinoma, places a patient at nearly the same risk for local recurrence (Table 4.4) (17). Failure of local control is not a certainty with such margins, but it is associated with an 80% incidence of recurrence. Looser et al. (17) found that 71% of patients with positive margins had recurrences at the primary site; compared with only 32% in patients with negative margins. Byers et al. (18) report similar findings. Extralaryngeal sites with significant recurrence rates after negative margin surgical excision are those in the oral cavity and pharynx. Looser et al. (17)

Table 4.4.
Histologic Status of Surgical Margins and Recurrence at Primary Site[a]

Lesion at Margin	No. Recurrence/Total (%)		5 Yr. Survival (%)	
Dysplasia	4/5	(80.0)	3/5	(60.0)
In situ carcinoma	11/13	(84.6)	3/13	(23.1)
Invasive carcinoma	16/25	(64.0)	7/25	(28.0)
Close, negative (within 0.5 cm)	14/19	(73.7)	4/19	(21.1)

[a]Modified from Looser KG, Shah JP, Strong EW: The significance of "positive" margins in surgically resected epidermoid carcinomas. *Head Neck Surg* 1:107–111, 1978.

Table 4.5.
Recurrence at Primary Site after Negative Margin Resection[a]

Site of Primary	No.	No. Recurrences (%)	
Tongue	510	166	(32.5)
Gingiva	134	42	(31.3)
Lip	81	7	(8.6)
Supraglottic larynx	167	42	(25.1)
Palate	137	57	(41.6)
Tonsil	147	61	(41.5)
Pharynx and pyriform sinus	183	68	(37.2)
Buccal mucosa	99	33	(33.3)
Floor of mouth	255	67	(26.3)

[a]Modified from Looser KG, Shah JP, Strong EW: The significance of "positive" margins in surgically resected epidermoid carcinomas. *Head Neck Surg* 1:107–111, 1978.

rank the palate, tonsil, and pharynx, including the pyriform sinuses, the highest with primary site recurrences of 41.6, 41.5, and 37.2%, respectively (Table 4.5).

Mucosal Margin

There is much ill-placed emphasis on mucosal margins. Submucosal extensions, spreading for a considerable distance, are seen especially in squamous cell carcinomas of the pharynx, hypopharynx, tongue and tonsil, and in adenoid cystic carcinomas (Fig. 4.2). In all sites, extension of the neoplasm into skeletal muscle is an adverse sign and should be noted.

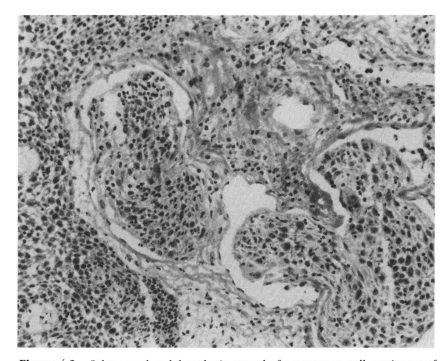

Figure 4.2. Submucosal endolymphatic spread of a squamous cell carcinoma of the hypopharynx.

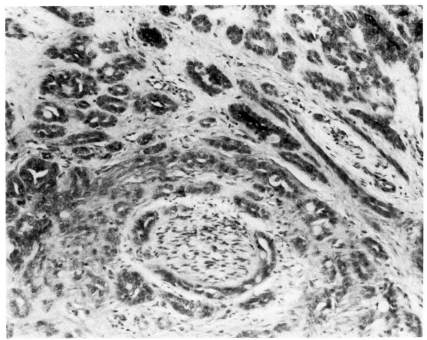

Figure 4.3. Perineurial invasion of a small nerve by a terminal duct adenocarcinoma of the soft palate.

Perineurial extension is required to be noted an all specimens and especially for large or "named" nerves (Fig. 4.3).

Margins After Radiotherapy or Chemotherapy

Margins of excision taken after radiotherapy or chemotherapy are the most difficult to interpret and least reliable to use as indicators because of the iatrogenic alterations. These occur more notably with radiotherapy. With the use of both therapeutic modalities, grossly visible tumor may actually disappear. Sectioning is nonetheless required to verify submucosal involvement or microscopic persistence of neoplasm.

Radiotherapy and most chemotherapeutic agents, like bleomycin, will cause a squamous cell carcinoma to "mature"—often leaving "tombstones" of keratin and a foreign body reaction with fibrosis. After therapy, the question is often asked, "How viable is the neoplasm?" This may be impossible to answer, since function and viability cannot be deduced with accuracy from a static, lifeless histologic preparation. Even after treatment, however, persistence of neoplasm is signified by the mere presence of keratinizing balls of a differentiated carcinoma.

Margins in Salivary Gland Tumors

Margins in salivary gland tumors are relative to the glands involved. For the parotid gland, margin selection is facilitated by the facts that nearly 80% of the tumors are in the superficial lobe (lateral to the facial nerve) and because the appropriate "biopsy" is a lateral lobectomy (Fig. 4.4). The

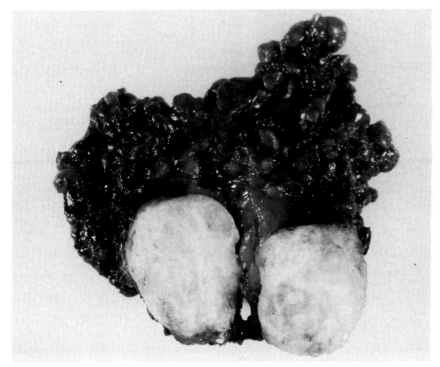

Figure 4.4. Pleomorphic adenoma of the superficial lobe of the parotid gland. Note the excision includes all of the superficial lobe.

deep surface must be examined, and any suspicious extension beyond the capsule of the gland proper is required to be sectioned. Since the facial nerve is preserved in nearly all instances, except when it is grossly non-dissectable from the tumor, the surgeon usually provides a specimen from near the nerve in order to discern any microscopic residual disease that would be treatable by postoperative irradiation.

The appropriate operation for a submandibular gland salivary tumor is at least total removal of the gland. Sections from the superior (nearest the floor of mouth), lateral and medial, deep and inferior margins are necessary for the evaluation of extraglandular extension into adjacent soft tissues (Fig. 4.5).

Margins for minor salivary gland tumors are like those for other mucosal lesions; depth and circumferential excision lines.

Meaning of Negative Margin

After an elusive carcinoma has been tracked by frozen section for a surgeon, the question may arise as to the clinical significance of the procedure. This is not easy to answer.

One of the putative indicators of complete surgical removal is a margin of uninvolved tissue around an excised malignancy. How generous the margin should be has not been, and probably cannot be, defined for all forms of cancer or for selected classes of malignancy. The anatomic site with its attendant restrictions, the presumed biologic characteristics of the

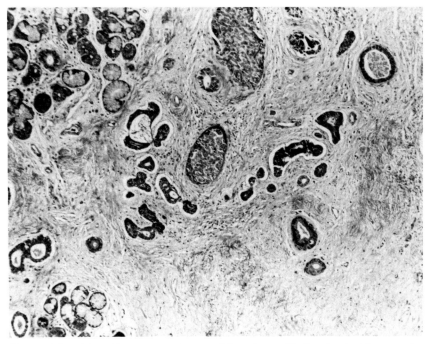

Figure 4.5. Adenoid cystic carcinoma of the submandibular gland with extension into periglandular soft tissues.

cancer, and conservation versus extended surgery, are just some of the factors that must be weighed in predetermining "adequate" margins of resection.

Gross residual neoplasm is locally persistent and nearly always associated with increased mortality. The clinical significance of residual microscopic cancer, on the other hand, has not been adequately defined, and there are a few pertinent retrospective studies of the problem.

Depending on the site of squamous cell carcinomas of the upper aerodigestive tracts the surgeon may or may not be able to obtain free margins from the tumor, and there is also the biologic significance of involved or uninvolved limits of the excision to consider. This variation relates more to the micro- and macroanatomic, biologic and epidemiologic environments of the sites of the carcinomas than to any intrinsic histologic differences among the squamous cell carcinomas themselves. These factors strongly infer that one cannot extrapolate margins in carcinomas of the larynx to carcinomas of the oral cavity and pharynx.

It has been claimed that microscopic accuracy of an adequate surgical margin is at least 50%; as judged by local recurrences (19). In part, this rather low assessment is due to pathologic and clinical difficulties coincident with the evaluation of tissues and submucosal extension or skip areas irradiated prior to surgery; this is especially noted in cases of hypopharyngeal and postcricoid carcinomas. Another contributing factor must be the lack of close cooperation between surgeon and pathologist.

A negative surgical margin is certainly not an assurance for successful local control. In fact, T-stage appears to be a more predictable determinant;

the smaller the carcinoma with free surgical margins, the higher the local control rate. Survival of patients with negative margins is almost linearly related to T-stage of the carcinoma.

Prognostic implications of a positive microscopic margin are also related to stage of the disease. The higher the stage, the higher the recurrence rate; and two, five, and more years survival is more dependent on stage, especially for patients with stage III and IV malignancies.

A significantly lower rate of local recurrences is reported in patients with primary squamous cell carcinomas of the larynx who have positive surgical margins after conservation laryngeal surgery. Thirty-nine of 111 patients who underwent hemilaryngectomy and were studied by Bauer et al. (20) had positive surgical margins; defined as close, gross, or microscopic involvement. Only 7 of the 39 developed a local recurrence. This certainly supports the axiom that the significance of margins is largely dependent on site and also points to the fact that patients who are candidates for conservative laryngeal surgery generally have early, and hence more favorable, carcinomas.

Despite the fact that the significance of surgical margins has an apparently aleatoric quality, the margins still provide therapeutic and prognostic guidelines. Vikram and associates (21) have shown a decrease in the failure rate at the primary site when postoperative irradiation therapy is provided; and they found more recurrences in patients who had microscopically positive margins.

Diagnosis

Except for cases in which salivary gland tumors and clinically positive (without prior needle aspirate diagnosis) lymph nodes are involved, most patients with head and neck cancer will have had prior conventional biopsy diagnosis, thereby negating a repeat confirmatory frozen section. Other exceptions are parapharyngeal space lesions, middle ear tumors, and lesions in inaccessible paranasal sites.

Frozen sections for diagnosis of major salivary gland tumors should in fact be limited. Surgeons who write on this topic give the impression that they have the uneasy task of navigating between Scylla and Charybdis when seeking frozen section consultations on salivary gland tumors, particularly tumors of the parotid gland; e.g., "the surgeon must be prepared for changes in microscopic diagnosis in approximately 18% of cases" (22); "to freeze, or not to" (23).

The single most important purpose of any frozen section diagnosis is to make a therapeutic decision; decisions that involve major salivary gland lesions require special introspection by the surgeon. Unless a precise diagnosis of a salivary tumor causes a surgical procedure to be modified, frozen section evaluation is an epiphenomenon; statements to the contrary are captious. Resection of the facial nerve is not dependent on the histologic subtype of a parotid neoplasm. It is based on the gross anatomic intimacy of a parotid neoplasm to the nerve (Fig. 4.6). Extent of parotidectomy is also less guided by histologic type than by size and extensions, especially when a definitive biopsy specimen is obtained by subtotal parotidectomy with removal of the tumor. To seek guidance on the basis of a frozen section

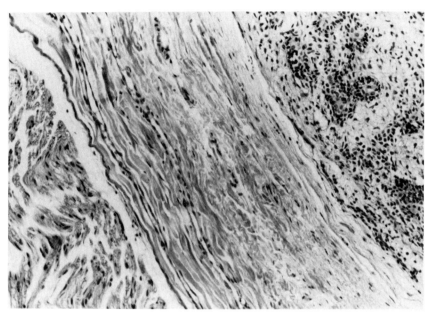

Figure 4.6. Pleomorphic adenoma (right) is separated only by its capsule from a branch of the facial nerve.

of salivary gland tumor in order that a neck dissection might be performed in a patient with a clinically negative neck is to lack an appreciation and knowledge of the frequency of nodal metastasis in the more commonly encountered salivary gland malignancies: adenoid cystic carcinoma, acinic cell carcinoma, low-grade mucoepidermoid carcinoma. None of this trio exhibits a high incidence of metastases to regional lymph nodes. High-grade carcinomas, such as the far less common primary squamous cell carcinoma, ductal carcinoma, and high-grade mucoepidermoid carcinoma, may warrant elective dissections of the neck; but this decision is principally surgical, not pathological.

Gates (23), in a thoughtful essay, has placed frozen sections for salivary gland tumors in appropriate context for head and neck surgeons. This message has not filtered down to all surgeons and certainly has not been given to surgical pathologists. The omission may be responsible for a certain degree of diffidence when a pathologist deals with salivary gland tumors. A precise histologic classification cannot always be given with permanent sections, let alone frozen section preparations. There is a finite number (approaching 2 to 3%) of salivary gland tumors that defy classification.

Some interrelated principles of surgery and pathology are essential for a pathologist to know when dealing with a request for frozen section sampling of salivary gland tumors:

1.) The smaller the salivary gland, the more likely a tumor will be malignant: 20% of parotid tumors, 50% of submandibular gland tumors, 55% of oral minor salivary gland tumors, and 80% of sublingual gland tumors will be malignant.

2.) Bilateral major salivary gland enlargement usually denotes benign disease or lymphoma. Only a grand total of 2 to 5% of salivary tumors are bilateral in a synchronous development; i.e., Warthin's tumor, lymphoepithelial lesion, and acinic cell carcinoma.

3.) Below the age of 1 yr, epithelial tumors of salivary glands are rare. The most common childhood salivary gland tumor is the pleomorphic adenoma, followed by mucoepidermoid and acinic cell carcinomas.

4.) Deep lobe parotid tumors make up 10% of tumors of the parotid gland. Regardless of the histologic type of neoplasm, a total parotidectomy is required. The pleomorphic adenoma is the predominant tumor found in the deep lobe.

5.) Sampling error is accountable for the largest number of changed diagnoses.

6.) Subclassification into low-grade or high-grade malignancies should be done if possible (Table 4.6).

7.) A tumor of the submandibular gland is minimally treated by a complete removal of the gland.

8.) Be wary of metastases to parotid nodes from extraparotid primaries. The most common are situated in areas drained by the parotid nodes, for example, facial and scalp skin (basal cell and squamous cell carcinomas and melanomas). Carcinomas from the breast and kidney are the most frequent infraclavicular malignancies with metastases to parotid nodes (Figs. 4.7 and 4.8).

Table 4.6.
Classification of Malignant Salivary Gland Neoplasms According to Clinicopathologic Grades

Low-Grade Carcinomas
    Terminal duct adenocarcinoma ("polymorphous low-grade adenocarcinoma")
    Tubular variant of adenoid cystic carcinoma
    Acinic cell carcinoma
    Epimyoepithelial carcinoma of intercalated ducts
    Low-grade mucoepidermoid carcinoma
    Noninvasive carcinoma in pleomorphic adenoma (carcinoma in situ)
Intermediate-Grade Carcinomas
    Cribriform and cylindromatous variants of adenoid cystic carcinoma
    Intermediate-grade mucoepidermoid carcinoma
    Myoepithelial carcinoma
    Well-differentiated papillary adenocarcinoma
    Malignant basaloid carcinoma
High-Grade Carcinomas
    Salivary duct adenocarcinoma
    High-grade mucoepidermoid carcinoma
    Squamous cell carcinoma
    Invasive carcinoma ex pleomorphic adenoma
    Malignant Warthin's tumor
    True malignant mixed tumors (carcinosarcoma)
    Undifferentiated carcinoma
      Small cell
      Large cell
      Neuroendocrine
      "Lymphoepithelial carcinoma"

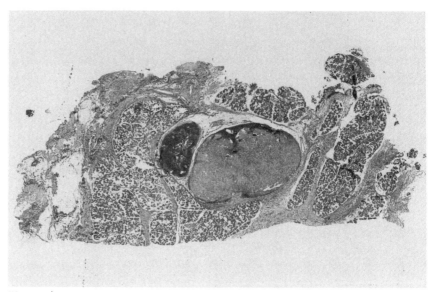

Figure 4.7. Metastatic renal cell carcinoma to an intraparotid lymph node. The primary was clinically occult. Note the confinement of the neoplasm to the lymph node.

9.) The frozen section "error rate" is higher in minor salivary gland tumors. Here also, nonrepresentative specimens are primarily responsible. This also applies to permanent sections.

10.) The most difficult differential diagnoses, regardless of the salivary sites are: *a*) distinguishing mucoepidermoid carcinomas from chronic sialadenitis or necrotizing sialometaplasia; *b*) distinguishing some mono-

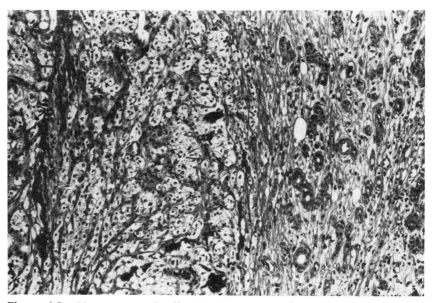

Figure 4.8. Metastatic renal cell carcinoma in parenchyma of parotid gland, indicating hematogenous metastasis.

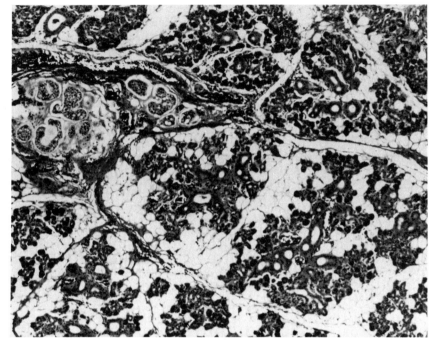

Figure 4.9. Adenoid cystic carcinoma infiltrating into parotid parenchyma at a distance removed from the primary mass.

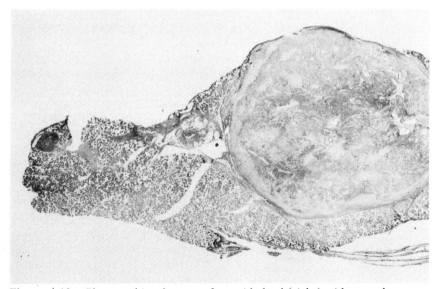

Figure 4.10. Pleomorphic adenoma of parotid gland (right) with a synchronous, smaller monomorphic adenoma (left). Note the superior margin of the pleomorphic adenoma is made only by the adenoma's capsule.

morphic adenomas from adenoid cystic carcinomas; _c_) distinguishing some low-grade adenoid cystic carcinomas from pleomorphic adenomas.

_11._) Primary (intrasalivary) supporting tissue tumors, except for the unique infantile hemangioma are very rare.

_12._) Frozen section of a salivary mass is indicated if the surgeon considers the lesion to be other than a neoplasm, such as lymph node, inflammatory disorder, or for margins as outlined above (Figs. 4.9 and 4.10).

Validation of Appropriate Tissue

This use of the frozen section is less for diagnosis than for the judicious selection of tissue for ancillary, if not diagnostic, procedures; these include tissue culture for micro-organisms and for special studies, such as electron microscopy or immunocytochemistry.

Resectability of Tumor

Since clinical staging of a neoplasm is fallible, especially in the complex anatomic structures of the head and neck, this use of the frozen section is probably the most appropriate of all. Specimens are the surgeon's responsibility and precede the performance of major resection. This form of frozen section is most often applied to the larynx in candidates for conservation surgery, but it is useful for suspected deep extensions, such as to the base of the skull or periosteum of bone.

SPECIFIC PROBLEMS IN HEAD AND NECK FROZEN SECTION DIAGNOSIS

Necrotizing Sialometaplasia Versus Carcinoma

Necrotizing sialometaplasia mimics carcinoma clinically and histologically. Failure to recognize the lesion has resulted in several instances of unnecessary radical surgery. The "overdiagnoses" are most often mucoepidermoid and squamous cell carcinomas.

Although it is preponderantly an oral lesion, necrotizing sialometaplasia is found anywhere salivary tissue is present; sinonasal tract, major salivary glands, larynx (24–26). In the extraoral sites, it is nearly always secondary to surgical manipulation and hence to compromise of the local blood supply (Figs. 4.11 and 4.12). The oral forms are usually spontaneous with the most common site of involvement being the junction of the hard and soft palates. The lesion may be present as a nonulcerated swelling but more often as an ulcer, deep seated and sharply demarcated from the surrounding mucosa. The lesions may be unilateral, bilateral, or midline.

The essential features of necrotizing sialometaplasia are prominent ductal squamous metaplasia with surface pseudoepitheliomatous hyperplasia, lobular necrosis of acini with mucous pooling, and an acute and chronic sialadenitis (Fig. 4.13). Importantly, the lobular architecture of the salivary tissue is preserved even in the presence of extensive inflammatory changes.

In contrast, mucoepidermoid carcinomas are never confined to lobules, nearly always manifest either a pushing or more often aggressive infiltration, and rarely show either pseudoepitheliomatous hyperplasia or well devel-

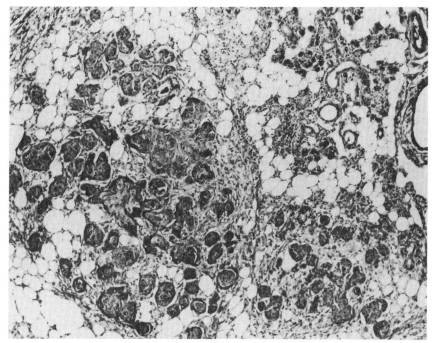

Figure 4.11. Necrotizing sialometaplasia in parotid gland. Note lobular confinement of the metaplastic islands. This lesion, like all observed by the author in the major salivary glands, followed surgical intervention.

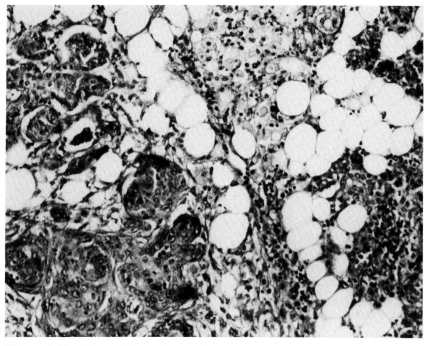

Figure 4.12. Necrotizing sialometaplasia of parotid gland. Higher magnification field of fig. 4.11.

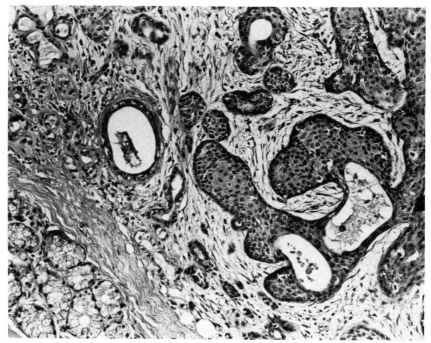

Figure 4.13. Necrotizing sialometaplasia of palate in near end-stage manifesting squamous metaplasia of ducts.

oped epidermoid characteristics (Fig. 4.14). Low-grade mucoepidermoid carcinomas are noted for their cystic architecture and tripartite differentiation: mucous, epidermoid, and intermediate cells (Fig. 4.15). Higher grades manifest increased numbers of intermediate cells, rarely keratinizing squamous cells and a solid (noncystic) architecture.

Oral Epithelial (Odontogenic) Residues and the Juxtaoral Organ Versus Margin of Resection Positive for Squamous Carcinoma

Odontogenic epithelial cell residues are derived from the dental lamina and are thought to be the origin of gingival cysts (lesions rarely seen after the age of 3 months) in infants. In adults, the epithelial remnants resemble cell nests of Malassez (27). Hodson (28) found residues in the anterior incisor areas in 58% of 26 necropsies and in 14% of 58 edentulous third molar regions.

It is not unusual to find such benign epithelial nests in close association with nerves at various sites in the orofacial region. Epithelial residues of odontogenic origin (dental laminae, sheath of Hertwig), remnants of surface mucosa in the depths of the mucosa of edentulous jaws, and the juxtaoral organ of Chievitz are those most often encountered (29–31).

The epithelial residues are found around teeth and also in the eruption tract along the neurovascular bundle supplying the teeth. They may be localized within bone, within gingival mucoperiosteum, and along dental nerves.

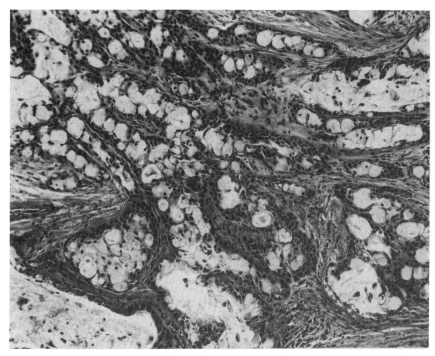

Figure 4.14. Intermediate grade mucoepidermoid carcinoma of oral cavity. Note the different cell types and invasive quality of the carcinoma.

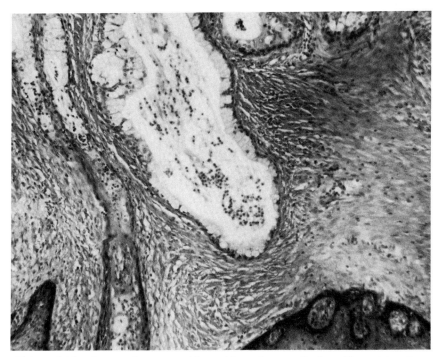

Figure 4.15. Low-grade mucoepidermoid carcinoma of palate. The origin of mucoepidermoid carcinomas from the excretory duct portion of the salivary duct unit is evident.

The juxtaoral organ lies in the buccotemporal space where fibroadipose tissue, the stem of the buccal nerve and its proximal branches, the buccal artery and associated venous plexus, several buccal glands, and on occasion, lymph nodes, form its environment. The organ is closely related to the buccotemporal fascia, either within the lower leaflets or between them.

The odontogenic nests and the juxtaoral organ need to be differentiated from foci of squamous carcinoma at the margin of resection. This differential diagnosis is even more difficult with the juxtaoral organ, due to its perineural location. The well circumscribed appearance of the groups of cells, lack of atypia, and presence of retrogressive changes are all features that favor the benign nature of the area in question. The diagnosis can be further confirmed by comparing these structures with a section from the carcinoma and by defining the precise location of these foci.

Microscopically, the residues can be described in two groups: I. small nests of basal cells with deeply staining nuclei and only a moderate amount of cytoplasm. They occur as small spherical groups of cells, larger cell nests, or in long or short chains or columns (like the sheath of Hertwig); II. larger cell nests with basal type cells and evidence of squamous differentiation. Palisading may be present at the periphery. In some instances, the residue may be entirely squamous in composition (Fig. 4.16).

In both types, retrogressive changes can be found; e.g., pyknosis, hydropic change, calcification, and cyst formation.

Verrucous Carcinoma Versus Hyperplasia

The two favored sites of this low-grade squamous cell malignancy are the buccal mucosa and the laryngeal glottis (32). It is likely that verrucous carcinoma evolves through a histologic spectrum (32–34). Perhaps it starts as a human papilloma virus-associated papilloma, further progresses to an intermediate histologic stage (verrucous hyperplasia), then to verrucous

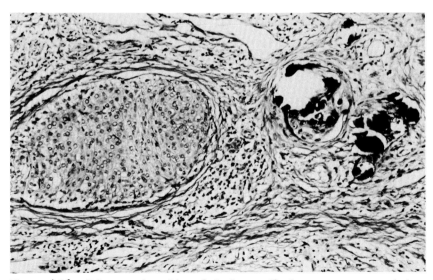

Figure 4.16. Odontogenic residue of gingiva manifesting squamous metaplasia.

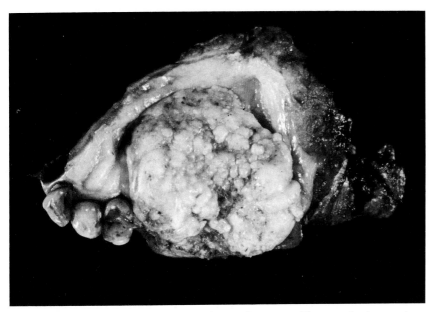

Figure 4.17. Verrucous carcinoma of buccal mucosa. The exophytic neoplasm arises in a clinical "leukoplakia."

carcinoma (Fig. 4.17). The pertinent clinicopathologic features of verrucous carcinoma are presented in Table 4.7.

There are few squamous lesions that histologically mimic verrucous carcinoma. In the fully developed carcinoma, pseudoepitheliomatous hyperplasia should not be a source of confusion because of the carcinoma's triad of keratosis, church spire arrangement of the outgrowth and the blunt, cytologically nonmalignant deep portions (Figs. 4.18 and 4.19). Verrucous hyperplasia can be used as a diagnostic term to indicate a mucosal lesion with all, or most, of the criteria for verrucous carcinoma but for which the depth of extension is less. If used as diagnosis rather than as descriptive designation, the surgeon should be told that biologically the behavior will not be unlike a verrucous carcinoma and more than two-thirds will eventuate into verrucous carcinoma or well-differentiated, nonsquamous carcinoma. In regard to the latter, it should also be appreciated that a significant number of verrucous carcinomas will manifest a different histologic form of squamous carcinoma within the same lesion. This has been termed hybrid verrucous squamous carcinoma.

Surgical removal, at times conservative, depending on the site and size of the carcinoma is the preferred treatment. This is not because radiotherapy carries without it the possible threat of "conversion" to an anaplastic carcinoma, but because radiotherapy fails to control local disease in nearly two-thirds of patients.

A "nibbler biopsy" of the surface of a verrucous carcinoma is an unsatisfactory specimen for either frozen section or permanent section diagnosis of verrucous carcinoma. It is the depth of the lesion which will show the characteristic pushing invasion by bland appearing squamous cells. Ex-

Table 4.7.
Clinical and Pathologic Features of Verrucous Squamous Cell Carcinoma

Patients
  Tobacco users
  Elderly men or women with history of snuff or smokeless tobacco use
  Poor oral and general hygiene
Sites of Predilection
  Buccal and gingival mucosa; glottis
Gross Appearance
  Arises usually in background of diffuse clinical leukoplakia
  Lesion is fungating or exophytic; usually well keratinized surface
Microscopic Appearance
  High degree of cellular differentiation without usual cytologic features of malignancy
  Pushing, blunt deep borders with bulbous configuration of rete ridges
  Deep, verruciform projections, often arranged in a "church spire" or "soldier in a file" architecture
  Prominent chronic inflammatory reaction in surrounding stroma
  Absence of vascular or perineural extension
Biologic Behavior
  No metastases in bona fide examples
  May exist in hybrid form, i.e., verrucous carcinoma and other non-verrucous squamous cell carcinoma in same lesion
  Multifocal or second primary in head and neck or same anatomic region in nearly 20% of oral verrucous carcinomas
  Surgical removal (may be conservative) is preferred therapy. Radiotherapy exhibits significant inability to control locally and requires high dose irradiation

cessive keratin formation is not specific and may in fact not be shown by some verrucous carcinomas.

Sarcomatoid Carcinoma Versus Pseudosarcomatous Stromal Reaction

This differential diagnosis can be one of the most difficult, if not impossible, of all lesions in the head and neck (35, 36). Primarily an oral and glottic or supraglottic lesion, the sarcomatoid carcinoma is defined as a squamous cell carcinoma in which the cells have assumed a metaplastic sarcomatoid phenotype (Figs. 4.20 and 4.21). If on frozen section, there is found a definable squamous cell carcinoma (usually well differentiated or even verrucous), the diagnosis is made without concern for the nature of the composition of the stromal component. Most sarcomatoid carcinomas are polypoid in configuration and have an ulcerated surface. The carcinoma should be sought at the cuff of the polypoid mass or at the depth. A single section may not be sufficient. If one fails to find carcinoma, a presumptive diagnosis or deferred diagnosis should be rendered so that permanent sections and cytokeratin immunocytochemistry can be performed to identify keratin immunoreactive stromal-like cells in the tumor.

The diagnostic problem is compounded when there has been prior radiotherapy. In such instances, it may be impossible to identify carcinoma cells in an irradiated matrix. The same principles of requiring definable carcinoma in the lesion should be applied.

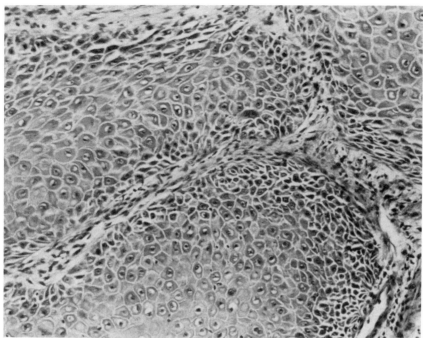

Figure 4.18. Verrucous carcinoma at its invasive border. Note the bulbous, pushing, very well differentiated features.

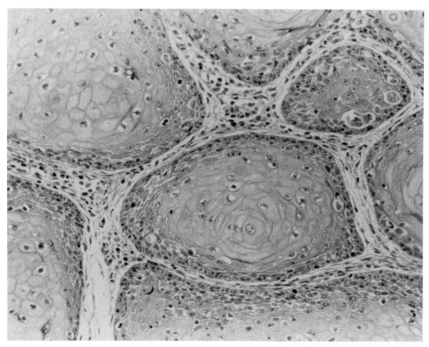

Figure 4.19. Verrucous carcinoma with characteristic bland cytomorphologic appearance.

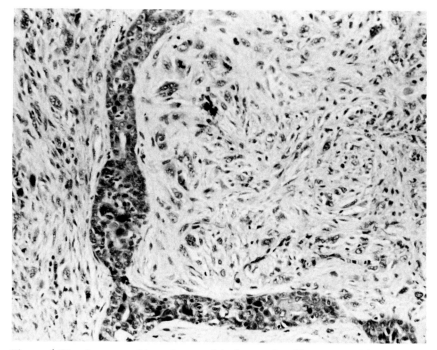

Figure 4.20. Sarcomatoid carcinoma of the larynx. Readily recognizable squamous cell carcinoma is surrounded by pleomorphic, metaplastic, and sarcoma-like carcinoma cells.

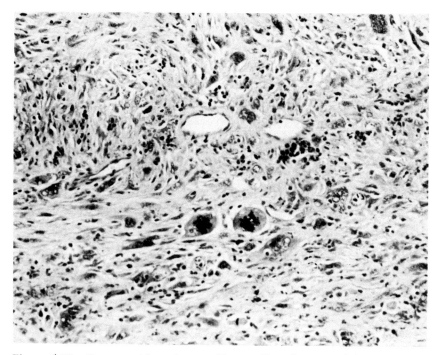

Figure 4.21. Sarcomatoid carcinoma of larynx. Note the atypical division figures. The latter are not found in reactive stromal cells.

Monomorphic Salivary Gland Adenoma Versus Adenoid Cystic Carcinoma

Both of these salivary gland tumors arise from the intercalated duct portion of the salivary duct unit and can share some histologic features as a consequence (37, 38). In the oral cavity, adenoid cystic carcinomas have a predilection for the palate, whereas monomorphic adenomas prefer the upper lip, buccolabial sulcus, or buccal mucosa. A capsule is usually not present in intraoral monomorphic adenomas, but they are more circumscribed than adenoid cystic carcinomas. There is, however, a tendency for multifocal origin in monomorphic adenomas at any site; 10% in the major salivary glands and more than that in the labial region.

The classic cribriform, cylindromatous, or solid architecture of the adenoid cystic carcinoma sets the carcinoma apart from most monomorphic adenomas (Fig. 4.22). This is especially pertinent when the constituent cells are examined. The monomorphic adenoma has uniform and regular small cuboidal cells, sometimes in a double layer (Fig. 4.23). Squamous or less well defined epidermoid metaplasia is rare in adenoid cystic carcinomas, but is quite often encountered in monomorphic adenomas, and takes the form of an abrupt island or focus. A similar cytomorphologic feature is also seen in ameloblastoma.

Invasion of small nerves is not seen with any monomorphic adenoma, but islands of tumor may abut onto the outer sheath of small nerve branches. Necrosis of neoplastic islands is not seen in monomorphic adenomas, but ischemic, cystic necrosis may be present in the center of a tumor nodule.

Like Warthin's tumor, some acinic cell carcinomas (and rarely a mucoepidermoid carcinoma) and monomorphic adenomas may take origin from enclaved salivary tissue within intra- or periparotid lymph nodes (Fig. 4.24). The frequency of such an event is highest in the subgroup of monomorphic adenomas known as dermal analogue tumors (37, 38). These lesions should not be misinterpreted as metastatic lesions.

Nonepidermoid Lesions of the Middle Ear

Space-occupying lesions of the middle ear have the following differential diagnosis: *a*) cholesteatoma or cholesterol granuloma, *b*) paraganglioma (jugulare, tympanicum), *c*) squamous cell carcinoma, *d*) adenomatous tumor of the middle ear, *e*) tumor of neural origin (schwannoma, meningioma), and *f*) a high jugular bulb (39–44).

A diagnosis of cholesteatoma requires the finding of squamous epithelium, usually keratinizing. In the absence of the squamous epithelium but with lipidic granulomas and acute and chronic inflammation, only a diagnosis of cholesterol granuloma can be applied.

Vascular lesions may be inflammatory, such as granulation tissue or an aural polyp. In view of the fact that true hemangiomas of this region are rare, vascular tumors should be regarded as paragangliomas until proven otherwise.

The adenomatous tumors of the middle ear are usually circumscribed, nondestructive tumors with origin from the middle ear mucosa. Patients with these lesions often give a history of what passes for chronic middle

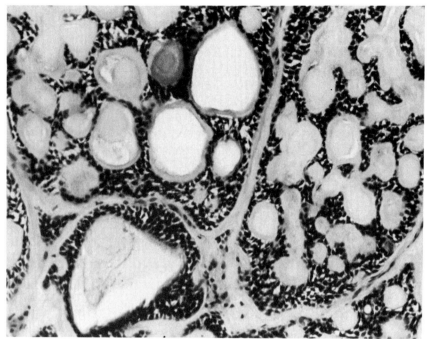

Figure 4.22. Adenoid cystic carcinoma having a cylindromatous architecture. Compare with the monomorphic adenoma in Fig. 4.23.

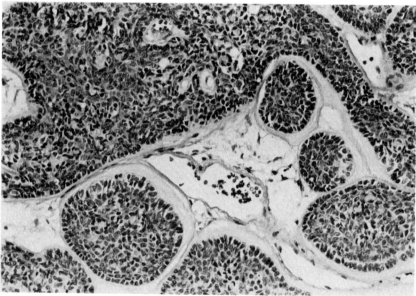

Figure 4.23. Monomorphic adenoma of parotid gland. This membranous variant may histologically resemble cutaneous adnexal tumors such as the dermal cylindroma or eccrine spiradenoma.

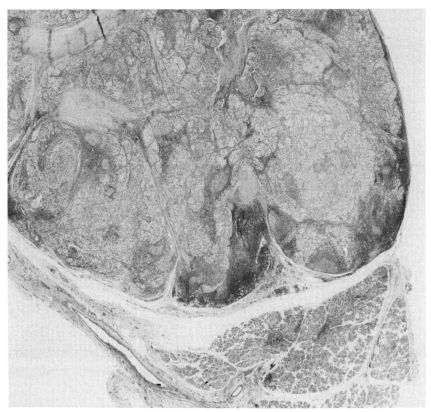

Figure 4.24. Intranodal acinic cell carcinoma. This is not a metastasis but represents origin from enclaved salivary tissue in an intraparotid lymph node.

ear inflammatory disease. A number of these tumors qualify for the designation of adenocarcinoma, based not only on their cytoarchitecture, but also on radiographic evidence of bone destruction. In all such instances, a metastasis to the temporal bone from another primary has to be excluded (43).

The adenomatous tumors can present several histologic appearances (Figs. 4.25–4.27), ranging from a benign proliferation of small glands admixed with sheets of uniform round to oval cells, to one simulating a glandular carcinoid or papillary and follicular carcinoma of the thyroid gland (40, 42, 43). Although there is a superficial resemblance to ceruminous tumors, the typical double layered epithelum of the latter is not found, nor is the iron-containing lipofuchsin-like pigment present. If the tympanic membrane is intact, a ceruminous gland tumor is automatically excluded, since the external auditory canal adjacent to the ear drum is devoid of ceruminous glands. Neither should the tumor be confused with a primary salivary gland tumor. Choristomatous salivary tissue in the middle ear cleft is rare, and even more are salivary gland tumors.

Ultrastructural study has demonstrated neuroendocrine differentiation in some of the adenomatous tumors of the middle ear (42). It is the author's

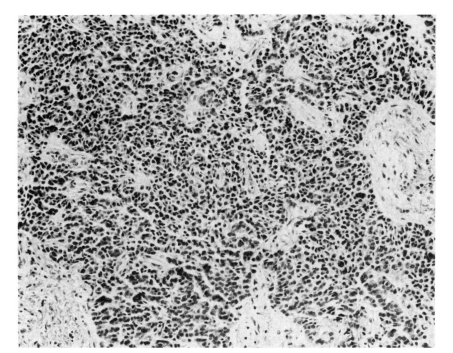

Figure 4.25. Adenomatous tumor of the middle ear manifesting attempts at tubular formation but with a preponderant cell pattern of isolated or groups of cells.

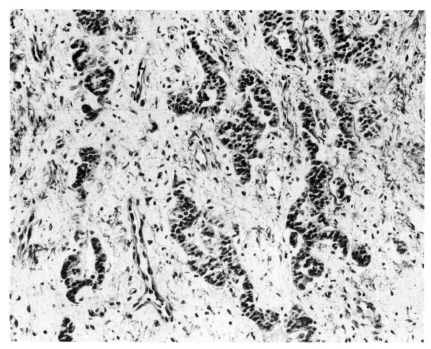

Figure 4.26. Adenomatous tumor of the middle ear with a tubuloductular formation.

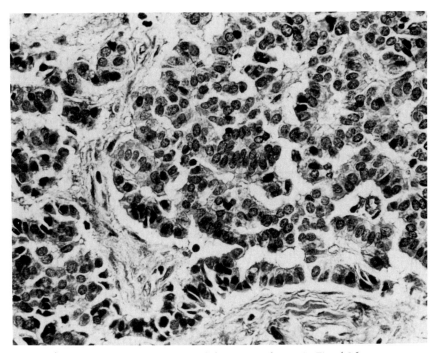

Figure 4.27. Higher magnification of the tumor shown in Fig. 4.26.

opinion that this is not unlike the neuroendocrine differentiation found in any other mucosal neoplasm in the head and neck and respiratory tract, a locally mediated differentiation of cells.

Mucosal Melanoma Versus Extramedullary Plasmacytoma

Although it would not seem to be a problematic differential diagnosis, the distinction between these two mucosal lesions may, at times, be difficult, particularly for those lesions in the sinonasal tract. In the nasal cavity and paranasal sinuses both lesions share common sites of predilection, such as the nasal septum, lateral wall, particularly the turbinates, or the adjacent sinuses (45, 46).

Each of the tumors may be polypoid or sessile and each may be solitary or multinodular and expansive. In the absence of melanin pigment, the monomorphic, "pure culture" array of cells seen in many mucosal melanomas and in plasmacytomas may be deceptively similar (Fig. 4.28). The presence of amyloid stroma cannot be used as a distinguishing factor, since only 15% of extramedullary plasmacytomas manifest this extracellar component (45).

The finding of a spindle cell or pleomorphic cell component in the putative melanoma separates it from the plasmacytoma (Fig. 4.29). Imprint cytologic study will also facilitate the differential diagnosis.

Figure 4.30 illustrates one other lesion that may be confused with plasmacytoma or melanoma, the plasmacytoid or hyaline cells found in myoepithelial-dominant pleomorphic adenomas or myoepitheliomas.

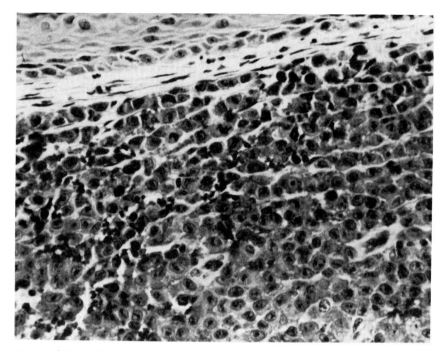

Figure 4.28. Mucosal melanoma of the nasal septum. In this growth pattern, there is a possibility of confusion with an extramedullary plasmacytoma.

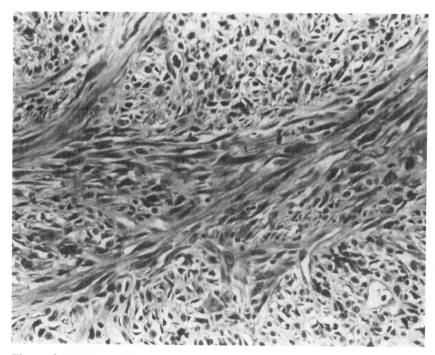

Figure 4.29. Mucosal melanoma of the nasal cavity. In this lesion, the spindle cell component is prominent.

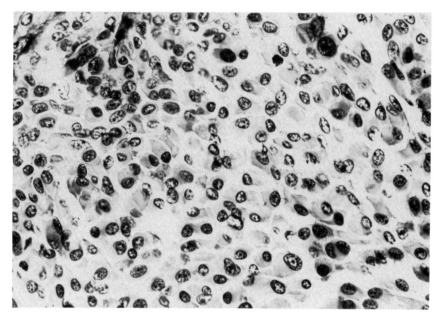

Figure 4.30. Myoepithelial cells of an intraoral pleomorphic adenoma exhibiting plasmacytoid or hyaline features.

Frozen Section Diagnosis of In Situ Carcinoma

The diagnosis of in situ squamous cell carcinoma in the upper aero-digestive tract is made with the same criteria applied at other mucosal sites. Usually, however, the diagnosis implies adjacent unsampled invasive carcinoma. This is especially true in the sinonasal tract and oral cavity. The true vocal cord is an exception; but even at this site, up to 40% will also show invasive carcinoma near by.

The Deferred Diagnosis in Head and Neck Frozen Sections

A deferred diagnosis given to a surgeon should not be viewed as either timidity or inexperience on the part of a surgical pathologist. There is an irreducible number of frozen section impressions that fall into the category of "defer to permanent sections." Lesions in the head and neck pose special problems. Although squamous cell carcinomas dominate the malignant neoplasms, the head and neck lesions run the gamut from those which are peculiar to the region, such as salivary gland tumors, to any of the soft tissue or bone tumors found elsewhere in the body.

Because of the complex anatomy of the head and neck and the type of extirpative surgery used for malignancies in that region, every effort to secure a preoperative, nonfrozen section biopsy, should be made. The burden should not fall to the pathologist and the frozen section mechanism. Preoperative diagnosis is far superior to an intraoperative one; it allows the surgeon to plan the surgery; it prepares the patient for what is to occur; and it places the frozen section in its appropriate role of guiding the surgeon by microscopically controlled surgery.

REFERENCES

1. Dehner LP, Rosai J: Frozen section examination in surgical pathology. *Minn Med* 60:83–94, 1977.
2. Pitts HH, Sturdy JH, Coady, CJ: Frozen sections. II. *Can Med Assoc J* 79:110–113, 1958.
3. Winship T, Rosvoll RV: Frozen sections: An evaluation of 1810 cases. *Surgery* 45:462–466, 1959.
4. Ackerman LV, Ramirez GA: The indications for and limitations of frozen section diagnosis: A review of 1269 consecutive frozen section diagnoses. *Br J Surg* 46:336–350, 1959.
5. French AJ, Lafler CJ: Frozen sections: Rapid tissue diagnosis. *Mich Med* 59:591–595, 1960.
6. Nakazawa H, Rosen P, Lane N: Frozen section experience in 3000 cases. *Am J Clin Pathol* 49:41–51, 1968.
7. Remsen KA, Lucente FE, Biller HF: Reliability of frozen section diagnosis in head and neck neoplasms. *Laryngoscope* 94:519–525, 1984.
8. Bauer WC: The use of frozen sections in otolaryngology. *Trans Am Acad Ophth Otol* 78:88–97, 1974.
9. Miller RH, Calcaterra TC, Paglia DE: Accuracy of frozen section diagnosis of parotid lesions. *Ann Otol Rhinol Laryngol* 88:573–576, 1979.
10. Hillel, AD, Fee WE, Jr: Evaluation of frozen section in parotid gland surgery. *Arch Otolaryngol* 109:230–232, 1983.
11. Dindzans LJ, van Nostrand AWP: The accuracy of frozen section diagnosis of parotid lesions. *J Otolaryngol* 13:382–386, 1984.
12. Davidson TM, Naum AM, Haghighi P, Astarita RW, Saltzstein SL, Seagren S: The biology of head and neck cancer. Detection and control by parallel histologic sections. *Arch Otolaryngol* 110:193–196, 1984.
13. Tromovitch TA, Stegman SJ: Microscopic-controlled excision of cutaneous tumors. Chemosurgery, fresh tissue technique, *Cancer* 41:653–658, 1978.
14. Byers RM: The biology of head and neck cancer. *Arch Otolaryngol* 110:485, 1984.
15. Fletcher S, Smart GE, Livingstone JRB: Grading of cervical dysplasia by frozen section. *Lancet* 2:599–600, 1985.
16. Boonstra H, Oosterhuis JW, Oosterhuis AM, Fleuren GJ: Cervical tissue shrinkage by formaldehyde fixation, paraffin embedding, section cutting and mounting. *Virchows Arch (Pt A)* 402:195–201, 1983.
17. Looser KG, Shah JP, Strong EW: The significance of "positive" margins in surgically resected epidermoid carcinomas. *Head Neck Surg* 1:107–111, 1978.
18. Byers RM, Bland KI, Borlase B, Luna MA: The prognostic and therapeutic value of frozen section determinations in the surgical treatment of squamous carcinoma of the head and neck. *Am J Surg* 136:525–528, 1978.
19. Lee JG: Detection of residual carcinoma of the oral cavity, oropharynx, hypopharynx, and larynx: A study of surgical margins. *Trans Am Acad Ophth Otol* 78:49–53, 1974.
20. Bauer WC, Lesinski SG, Ogura JH: The significance of positive margins in hemilaryngectomy specimens. *Laryngoscope* 85:1–13, 1975.
21. Vikram B, Strong EW, Shah JP, Spiro R: Failure at the primary site following multimodality treatment in advanced head and neck cancer. *Head Neck Surg* 6:720–723, 1984.
22. Conley J: *Salivary Glands and the Facial Nerve.* New York, Grune & Stratton, 1975, p 85.
23. Gates GA: To freeze, or not to . . . *Arch Otolaryngol* 109:229, 1983.
24. Grillon GL, Lally ET: Necrotizing sialometaplasia: Literature review and presentation of five cases. *J Oral Surg* 39:747–753, 1981.
25. Fechner RE: Necrotizing sialometaplasia. A source of confusion with carcinoma of the palate. *Am J Clin Pathol* 67:315–319, 1977.
26. Batsakis JG: *Tumors of the Head and Neck: Clinical and Pathological Considerations,* ed 2. Baltimore, Williams & Wilkins, 1979, p 34–39.
27. Shear M: *Cysts of the oral regions,* ed 2. Bristol, Wright PSG, 1983, p 44.
28. Hodson JJ: Epithelial residues of the jaw with special reference to the edentulous jaw. *J Anat* 96:16–28, 1962.
29. Lutman GB: Epithelial nests in intraoral sensory nerve endings simulating perineural invasion in patients with intraoral carcinoma. *Am J Clin Pathol* 61:275–284, 1974.

30. Jensen JL, Wuerker RB, Correll RW, Erickson JO: Epithelial islands associated with mandibular nerve: Report of two cases in the walls of mandibular cysts. *Oral Surg Oral Med Oral Path* 48:226–230, 1979.
31. Tschen JA, Fechner RE: The juxtaoral organ of Chievitz. *Am J Surg Pathol* 3:147–150, 1979.
32. Batsakis JG, Hybels R, Crissman JD, Rice DH: The pathology of head and neck tumors: Verrucous carcinoma, part 15. *Head Neck Surg* 5:29–38, 1982.
33. Slootweg PJ, Muller H: Verrucous hyperplasia or verrucous carcinoma. *J Max Fac Surg* 11:13–19, 1983.
34. Hansen LS, Olson JA, Silverman S: Proliferative verrucous leukoplakia. A long-term study of thirty patients. *Oral Surg Oral Med Oral Path* 60:285–298, 1985.
35. Batsakis JG, Rice DH, Howard DR: The pathology of head and neck tumors: Spindle cell lesions (sarcomatoid carcinomas, nodular fasciitis, and fibrosarcomas) of the aerodigestive tracts. *Head Neck Surg* 4:499–513, 1982.
36. Batsakis JG: "Pseudosarcoma" of the mucous membranes of the head and neck. *J Laryngol Otol* 95:311–316, 1981.
37. Batsakis JG, Brannan RB, Sciubba JJ: Monomorphic adenomas of major salivary glands: A histologic study of 96 tumors. *Clin Otolaryngol* 6:129–143, 1981.
38. Batsakis JG, Brannon RB: Dermal analogue tumours of major salivary glands. *J Laryngol Otol* 95:155–164, 1981.
39. Stell PM: Carcinoma of the external auditory meatus and middle ear. *Clin Otolaryngol* 9:281–299, 1984.
40. Schuller DE, Conley JJ, Goodman JH, Clausen KP, Miller WJ: Primary adenocarcinoma of the middle ear. *Otolaryngol Head Neck Surg* 91:280–289, 1983.
41. Sinnreich AI, Parisier SC, Cohen NL, Berreby M: Arterial malformations of the middle ear. *Otolaryngol Head Neck Surg* 92:194–206, 1984.
42. Riches WG, Johnston WH: Primary adenomatous neoplasms of the middle ear. Light and electron microscopic features of a group distinct from the ceruminomas. *Am J Clin Pathol* 77:153–161, 1982.
43. Hyams VJ, Michaels L: Benign adenomatous neoplasm (adenoma) of the middle ear. *Clin Otolaryngol* 1:17–26, 1976.
44. Dayal VS, Lafond G, von Nostrand AWP, Holgate R: Lesions simulating glomus tumors of the middle ear. *J Otolaryngol* 12:175–179, 1983.
45. Batsakis JG: Plasma cell tumors of the head and neck. *Ann Otol Rhinol Laryngol* 92:311–313, 1983.
46. Batsakis JG, Regezi JA, Solomon AR, Rice DH: The pathology of head and neck tumors: Mucosal melanomas, part 13. *Head Neck Surg* 4:404–413, 1982.

5

Gynecologic Specimens

Elvio G. Silva, M.D.

Of all frozen sections, 1 to 5% are from gynecologic specimens for which interpretation is highly accurate (1). Fifty percent of these sections are from the ovary, and the remainder are from the vulva, cervix, and endometrium.

VULVA

Frozen section is requested for specimens from the vulva to examine the margins of resection in patients operated on for carcinoma, melanoma, and Paget's disease. The principles regarding margins of resection are similar to those discussed in Chapter 1. Carcinomas and Paget's disease are usually multicentric lesions, and it is not unusual to see microscopic foci of neoplasm in areas not grossly involved. We have successfully stained margins in which Paget's disease was suspected with rapid alcian blue (see Chapter 1). In these cases, mucin is usually easy to identify because the tumor cells are in the epithelium, and there is no interference with stromal or connective tissue mucin.

CERVIX

We evaluate frozen section cone biopsy specimens of the cervix from patients with squamous carcinoma or extensive high-grade dysplasia who will undergo hysterectomy after biopsy. The purposes of freezing the cone biopsy specimen are to determine the extent of disease, the presence of invasive carcinoma, and the depth of tumor infiltration, but not to grade the dysplasia. The information will then determine what type of hysterectomy is to follow. We have used this method since 1960, a few years after the closed-chamber cryostat was introduced in frozen section procedures (2). Advantages of performing a frozen section cone biopsy are that the patient will undergo only one hospital admission, one course of anesthesia, and one postoperative period. Patients who have a hysterectomy performed after frozen section cone biopsy of the cervix are those with a carcinoma in situ who no longer want to conceive, those who have microinvasive or invasive carcinoma, and patients whose cone biopsy specimen demonstrates involvement of the endocervical margin. When dysplasia has already been diagnosed in a patient but no hysterectomy is to be done, we do not freeze the cone biopsy specimen. The depth of invasion of frozen and permanent sections is almost the same, the frozen tissue section usually being no more than 0.1 to 0.2 mm thicker.

ENDOMETRIUM

Rarely, an endometrial curettage specimen may be submitted for frozen section immediately before a hysterectomy to be certain that the endometrium is free of malignancy. Such a request is most likely when benign disease such as leiomyomata or adenomyosis is present in the uterus.

If a frozen section diagnosis of malignancy is made on the basis of a curettage specimen alone, the surgical strategy and intraoperative staging procedure may be modified. In rare instances, the pathologist may be placed in the position of trying to distinguish atypical adenomatous hyperplasia from well differentiated adenocarcinoma, a distinction that is difficult, if not impossible to make on the basis of frozen section. The pathologist should remain conservative in this kind of situation, and the surgeon should rely on clinical judgment in deciding whether the procedure should be modified.

OVARY

A frozen section of an ovarian neoplasm must first be classified as one of the three main types of tumor: sex cord stromal tumor, germ cell tumor, or epithelial neoplasm.

Sex Cord Stromal Tumors

Diagnosis of sex cord stromal tumors is usually not difficult, except when a tubular pattern predominates (Fig. 5.1), which might be confused with an epithelial tumor, mainly endometrioid carcinoma (Fig. 5.2). Table 5.1 shows the main histologic features in the differential diagnosis.

The differential diagnosis may, however, turn out to be difficult and, in the opinion of some authors, impossible (3). Although these two entities are usually treated similarly, differential diagnosis of frozen section is still necessary for gathering needed information: If the lesion is a Sertoli cell

Table 5.1.
Sertoli Cell Tumor Versus Ovary Carcinoma

Characteristic	Sertoli Cell Tumor	Primary Ovarian Carcinoma
Size of glands	Usually small, uniform	Mixture of small and large
Pattern	Usually a mixture—glandular, sarcomatoid, trabecular, retiform, heterologous	Only glandular
Solid tubules	Frequent	Rare
Mucin	Negative	Positive
Squamous metaplasia	Absent	Frequent

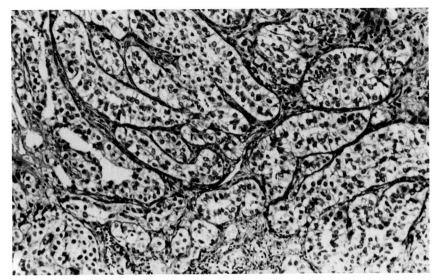

Figure 5.1. Sertoli cell tumor. Small, uniform tubules lined by cells with clear cytoplasm.

tumor, the primary will be in the ovary, and if it is an endometrioid carcinoma, metastasis to the ovary will have to be investigated (see Epithelial Tumors, this chapter).

GERM CELLS TUMORS

Germ cell tumors in the ovary are usually teratomas, dysgerminomas, endodermal sinus tumors, or a mixture of the three. The infrequent em-

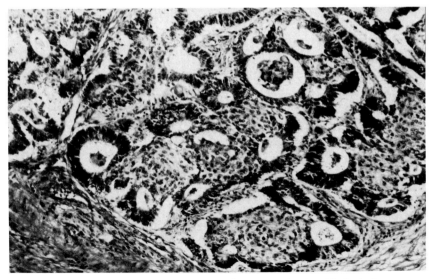

Figure 5.2. Endometrioid carcinoma. Medium size glands with foci of squamous metaplasia.

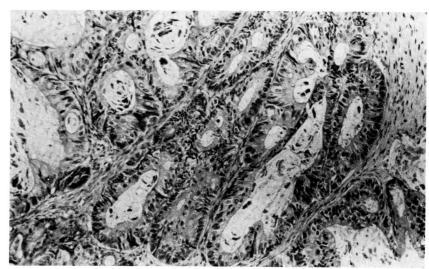

Figure 5.3. Metastatic colonic carcinoma in ovary. Uniform glands lined by epithelium of similar thickness.

bryonal carcinoma of the ovary (4) might be confused with primary or metastatic adenocarcinoma. Embryonal carcinoma affects patients younger than 30 yr and is unilateral. Probably the most important histologic feature in the differential diagnosis is the identification of other germ cell tumor components.

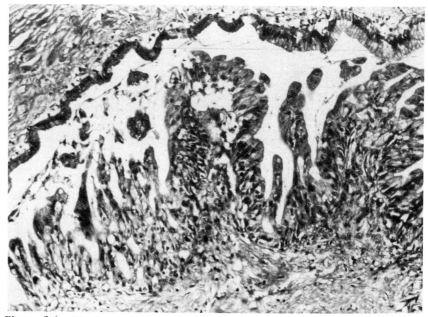

Figure 5.4. Mucinous carcinoma, primary in ovary. Marked variation in the thickness of the neoplastic epithelium. Adjacent area of low grade tumor is present.

EPITHELIAL TUMORS

Of all gynecologic neoplasms in which frozen section diagnosis is crucial for surgical management, epithelial tumors of the ovary are among the most important.

Serous neoplasms, mesonephroid (clear cell) tumors, and Brenner tumors usually do not present a problem in diagnosis. Mesonephroid carcinoma might be confused with metastatic clear cell carcinoma from the kidney; however, the combination of papillary, glandular, solid, and cystic patterns with hobnail cells are characteristic of mesonephroid carcinoma. Malignant Brenner tumor might be confused with metastatic transitional cell carcinoma from the urinary tract, but it is extremely unusual to encounter transitional cell carcinoma metastatic to the ovary when the bladder primary is unknown. The most common problem in differential diagnosis is distinguishing mucinous and endometrioid carcinoma primary in ovary from metastatic carcinoma from the gastrointestinal tract (Figs. 5.3 and 5.4). This differential diagnosis is of paramount significance. If the tumor in question is primary in the ovary, the surgeon will, after its excision, stage the patient with biopsy specimens from multiple sites. If the pathologist interprets the tumor in the ovary as metastatic, however, or if the question of whether the tumor is primary or metastatic is not resolved by frozen section examination, the surgeon must search for another primary site in the stomach, small and large bowel, and pancreas. Failure to recognize the tumor in the ovary as metastatic during the operative procedure will result in a lengthy and costly search for a primary carcinoma postoperatively, and probably in a second operation. Table 5.2 includes features useful for making the diagnosis between primary and metastatic epithelial tumors in the ovary.

Carcinoid tumors are another histologic type of neoplasm that may create problems in determining whether they are primary or metastatic. In this situation, neither pattern nor cytologic characteristics will be useful. Primary ovarian carcinoid tumors are unilateral (5) and usually associated with teratomas (6), Sertoli-Leydig cell tumors (7), or mucinous epithelial tumors (8).

Table 5.2.
Primary Versus Metastatic Carcinoma in Ovary

Characteristic	Primary Epithelial Ovarian Tumor	Carcinoma Metastatic to the Ovary
Cellularity	Variation in thickness of the epithelium lining glands	Uniform
Cell type	Commonly, areas of mucinous, endometrioid, mesonephroid, transitional, serous cells	Uniform
Areas of low-grade tumor	If present, they are diagnostic of primary ovarian neoplasm	Absent
Miscellaneous	Liver metastases are rare, occur late in course of disease	Liver metastases are frequent and early in course of disease

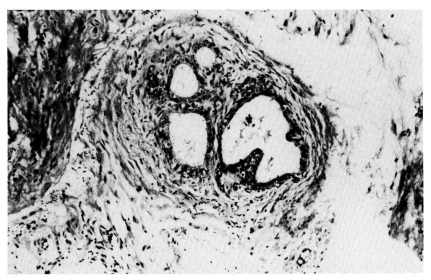

Figure 5.5. Endosalpingiosis in peritoneum, found during a second look operation.

SEROUS PAPILLARY PROLIFERATIONS OF PERITONEAL ORIGIN (ENDOSALPINGIOSIS)

It is not unusual during an exploratory laparotomy in a female patient to find one or more small discrete epithelial, usually papillary lesions arising from the peritoneal surface and having the histologic features of serous or endosalpingeal type epithelium. The criteria for separating serous carcinoma, serous tumors of low malignant potential (borderline serous tumor), and benign serous tumors are clearly established when the tumor is primary

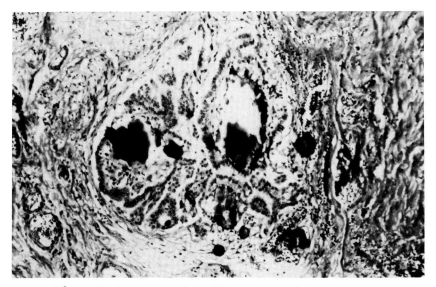

Figure 5.6. Endosalpingiosis with proliferative hyperplastic epithelium and multiple psammoma bodies.

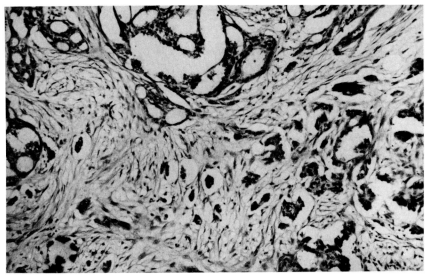

Figure 5.7. Metastatic serous carcinoma in omentum. Note stromal invasion.

in the ovary. The same criteria, however, do not necessarily apply to extraovarian serous papillary proliferations. The situation becomes problematic for the pathologist when the patient has a primary serous ovarian neoplasm and is found to have one or more serous papillary proliferations outside the ovary involving the peritoneal surface. It is important to be aware that the grade of the tumor must be based on the appearance of the lesion in the ovary. An implant in the peritoneum, associated with a tumor of borderline malignancy in the ovary, might elicit a marked desmoplastic reaction. This desmoplasia should not be used to upgrade the borderline neoplasm in the ovary. When the ovarian tumor is a carcinoma, the interpretation of these epithelial proliferations is of paramount significance, since it will determine the stage of the disease. It has been our policy to classify these papillary lesions as benign proliferations (Figs. 5.5 and 5.6) unless mitotic figures, necrosis, significant cytologic atypia, and stromal invasion with desmoplasia can be identified (Fig. 5.7). It is important also to bear in mind that these patients are usually young and in their reproductive years. Rendering a diagnosis of malignancy could potentially result in a radical surgical procedure. We believe that this situation represents one of the most explicit examples where a diagnosis must be objectively based on the unquestionable presence of all the morphologic criteria outlined above.

REFERENCES

1. DiMusto JC: Reliability of frozen sections in gynecologic surgery. *Obstet Gynecol* 35:235–240, 1970.
2. Rutledge F, Ibanez MI: Use of the cryostat in gynecologic surgery. *Am J Obstet Gynecol* 83:1208–1213, 1962.
3. Scully RE: *Atlas of Tumor Pathology.* Washington, DC, Armed Forces Institute of Pathology, 1978, p 202.
4. Kurman RJ, Norris NJ: Embryonal carcinoma of the ovary: A clinicopathologic entity distinct from endodermal sinus tumor resembling embryonal carcinoma of the adult testis. *Cancer* 38:2420–2433, 1976.

5. Talerman A: Carcinoid tumors of the ovary. *J Cancer Res Clin Oncol* 107:125–135, 1984.

6. Robboy SJ, Norris HJ, Scully RE: Insular carcinoid primary in the ovary: A clinicopathologic analysis of 48 cases. *Cancer* 36:404–418, 1975.

7. Young RH, Prat J, Scully RE: Ovarian Sertoli-Leydig cell tumors with heterologous elements. I. Gastrointestinal epithelium and carcinoid: A clinicopathologic analysis of 36 cases. *Cancer* 50:2448–2456, 1982.

8. Robboy SJ: Insular carcinoid of ovary associated with malignant mucinous tumors. *Cancer* 54:2273–2276, 1984.

6

Lung

B. Balfour Kraemer, M.D.

The pathologist plays a pivotal role as intraoperative consultant when rendering a frozen section diagnosis on a lung mass or a mediastinal lymph node. He has great power in determining the intraoperative course of events. A particular frozen section diagnosis can give the surgeon license to proceed with a pneumonectomy, whereas a different frozen section interpretation will direct him to immediately terminate the procedure.

The intraoperative approach to a lung mass is closely related to the clinical stage, anatomic site of the mass, and the patient's pulmonary reserve. The surgeon relies on accurate frozen section guidance in determining the most appropriate surgical management. Since staging for lung carcinoma is often carried out by frozen section, the pathologist must be cognizant of the therapeutic implications every frozen section diagnosis carries. In the sequence from one frozen section to the next, the pathologist should be able to predict the surgeon's next move in the operating suite, anticipating which additional tissues, if any, will be submitted for frozen section.

INDICATIONS FOR FROZEN SECTION

There are three main indications for requesting a frozen section diagnosis of a lung or lung-related specimen.

Mediastinal Lymph Node Evaluation in Staging of Bronchogenic Carcinoma

The choice of therapy for bronchogenic carcinoma depends to a great extent upon whether there is mediastinal lymph node involvement (1–4). The location of the lung primary determines the type of mediastinal exploration that will be performed (5,6). If lymph nodes are negative, a thoracotomy is undertaken, either during the same anesthesia or within a week following the procedure. If lymph nodes are positive, the location of the involved lymph node(s) combined with the histologic type of the metastasis will determine the potential for resectability (1,7–10).

Evaluation of Lung Parenchymal Disease

Frozen section of a lung mass is often requested to confirm the clinical impression of malignancy. If the patient has a history of an extrapulmonary primary, frozen section may be requested to confirm that the lung mass is metastatic rather than primary.

Two additional situations in which a frozen section is often requested include open lung biopsy in an immunocompromised patient and lung biopsy in the patient with congenital heart disease who may be a candidate for corrective surgery. Pediatric patients with pulmonary hypertension secondary to congenital cardiovascular defects may have potentially reversible disease. The degree of morphologic hypertension is graded (11–13), and the severity of the vascular change helps the surgeon to decide whether a corrective or palliative operation should be performed (11). This specialized use of frozen section is usually performed in tertiary pediatric centers with an active pediatric cardiology service.

Evaluation of Lung, Bronchial, and Pleural Margins

Since the goal of resection is to remove all or as much neoplasm as possible, the surgeon will often request frozen sections of the above tissues to confirm that tumor-free surgical margins have been obtained. Frozen section of a lung margin is often indicated in segmental or wedge resection of a peripheral lung mass in order to determine if a more extensive procedure should be performed. A positive bronchial margin in a lobectomy specimen usually prompts a second bronchial resection, or may lead to a more radical procedure. Involvement of the visceral pleura changes the TMN classification from T1 to T2 (14), and the surgeon may wish to confirm such a finding at the time of resection.

TYPES OF SPECIMENS

Staging

Mediastinal Lymph Nodes

As already discussed, frozen section evaluation of mediastinal lymph nodes aids in determining resectability or nonresectability of a lung primary. The anatomic location of the lung primary determines its lymphatic drainage route, and thus dictates which mediastinal lymph nodes are biopsied in preoperative staging. Right lung lymphatics drain into the right pretracheal, paratracheal, and tracheobronchial lymph node chains. A major part of the lymphatics of the left lower lobe demonstrates crossover, emptying into the inferior tracheobronchial (subcarinal) lymph nodes, which in turn drain into the right paratracheal chain(s) (15). Carcinomas arising either within the right lung or left lower lobe may be staged preoperatively via transcervical (Carlen's) mediastinoscopy (16). This procedure provides access to right-sided, central, and left paratracheal lymph node groups (16,17). In mediastinoscopy, a rigid scope having a luminal caliber slightly larger than 10 mm is inserted along the pretracheal fascial plane. Lymph nodes are retrieved via biting forceps, pulled through the mediastinoscope, and then submitted for frozen section. Mediastinal lymph nodes travel a perilous journey from their origin into the hands of the pathologist. Even in experienced surgical hands, atraumatic biopsy is difficult, and significant crushing and fragmentation are common sequelae.

The left upper lobe lymphatics drain into the left paratracheal and subaortic (Botallo's) lymph nodes. Carcinomas arising in the left upper lobe or hilum are usually staged via anterior (Chamberlain) mediastinotomy (3,6,17–19), a procedure which best visualizes these lymph node groups and exposes the lung root. The mediastinum is entered through a second or third costal cartilage incision, allowing exposure to the entire left paratracheal chain, aorticopulmonary window (subaortic lymph nodes), the mediastinal pleura, and lung hilum. The operative field is larger, and in contrast to mediastinoscopy, tissue retrieved for frozen section from this procedure is less likely to be subjected to biopsy trauma.

Parascalene Lymph Nodes

Palpable scalene lymph nodes are often biopsied for frozen section in the preoperative evaluation of patients with lung carcinoma. Some surgeons will biopsy nonpalpable scalene lymph nodes if the lung carcinoma is centrally located and the histology is either unknown, or classified as adenocarcinoma (20). Retroscalene dissection creates an anatomic passageway to the thoracic inlet and apex of the lung and is a suitable method for biopsy of a neoplasm in the superior sulcus (21,22).

Lung

Intraoperative Fine Needle Aspiration

Intraoperative cytologic evaluation of needle aspirates from lung and mediastinal lymph nodes has been reported to be a useful adjunct in the diagnosis and staging of lung neoplasms (23,24). Our experience and reliance on rapid intraoperative fine needle aspiration interpretation is limited and is supplemented by frequent evaluation of touch imprints, which are prepared at the time of frozen section (see Chapter 1).

Flexible Bronchoscopy

The practice of submitting transbronchial biopsies for frozen section should be discouraged. The small volume of material combined with crush and frozen section artifact makes frozen section interpretation difficult or impossible. Leveling the frozen section block in an effort to obtain an adequate section often leaves no tissue for paraffin embedding. Rarely, the clinician may submit a transbronchial biopsy for frozen section from an immunocompromised patient, especially an acquired immunodeficiency syndrome (AIDS) patient. As the etiology for the patient's respiratory distress is often due to *Pneumocystis carinii* (25,26), in this situation, the pathologist should inquire whether a bronchoalveolar lavage has been performed. Routinely processed transbronchial biopsy combined with bronchoalveolar lavage has been reported to have a very high diagnostic yield (91%) for *P. carinii* (27). Touch imprints from the biopsy and the pellet from the centrifuged lavage fluid can be stained with special stains for identification of the organism (28). If negative, open lung biopsy will probably be performed.

Needle Biopsy

Percutaneous lung needle biopsy is most often used to diagnose clinically suspicious peripheral nodules or lobar consolidations which are believed to be infectious. When neoplasm is suspected, touch imprints should be performed before the tissue core is frozen. Rarely, a tissue core needle biopsy may be submitted for frozen section, with the request that it be handled as an open lung biopsy. In this situation, the pathologist should be aware of the limitations imposed by such a request. The amount of tissue is obviously less than that usually received from an open lung biopsy procedure, and the diagnostic yield will be lower than that expected from an open lung biopsy (29). If more than one needle biopsy is submitted, one biopsy may be submitted for frozen section and handled as an open lung biopsy (see Open Lung Biopsy, this Chapter). The second needle biopsy can be submitted for routine processing.

Thoracotomy Tissue

A thoracotomy may be either limited, confining the surgeon to a small operative field, or exploratory, allowing access to the entire hemithorax.

Open Lung Biopsy

Open lung biopsy is performed via limited thoracotomy, through which one or more representative regions are biopsied. The lung biopsy is delivered in a sterile condition to the frozen section suite.

The recommended procedure for handling an open lung biopsy is outlined in a separate section (see p. 132).

Wedge and Segmental Resection

A simple wedge resection is performed for a peripherally located lung mass measuring less than 2 cm in diameter without evidence of lymph node metastasis in a patient with limited pulmonary reserve. In addition, wedge resection is the usual procedure for resection of pulmonary metastatic disease. Segmentectomy is carried out when a peripheral lung mass is greater than 2 cm in diameter and shows no evidence of lymph node metastasis. The lung mass may be either primary or metastatic. Segmental resection for a lung primary may be performed if the patient cannot tolerate a more extensive procedure (30).

Lobectomy

Lobectomy is undertaken when a lung mass is 3 cm or greater in diameter, but remains within the anatomic confines of the involved lobe. Completion lobectomy is carried out when frozen section margins of a wedge or segmental resection are positive and the patient is considered a suitable candidate for this more radical procedure. Similarly, if the histology of a lung mass in a wedge or segmental resection is strongly suggestive of a lung primary, a completion lobectomy may be performed so that bronchopulmonary and hilar lymph nodes and the lobar bronchial margin may be evaluated. Rarely, a stage III patient (positive mediastinal lymph nodes) is a candidate for lobectomy. In such a situation, the primary and lymph node metastasis are of squamous histology, and the lymph node metastasis is located in the low ipsilateral paratracheal chain (9).

Pneumonectomy

The standard pneumonectomy is performed when the primary or involved bronchopulmonary lymph nodes cannot be encompassed by a lesser procedure. A completion pneumonectomy is often performed if frozen section margins of the lobectomy are positive and if the patient is considered a suitable candidate for such a resection. Extended pneumonectomy may be performed when there is extension of carcinoma into the adventitia of great vessels and/or chest wall. Such en bloc resections usually require multiple frozen sections to evaluate margins.

Bronchial Margin

The Standard Bronchial Margin

One type of bronchial margin is that which the surgeon separately submits. The cut surface, which represents the true surgical margin, may or may not be designated by the surgeon. The other type of bronchial margin is that which the pathologist submits, requiring a circumferential trimming off the proximal aspect of the lobar or main stem bronchus. Either method is acceptable for evaluation of the bronchial margin.

The Bronchial Margin in Sleeve Resections (Lobectomy and Pneumonectomy)

Bronchoplastic procedures are performed on selected patients who have carcinomas localized to the carina, mainstem, or secondary bronchus (31–34). In a sleeve lobectomy, a wide resection of the involved primary bronchus and corresponding lobe is performed. The stump of the primary bronchus is reanastomosed, either to an adjacent secondary bronchus or to the remainder of the primary bronchus that was not initially resected (31–33). In a sleeve pneumonectomy, the tracheobronchial bifurcation (carina) and involved primary bronchus with the corresponding lung are removed. A circumferential reanastomosis of the trachea to the contralateral primary bronchus is performed (34).

The pathologist should be familiar with bronchoplastic procedures, since the surgeon may submit the sleeve as a separate specimen and request that both bronchial margins be examined by frozen section (34). The pathologist should request that the specimen be oriented by the surgeon in order to prevent confusion at the time of frozen section.

Pleural Biopsy

Frozen section diagnosis of a pleural needle biopsy may be requested, and is often undertaken when there is a clinical suspicion of granulomatous pleuritis (such as tuberculosis) or neoplastic disease. The overall diagnostic reliability of pleural needle biopsy is variable (35), and this procedure is often followed by open biopsy. Thoracoscopy is often used in the evaluation of malignant effusions, and allows for biopsy of the pleural lining of the entire hemithorax. Transdiaphragmatic liver biopsy may be performed using this technique (36).

FROZEN SECTION DIAGNOSIS OF LUNG AND LUNG RELATED TISSUES

Mediastinal Lymph Nodes

There are four main diagnostic difficulties the pathologist should anticipate in the frozen section evaluation of mediastinal lymph nodes:

Pseudomalignant Crush Artifact or Metastatic Small (Oat) Cell Carcinoma?

As described in a previous section (see p. 112), the method of mediastinoscopic biopsy is less than optimal for lymph nodes, often introducing crush artifact. Unfortunately, the crush artifact found in tissues permeated by small cell carcinoma may also be extensive. Mediastinal lymph nodes involved by metastatic small cell carcinoma generally have effacement of the lymph node architecture. Identification of extensive crush artifact alone is not diagnostic of metastatic small cell carcinoma (Fig. 6.1). The pathologist must unequivocally identify other features characteristic of small cell carcinoma to make a definitive diagnosis. The most helpful features include identification of noncrushed viable neoplastic cells with hyperchromatic nuclei, finely stippled chromatin and inconspicuous nucleoli, extensive necrosis, and Azzopardi effect (37,38). If the pathologist is uncertain about

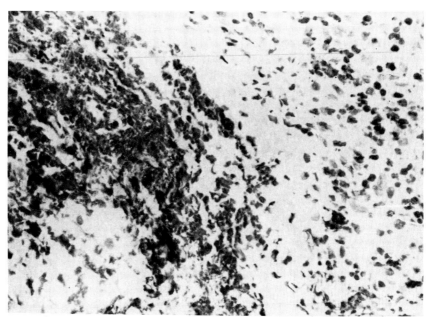

Figure 6.1. Frozen section of mediastinal lymph node with crush artifact.

the diagnosis, additional levels of the frozen section block should be examined. Since small cell carcinoma has a tendency to infiltrate mediastinal fat, clusters of viable neoplastic cells within extranodal fat should be identified. A second lymph node biopsy should be requested if uncertainty persists.

Pseudomalignant Crush Artifact or Malignant Lymphoma?

In general, lymphomatous infiltrates display less crush artifact than small cell carcinoma. If a lymphoproliferative process is suspected at the time of frozen section, the diagnosis should be deferred.

Sclerotic and/or Granulomatous Mediastinal Lymph Nodes

These problems are discussed in detail in Chapter 10, **Mediastinum.**

Metastatic Keratinizing Squamous Carcinoma or Involuted Thymus?

With aging, the lymphoid component of the thymus decreases, and the relative amount of thymic epithelium becomes increased. Hassall's corpuscles become unusually prominent, and medullary epithelial cells assume a spindled configuration. If a portion of involved thymus is submitted for frozen section, its appearance may closely resemble lymph node having foci of metastatic keratinizing squamous carcinoma (Fig. 6.2). If the patient has a previous proven diagnosis of bronchogenic squamous carcinoma, this diagnosis becomes even more plausible. A detailed study of Hassall's corpuscles by high power examination may add to the diagnostic confusion. Hassall's corpuscles are concentric proliferations of keratinizing epithelial cells set within a lymphoid stroma, and may demonstrate some degree of cytologic atypia. It is not surprising that small biopsies of involuted thymic

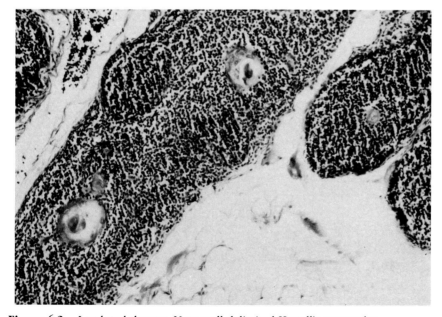

Figure 6.2. Involuted thymus. Note well delimited Hassall's corpuscles.

tissue can be misinterpreted as metastatic squamous carcinoma. This diagnostic pitfall is common and is a serious error. To most surgeons, a diagnosis of carcinoma metastatic to mediastinal lymph nodes implies unresectability.

To make this important distinction, specific features must be sought. Even with atrophy, the thymus maintains its lobular architecture; low power examination is helpful in assessing this architectural feature. The location of the foci of squamous differentiation in relation to the lymphoid tissue is also important. Hassall's corpuscles reside within the thymic medulla, found within the deep lymphoid stroma of the involuted thymus, often within areas of fatty infiltration. Although Hassall's corpuscles may display focal cytologic atypia, they are architecturally discrete, with no associated desmoplasia or necrosis.

Lung

Small Cell Carcinoma

The majority of small cell carcinomas are diagnosed on the basis of cytology, bronchoscopic or needle biopsy (39). Occasionally, an unsuspected small cell carcinoma may be encountered at the time of frozen section. As with mediastinal lymph nodes, small cell carcinoma in the lung may display extensive crush artifact. Confusion with malignant lymphoma may arise. In addition to the features already described for small cell carcinoma, the identification of pagetoid spread of small cell carcinoma through and along the bronchial epithelium has been reported to be a helpful finding in confirming the diagnosis of small cell carcinoma (40).

Although chemotherapy is the conventional therapy for small cell lung carcinoma (39,41), if the pathologist renders a frozen section diagnosis of small cell carcinoma, the surgeon may proceed with a debulking procedure. Surgical margins will probably be of little concern.

The main differential diagnosis is atypical carcinoid. The histologic distinction between small cell carcinoma and atypical carcinoid on frozen section may be exceedingly difficult. As the overall 5-yr survival for atypical

Table 6.1.
Histologic Features of Atypical Carcinoid and Small Cell Carcinoma

Atypical Carcinoid	Small Cell Carcinoma
Disordered trabecular or insular architecture	Sheets of cells
Moderate cellularity	Increased cellularity
Patchy mitoses	Abundant mitoses
Patchy necrosis	Prominent necrosis
Variable nuclear pleomorphism	Marked nuclear pleomorphism
Nucleic acid deposits in vessel wall absent	Nucleic acid deposits on vessel wall present
Lymph node metastasis—present (15 to 60%)	Lymph node metastasis present in more than 60%
Micrometastases	Most are macrometastases
Organoid pattern	Nonorganoid pattern

carcinoid is approximately 50% (42,43), most surgeons will attempt to completely resect such a neoplasm and sample the regional lymph nodes. Some of the major histologic features for atypical carcinoid and small cell carcinoma are outlined in Table 6.1.

Carcinoid (Typical and Spindled)

"Typical" carcinoid may arise centrally or peripherally. In its more common central (endobronchial) form, the classical trabecular arrangement is usually maintained (Figs. 6.3 and 6.4). A peripheral carcinoid may have a variety of histologic patterns, the most common of which is spindled (44). Spindled carcinoids have an unexplained predilection for the right middle lobe (44). Although a spindled pattern may predominate, the remaining organoid framework is usually preserved. A rapid reticulin strain helps to emphasize this feature (see Chapter 1).

The differential diagnosis for spindled carcinoid is localized fibrous mesothelioma (Fig. 6.5) (45–47). Although both neoplasms are peripheral in location, localized fibrous mesothelioma is intimately associated with the pleura. Spindled carcinoid rarely involves it (44). When the cytologic characteristics of a spindled cell neoplasm favor one or the other of the above entities, its relationship to the pleura should be defined.

Two other histologic variations reported to occur in lung carcinoids are papillary (48) and clear cell (49) patterns, which are discussed in separate sections of this chapter (see *Clear Cell Histology* and *Papillary Pattern*).

Carcinoid may be easily confused with metastatic neoplasms, especially those that tend to have an acinar arrangement, such as prostatic adenocar-

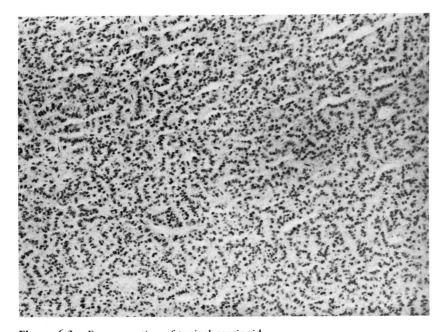

Figure 6.3.   Frozen section of typical carcinoid.

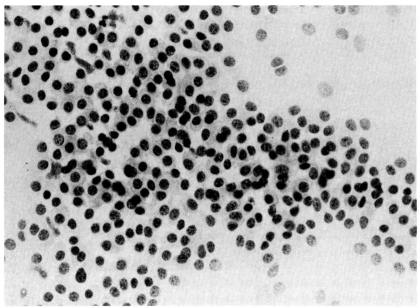

Figure 6.4. Touch imprint of carcinoid. Hematoxylin and eosin.

cinoma (Fig. 6.6). The presence of mitosis and nuclear pleomorphism are helpful in making the distinction (Fig. 6.7).

Lung Tumorlets

By definition, a tumorlet is less than 5 mm in diameter (50). A tumorlet is usually an incidental finding on frozen section, often found in heavily

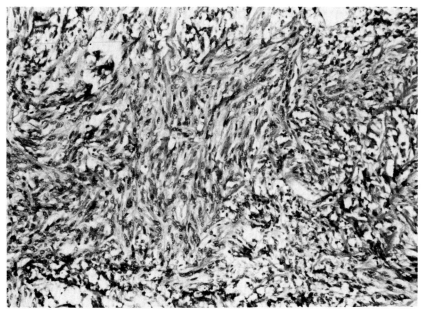

Figure 6.5. Localized fibrous mesothelioma.

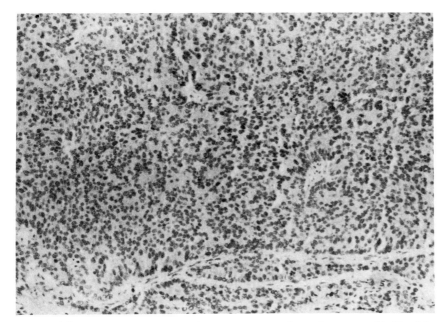

Figure 6.6.   Metastatic prostatic adenocarcinoma in lung. Compare with Fig. 6.3.

scarred lung tissue, and may be of squamous or carcinoid-type histology. A squamous tumorlet is simply a focus of metaplastic bronchiolar epithelium which partially plugs alveolar ducts (51). This type of metaplastic change should be easily distinguished from squamous carcinoma.

   Carcinoid tumorlets are bronchocentric and arise from either peri-bronchiolar soft tissues or the bronchiolar wall (Fig. 6.8). They are often

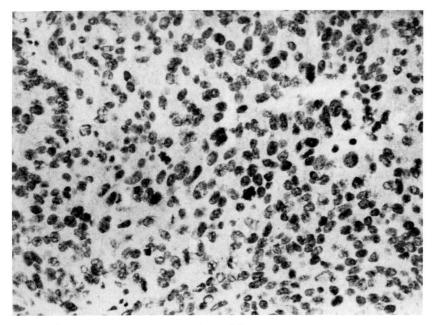

Figure 6.7.   Higher magnification of Fig. 6.6.

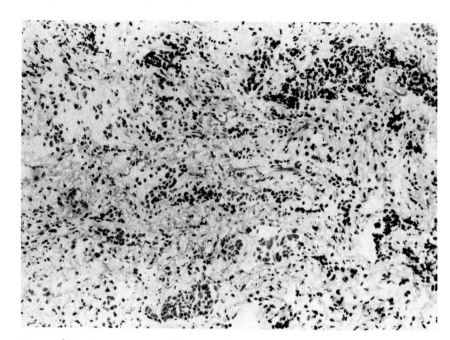

Figure 6.8. Frozen section of carcinoid tumorlet. Its bronchocentric relationship may be obscured in scarred or collapsed lung.

multiple and may be associated with a peripheral carcinoid or other types of primary lung neoplasms (44,52). On frozen section, carcinoid tumorlets may be misinterpreted as metastatic carcinoma (44), especially if they are found in association with another neoplasm and if there is extensive crushing of the lung tissue. Lymphatic invasion should be sought to confirm a diagnosis of metastasis. Deeper sections of the frozen section block may be helpful in characterizing a tumorlet.

Primary or Metastatic?

Frozen section evaluation of a solitary peripheral lung nodule is often requested in a patient who has a history of an extrathoracic primary. The frozen section is requested in order to determine what type of resection should be performed. If a lung primary is favored on frozen section, lobectomy is the treatment of choice. If, on the other hand, metastatic disease is favored, wedge resection or segmental resection will be undertaken. Sometimes, it is impossible to classify a lung neoplasm as primary or metastatic; in this situation, the surgeon determines the type of operative management.

The following guidelines, arranged according to a predominant histology or pattern, may be helpful in distinguishing a primary from a metastatic neoplasm in the lung:

Squamous Histology. Pulmonary metastases from an extrathoracic squamous cell carcinoma may often display more keratinization than bronchogenic squamous carcinoma. Rarely, metastatic squamous carcinoma may erode through a bronchial wall and spread laterally along the surface epithelium, leaving the basal portion of the bronchial epithelium unaltered (53). This feature should not be confused with in situ carcinoma. Features favoring a lung primary include squamous carcinoma in situ of adjacent bronchial epithelium and an endobronchial origin, often demonstrated grossly in an intact specimen. A mixture of squamous and adenocarcinoma histology is common in lung primaries.

Adenocarcinoma Histology. If an adenocarcinoma is identified on frozen section, and if the patient has no history of an extrapulmonary adenocarcinoma, the probability that the adenocarcinoma is a lung primary is high. If, however, the patient has a history of an extrapulmonary adenocarcinoma, the situation becomes more complicated. Representative slides of the extrapulmonary primary should be available for the pathologist's review, and may be helpful at the time of frozen section.

A special problem in evaluating adenocarcinoma in the lung is the interpretation of a bronchioloalveolar carcinoma (54–58). Frozen section diagnosis of this special type of lung carcinoma lesion can be very treacherous, especially on a needle biopsy. Bronchioloalveolar carcinoma has a variety of gross and histologic appearances and closely mimics other nonneoplastic, benign and malignant entities. The frozen section differential diagnosis of bronchioloalveolar carcinoma is presented in Table 6.2.

Distinguishing primary bronchioloalveolar carcinoma from metastatic carcinoma with a bronchioloalveolar pattern of dissemination is often impossible. What is possible, and more important, is to distinguish bronchioloalveolar carcinoma from a nonneoplastic process, such as reactive pneumonitis. Injured or inflamed lung tissue may have exuberant alveolar pneumocytic hyperplasia. When found in atelectatic lung, this hyperplastic change can simulate invasive glands. In reactive processes, the degree of hyperplasia is variable, and the hyperplastic zones gradually blend into surrounding lung parenchyma without abrupt transition. This feature is best appreciated on low power magnification. Cytologically, reactive alveolar pneumocytes have a low nucleocytoplasmic ratio with small or inconspicuous nucleoli and few or no mitoses (Fig. 6.9).

Bronchioloalveolar carcinoma proliferates along distal air spaces, usually preserving the alveolar architectual framework. On low power magnification, bronchioloalveolar carcinoma may not even resemble a neoplasm. When superimposed on emphysematous lung, the alveolar pattern of spread is deceptively similar to reactive pneumocytic hyperplasia (Figs. 6.10 and 6.11). However, in contrast to reactive pneumonitis, the transition from normal alveolar lining cells to cells of bronchioloalveolar carcinoma is ab-

Table 6.2.
Frozen Section Differential Diagnosis of Bronchioloalveolar Carcinoma

Primary	Metastatic	Reactive
Sclerosing hemangioma	Carcinoma	Lipoid pneumonitis
Intravascular sclerosing tumor	Colon	Bronchopneumonia
Papillary carcinoid	Breast	Organizing infarct
Mesothelioma	Pancreas	Bronchiolitis obliterans
Pulmonary blastoma	Prostate	Drug pneumonitis
	Ovary	Radiation damage
	Kidney	
	Thyroid	

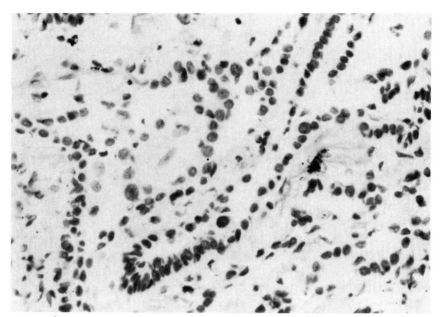

Figure 6.9. Frozen section of reactive pneumonitis. Alveolar lining cells are hyperplastic, but with relatively uniform nuclei.

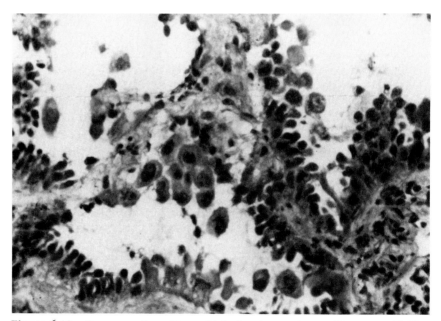

Figure 6.10. Frozen section of bronchioloalveolar carcinoma. Compare with Fig. 6.9.

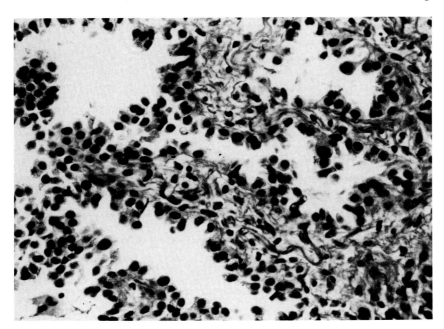

Figure 6.11. Bronchioloalveolar carcinoma. Hobnail pattern.

rupt, and is apparent even on low power magnification. Attention to cytologic detail is also helpful in confirming a diagnosis of bronchioloalveolar carcinoma. Two predominate histologic types are recognized (55). The nonciliated columnar mucinous epithelial type is usually well differentiated, with prominent, basally situated nuclei having prominent nucleoli. A papillary component may or may not be evident. The second histologic type is the peg-shaped or "hobnail" pattern which may form papillary tufts that exfoliate into alveolar spaces. Cytologic atypia may be patchy, but is uniformly present (Fig. 6.12). Atypical mitoses and single cell necrosis are often identified. Intranuclear inclusions are sometimes prominent. The hobnail variant is most easily confused with reactive alveolar pneumocytic hyperplasia, whereas the mucinous variant is most easily confused with metastatic adenocarcinoma (Fig. 6.13).

A special type of injury reaction in the lung is alveolar cell hyperplasia and dysplasia secondary to cytotoxic therapy, seen most commonly in patients treated with busulfan, bleomycin, or methotrexate (59–64). Radiation damage may also induce a significant alveolar dysplasia (65). Grossly, these types of pneumonitis rarely produce mass lesions, and the history is the most helpful evidence in making such a diagnosis at the time of frozen section.

Clear Cell Histology. Frozen section diagnosis of solitary lung neoplasms having a predominant clear cell patten is complicated by the fact that metastatic renal cell carcinoma must always be considered in the differential diagnosis. Approximately 2% of patients with renal cell carcinoma present with solitary lung metastases before the primary is discovered (66,67). When a clear cell neoplasm is examined on frozen section, a rapid Oil Red

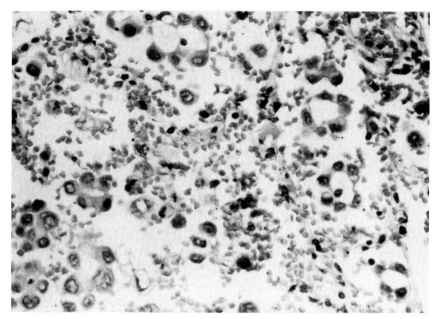

Figure 6.12. Bronchioloalveolar carcinoma. Papillary tufts have exfoliated into alveolar sacs.

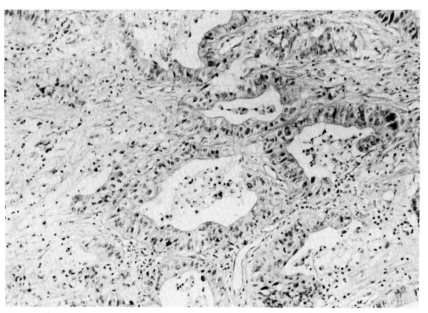

Figure 6.13. Metastatic colonic adenocarcinoma in bronchioloalveolar arrangement.

O stain for fat can be performed on frozen section material. If positive, this supports a diagnosis of metastatic renal cell carcinoma. Since renal cell carcinoma has fairly distinctive ultrastructural features (68), tissue should be reserved for electron microscopy.

Focal or extensive clear cell change is common in primary lung carcinomas, especially in squamous carcinoma (69). Foci of obvious squamous differentiation may be absent, and in such cases the other features characteristic of bronchogenic squamous carcinoma must be sought.

The rare benign clear cell tumor is entirely composed of clear cells and is usually devoid of necrosis or intracytoplasmic fat (70,71). Carcinoid and sclerosing hemangioma may also have a population of clear cells and may be confused with the above mentioned entities (49,52). Emphasis has been placed on the type of vasculature present in lung neoplasms with clear cell features. Thick-walled muscular arterioles are found in both metastatic renal cell carcinoma and in primary lung carcinomas (66,69). In contrast, benign clear cell tumors and carcinoid have a sinusoidal venous proliferation. Sclerosing hemangioma may have both an arterial and a venous supply (52). The vessels within a lung neoplasm may be difficult to evaluate on frozen section and may be obscured by cystic degeneration or necrosis.

Papillary Pattern. The differential diagnosis of papillary neoplasms in the lung is extensive. The most commonly encountered papillary lung neoplasms are listed in Table 6.3.

Of the primary neoplasms listed, sclerosing hemangioma, intravascular sclerosing tumor, and bronchioloalveolar carcinoma cause the greatest diagnostic difficulty. They are often confused with each other on frozen section. Bronchioloalveolar carcinoma may also be mistaken for reactive pneumonitis.

Sclerosing hemangioma typically presents as a solitary lower lobe nodule in the adult female. Grossly, it may range from 0.5 to 8 cm in diameter, and is often hemorrhagic. Histologically, four patterns have been described (52), and include papillary, sclerotic, hemorrhagic, and solid. One or more patterns may predominate. Satellite nodules of sclerosing hemangioma or carcinoid tumorlets may be present. The papillary component may initially

Table 6.3.
Frozen Section Differential Diagnosis of Papillary Lung Neoplasms

Primary	Metastatic
Tracheobronchial papillomatoisis	Carcinoma
Benign papilloma	Breast
Papillary tumors of surface epithelium	Colon
Sclerosing hemangioma	Pancreas
Carcinoid	Prostate
Mesothelioma	Ovary
Primary lung carcinoma	Thyroid
Papillary adenocarcinoma	Kidney
Bronchioloalveolar carcinoma	
Intravascular sclerosing tumor	
Pulmonary blastoma	

mislead the pathologist as he views frozen section, since it gives an epithelial overtone to the neoplasm (Figs. 6.14 and 6.15). The papillae in sclerosing hemangioma are usually located at the peripheral edge, are of variable size, and usually closely apposed. Attention to cytologic detail of the papillary component is the key in making the distinction between sclerosing hemangioma and bronchioloalveolar carcinoma. The alveolar lining cells overlying the papillae in sclerosing hemangioma are low cuboidal type, and without atypia. Foamy macrophages are usually present. Bronchioloalveolar carcinoma demonstrates obvious cytologic atypia. The alveolar framework of bronchioloalveolar carcinoma is usually preserved, whereas in sclerosing hemangioma, the architectural integrity of the lung in the area of the neoplasm is destroyed. A bronchiolar in situ component may be identified in bronchioloalveolar carcinoma (Fig. 6.16), a feature absent in sclerosing hemangioma.

Intravascular sclerosing tumor, also known as intravascular bronchioloalveolar tumor (72–75) or sclerosing angiogenic tumor (76), is a rare lung neoplasm which also has a predilection for adult females. In contrast to sclerosing hemangioma, which is usually solitary, intravascular sclerosing tumor typically has multiple nodules and appears grossly indurated. Histologically, a zonal phenomenon is observed. The central portion of the neoplasm consists of solid, hyalinized fibrous tissue which blends with interdigitating, closely apposed bands of sclerotic lung tissue. These sclerotic bands are lined by alveolar lining cells. The pattern and degree of sclerosis superficially resembles sclerosing hemangioma. The sclerotic component blends with the neoplastic cellular proliferation at the advancing edge of the neoplasm, which insinuates into and through alveolar pores. The re-

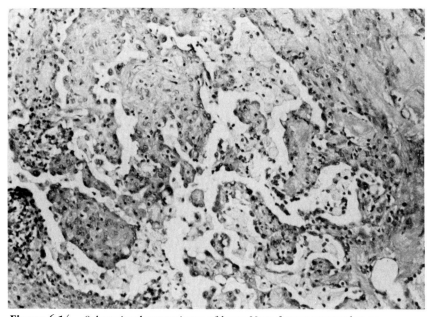

Figure 6.14. Sclerosing hemangioma of lung. Note foamy macrophages.

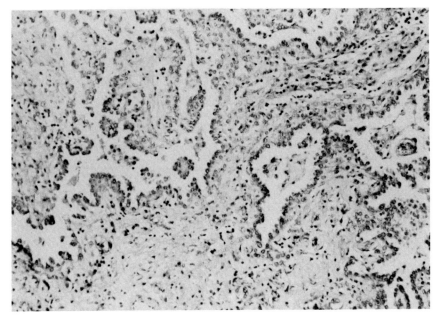

Figure 6.15. Sclerosing hemangioma with papillary component. Hyperplastic cells overlie papillae.

semblance to sclerosing hemangioma or even bronchioloalveolar carcinoma may be striking and is often difficult to distinguish on frozen section. In such a situation, the frozen section interpretation should be descriptive. Tissue for electron microscopy should be taken and may be helpful in the final diagnosis (73,75).

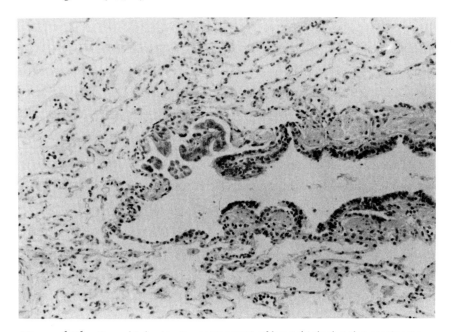

Figure 6.16. Bronchiolar in situ component of bronchioloalveolar carcinoma.

Spindled Pattern. The frozen section differential diagnosis for a spindled cell lung lesion is extensive. The most common entities are listed in Table 6.4 (see Carcinoid, this Chapter).

Accurate frozen section diagnosis can be exceedingly difficult. Electron microscopy is often necessary. If the clinical history is not helpful, in most cases, the frozen section interpretation should remain descriptive. The diagnosis of "spindle cell proliferation, possibly malignant" allows the surgeon to proceed with resection. The one reactive process most likely to be confused with a neoplasm on frozen section is plasma cell granuloma (inflammatory pseudotumor) (77–79). An inflammatory process which forms a mass lesion and typically affects children or young adults, it is usually encountered as a central mass associated with a major bronchus (Fig. 6.17). Histologically, a mixture of plasma cells, lymphocytes, eosinophils, and benign histiocytes is set within a fibroblastic, sclerotic, or hyalinized vascular stroma (Fig. 6.18). If the fibroblastic component is prominent, confusion with sarcoma may occur. The inflammatory cell population may be confused with Hodgkin's disease, or even plasmacytoma.

Chondroid Histology. Cartilagenous hamartoma and metastatic mature cystic teratoma can be confused with each other on frozen section. Bronchial hamartomas may be solitary or multicentric, centrally or peripherally located, and may undergo cystic degeneration (79–83). A peripheral hamartoma often self-enucleates during resection, thereby destroying its anatomic relationship to lung tissue. Mature cystic teratoma may also easily shell out from lung tissue. Grossly, the two may look very similar.

Cystic teratoma is rare as a primary lung neoplasm (84); it is more often found as one of the components in a metastatic mixed germ cell tumor. Post-therapy germ cell tumor metastases often display extensive zones of necrosis, admixed with viable cystic teratoma. On frozen section, the combination of endodermal, mesodermal, and ectodermal derivatives may be lacking. In this situation, the history is usually the only helpful distinguishing feature.

Table 6.4.
Frozen Section Differential Diagnosis of Spindled Cell Lesions Commonly Found in Lung

Reactive	Primary
Pleural plaque	Spindled carcinoid
Plasma cell granuloma	Localized fibrous mesothelioma
(inflammatory pseudotumor)	Sclerosing hemangioma
	Carcinoma
Metastatic	Spindled squamous
	Small cell
	Fibrosarcomatous mesothelioma
Sarcomas	Sarcoma
Carcinomas	Fibrosarcoma
Malignant melanoma	Leiomyosarcoma
	Angiosarcoma

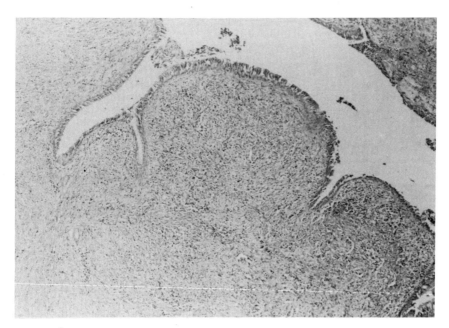

Figure 6.17. Plasma cell granuloma (inflammatory pseudotumor). Polypoid projection into bronchus.

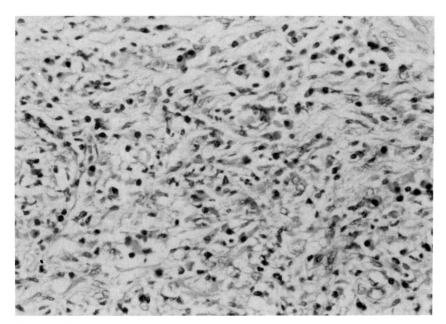

Figure 6.18. Plasma cell granuloma (inflammatory pseudotumor). Polymorphous collection of fibroblasts, plasma cells, and lymphocytes.

Lymphoid Processes

Any extranodal lymphoproliferative process should be handled as if it were a possible malignant lymphoma, reserving tissue for appropriate special studies (see Chapter 12, **Lymph Nodes**). With one exception (the intrapulmonary lymph node), frozen section diagnosis of lymphoid proliferations should routinely be deferred (see When to Defer a Frozen Section, this Chapter). Most intrapulmonary lymph nodes are located subpleurally or in the interlobular fissure and are found in 15% of adults (85,86). They may be detectable on a chest film and may rarely be present as coin lesions. On gross inspection, the lymph node is usually compressed against the pleura and has anthracotic pigment. From the pleural surface, it has a purple-grey hue and appears as a slight bulge. Histologically, intrapulmonary lymph nodes have architectural features similar to other lymph nodes, except that they may have an incomplete capsule. Histologically, enlarged intrapulmonary lymph nodes display benign reactive follicular hyperplasia and sinus histiocytosis.

Open Lung Biopsy

Bacterial, viral, fungal, and protozoan organisms can infect lung tissue and produce a wide variety of morphologic patterns of pneumonia. The pattern and type of pneumonia often provide clues as to the etiologic agent responsible. Evaluation of infectious processes in immunocompromised patients is often difficult, since the host response may be atypical or lacking altogether.

The open lung biopsy has been the standard method for evaluating possible infectious lung disease in selected immunocompromised patients with acute interstitial pneumonitis whose clinical workup has otherwise been negative. Acquired immunodeficiency syndrome (AIDS) patients with suspected *Pneumocystis carinii* pneumonia who have failed a course of trimethoprim-sulfamethoxazole may undergo open lung biopsy in an effort to establish a diagnosis of *P. carinii* pneumonia. The Center for Disease Control previously required biopsy confirmation of *P. carinii* to allow treatment with the alternative drug of choice, pentamidine isethionate (87). This restriction has since been lifted.

The recommended procedure for handling an open lung biopsy is outlined in Table 6.5.

A special problem at the time of frozen section from both the diagnostic and technical standpoint is the diagnosis of *Pneumocystis carinii* pneumonia (87,91,92). There are five main diagnostic problems the pathologist should be prepared to encounter when dealing with a possible *P. carinii* lung infection:

1.) The pathognomonic alveolopathy is absent in early infection. Most patients are biopsied early in the course of respiratory insufficiency. The classical frothy, cohesive intra-alveolar exudate (Fig. 6.19) is not usually seen. The interstitium may be only mildly edematous. Thin wisps of hyaline membranes may be present along the alveolar lining.

Table 6.5.
Procedure for Handling an Open Lung Biopsy

Sterile fresh lung tissue (5 to 10 g):

1. Submit a portion for frozen section and keep remaining lung tissue sterile
   a. One hematoxylin-eosin section
   b. Additional sections for:
      1. Rapid GMS
      2. Acid-fast
      3. Mucicarmine
2. Perform 10 touch preparations
   a. Five air dried
   b. Five fixed in 95% ethanol (use Carnoy's fixative if imprints are excessively bloody)
   c. When indicated, additional stains for:
      1. PAS (fixed)
      2. Mucicarmine (fixed)
      3. Rapid GMS (air dried)
3. Take aliquots for electron microscopy (gluteraldehyde fixation), microbiologic, viral, and fungal cultures.
4. When indicated submit tissue for immunofluorescent or chemical (asbestos) analysis (Refs. 88–90). (Snap freeze at − 70°C in liquid nitrogen.)
5. Routinely process remaining tissue in:
   a. 10% buffered formaldehyde solution
   b. B5 fixative (lymphoproliferative process)

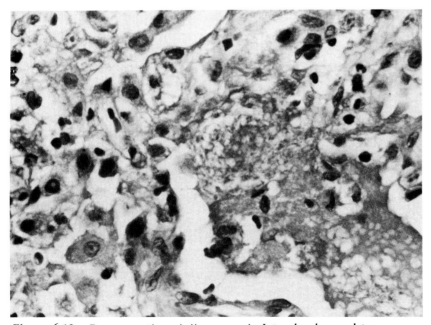

Figure 6.19. *Pneumocystis carinii* pneumonia. Intra-alveolar exudate.

2.) Atypical features may be present. A spectrum of histologic changes not classically associated with *P. carinii* have been reported (93) and include interstitial fibrosis, epithelioid granulomas, multinucleated giant cells, an interstitial infiltrate composed of lymphocytes, histiocytes and plasma cells, extensive accumulations of alveolar macrophages, and focal calcification.

In AIDS patients, trophozoites (excysted forms) tend to be numerous (94) and may significantly outnumber the cysts.

3.) Therapy may be instituted prior to biopsy. In patients with AIDS, trimethoprim-sulfamethoxazole may be empirically administered prior to biopsy. Several days after therapy, *Pneumocystis* organisms may still be present in lung (95) but become widely dispersed. Silver staining of the organism may be only faintly positive, or may even become negative (96).

4.) Multiple infectious agents may be present. Pulmonary disease in immunocompromised patients may take the form of single or multiple opportunistic infections. In the acquired immune deficiency syndrome, *Pneumocystis carinii* may coexist with Cytomegalovirus, *Mycobacterium avium intracellulare, Cryptococcus neoformans, Aspergillus, Nocardia,* and the enteric protozoan Cryptosporidium. Two studies have shown that touch imprints (Wright-Giemsa and Papanicolaou) are at least three times as sensitive in detecting Cytomegalovirus inclusions as is the routine frozen section (97,98). Another more recent study has reported that culture techniques for Cytomegalovirus are even more sensitive than cytologic methods in detecting Cytomegalovirus infection (99). Concurrent Cytomegalovirus and *Pneumocystis* infection have been reported to be associated with a poor prognosis (26). Identification of *M. avium intracellulare* in the lung implies extrapulmonary involvement of other tissues, usually liver and bone marrow (26,100,101).

5.) Special histochemistries may be capricious, difficult to interpret, and subject to variation by technical personnel.

The pathologist has a variety of special stains at his disposal which help visualize *P. carinii.* Each has advantages and disadvantages. These are listed in Table 6.6.

Many laboratories are converting to use of microwave ovens for more rapid silver impregnation. Incubation time is reduced to 70 seconds, the entire staining process takes 10 minutes, and there is minimal background precipitate (108).

On rapid silver stains, *Pneumocystis carinii* organisms can be confused with red blood cells, nonbudding yeast forms, and granulocytes. The distinctive morphology of the organisms helps to distinguish them from other silver-positive structures. *P. carinii* organisms have a delicate capsular wall which measures 4 to 6 μm in diameter (Fig. 6.20). The capsule is often collapsed, creating crescentic forms that resemble helmets or teacups. The trophozoite's presumed site of exit from the cyst is identified as a centralized pair of dots and can be detected with oil immersion.

Some simple variations in routine techniques have improved our diagnostic reliability of open lung biopsy detection of *P. carinii:*

1.) The frozen section slide is fixed in formaldehyde solution for 1 minute prior to staining. This improves cytologic detail without inducing significant artifact.

Table 6.6.
Stains for *Pneumocystis carinii*[a]

Stain	Advantages	Disadvantages
Wright-Giemsa	Fairly rapid (about 1 h)	Stains only trophozoite, sporozoite; staining artifact
Toluidine blue O (102)	Rapid; stains cyst	Hazardous reagent (ether/sulfuric acid); staining quality variable
10-min Gomori methenamine (103)	Rapid (10-min); stains cysts	Hazardous reagent (dimethylsulfoxide)
Cresyl echt violet (104)	Fairly rapid (about 1 h)	Toxic reagent (glacial acetic/sulfuric acid)
Gram-Weigert (91)	Fairly rapid (30 min)	Toxic reagent (aniline oil)
Rapid Gomori methenamine (105)	Fairly rapid (20 min); stains cyst wall and sporozoites	Expensive reagent; does not stain trophozoite; staining artifact
Grocott methenamine (106)	Stains cyst wall and sporozoites; shorter incubation than Gomori	Expensive reagent; does not stain trophozoite; staining artifact
Fluorescence epi-illumination (107)	Stains cyst wall and sporozoite	Use only on pap smear; erythrocytes also fluoresce

[a]Trophozoite = excysted form; sporozoite = encysted form.

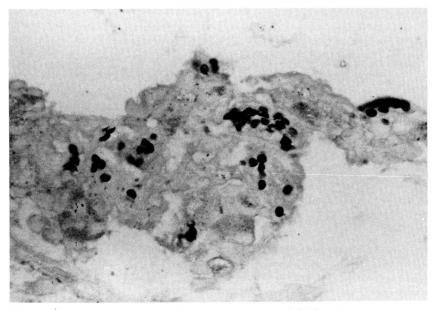

Figure 6.20. *Pneumocystis carinii* pneumonia. Rapid GMS stain.

2.) Grocott's modified method is used, since the incubation period is shorter than for the Gomori methenamine technique and the precipitate is slightly less.

3.) All slides are overstained for 10 min past the recommended time, using a *Pneumocystis carinii* control.

4.) Touch imprints are air dried rather than fixed in ethanol. Gentle swishing of the touch imprint in Coplin jar washes off a significant number of organisms. Cysts adhere much better if the touch imprint is allowed to air dry before staining.

Frozen Section Diagnosis of the Bronchial Margin

A positive bronchial margin should be classified into one (or more) of the following categories (109): *a*) in situ carcinoma; *b*) direct extension into the bronchial wall; *c*) positive peribronchial soft tissues; *d*) submucosal peribronchial lymphatic permeation.

A positive bronchial margin may create unexpected intraoperative management problems. Preoperative endoscopic biopsies may have been performed to help determine "safe" bronchial margins (110–113). The area most often biopsied by the bronchoscopist is the lobar spur, which represents the anatomic margin of the lobe and is the most convenient and easiest site to biopsy. The actual surgical margin may not correspond to the anatomic margin and in many cases may be distal to it, often by as much as 1 cm. A negative endoscopic biopsy contradicted by a positive bronchial margin at the time of resection complicates the planned procedure. The simple lobectomy is suddenly not so simple. The nature of the frozen section report will influence the surgeon's management. For categories *a* through *c* listed above, the surgeon will take a second bronchial margin if possible. If no additional margin is submitted, postoperative radiation may be given (114). If lymphatic involvement is identified, there is no rational basis for taking a second margin. Lymphatic involvement of the bronchial stump has been reported to be associated with a poor prognosis (109).

Repeated observations have shown that the natural history of in situ carcinoma of the bronchial epithelium has certain distinctive features (110). The pathologist who is familiar with these features will be able to interpret frozen sections more effectively and will be able to understand the reason for possible discrepancies between the preoperative and intraoperative diagnosis:

1.) Squamous carcinoma in situ of bronchial origin usually arises in the surface epithelium of a segmental bronchus and may spread proximally to involve the lobar or main stem bronchus.

2.) The transition from normal or metaplastic epithelium to in situ carcinoma is often abrupt, especially at the proximal leading edge.

3.) Submucosal glandular extension may simulate invasion, especially when there is deep involvement of the glands adjacent to cartilage.

4.) In situ carcinoma often demonstrates field effect (multicentricity).

The evaluation of bronchial margins from sleeve resections is discussed in a separate section of this chapter.

Artifactual sloughing of the bronchial epithelium should not be con-

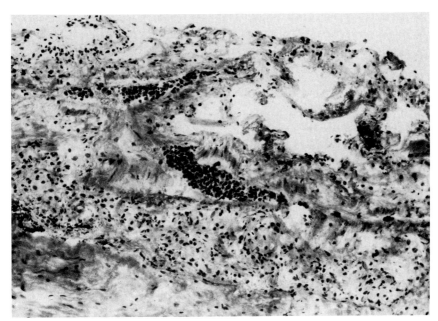

Figure 6.21. Frozen section of bronchial margin. Sloughing and distortion of bronchial epithelium simulate invasion.

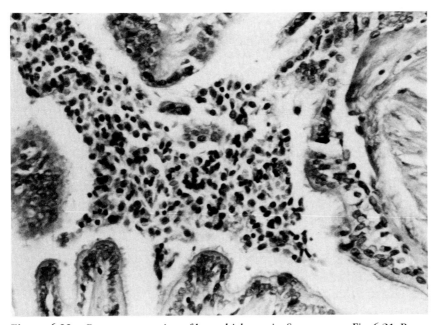

Figure 6.22. Permanent section of bronchial margin. Same case as Fig. 6.21. Bronchial epithelium is sloughed into lumen.

fused with a malignant infiltrate (Fig. 6.21). Such a finding is usually focal. Permanent sections reveal this process clearly (Fig. 6.22).

Frozen Section Diagnosis of the Pleura

Mesothelial Proliferations

Pathologists continue to struggle with the interpretation of mesothelial proliferations from the cytologic, histologic, immunocytochemical, and ultrastructural level (115–118). To this is added the dimension of frozen section diagnosis. Mesothelial proliferations are especially difficult to characterize on frozen section and are usually best left unclassified.

Reactive pleuritis may induce an exuberant mesothelial hyperplasia, especially if associated with an infarct, granulomatous inflammation (especially tuberculous), or bloody effusion. Reactive mesothelial cells may be epithelioid and/or spindled, may demonstrate cytologic atypia with mitoses, hypertrophic or double nuclei, and may even form papillary projections. Frozen section distinction between a reactive pleuritis and mesothelioma requires gross identification of an index mass; the cytologic distinction is often impossible. Distinction between malignant mesothelioma and pleural carcinomatosis is even more difficult, and usually requires histochemical, immunocytochemical, and electron microscopic study.

Localized fibrous mesothelioma (45–47), may create diagnostic problems at the time of frozen section. A potentially locally aggressive neoplasm, it may arise from the visceral pleura and invaginate into the lung, or take its origin from the parietal pleura and extend outward, involving the mediastinum or chest wall structures. Histologically, it may resemble a variety of other lung neoplasms, including spindled carcinoid (44), plasma cell

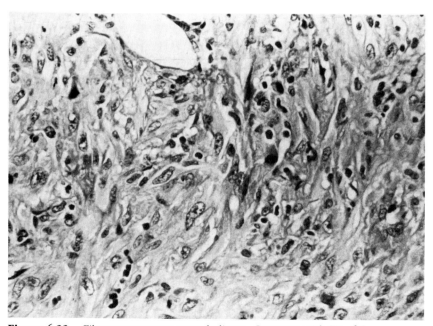

Figure 6.23. Fibrosarcomatous mesothelioma. Compare with Fig. 6.5.

granuloma (inflammatory pseudotumor) (77–79), and malignant meso-thelioma (Fig. 6.23). In its usual form, localized fibrous mesothelioma is grossly circumscribed, is in intimate contact with the pleura, and is covered by an intact layer of mesothelial cells. The frozen section distinction be-tween localized fibrous mesothelioma and spindled carcinoid has already been discussed in a previous section (see Carcinoid, p.119).

WHEN TO DEFER A FROZEN SECTION

The morbidity from thoracotomy is greater than with most other types of major surgical procedures, and the pathologist should not defer a frozen section diagnosis, except in special situations:

Lymphoproliferative Process

The diagnosis of any extranodal lymphoproliferative process should be routinely deferred. Representative tissue should be obtained for special studies, as when handling a lymph node containing a possible malignant lymphoma (see Chapter 12, **Lymph Nodes**). The treatment of lymphopro-liferative processes involving the lung is usually non-surgical, although some advocate surgical resection (119). Regardless of the planned treatment, diagnosis should be deferred.

If a mediastinal lymph node is suspicious for malignant lymphoma, or has extensive zones of sclerosis or necrosis, the diagnosis should be deferred (see Chapter 10, **Mediastinum**).

The special problem of the intrapulmonary lymph node is discussed in a separate section (see p. 132).

Papillary Lesions That Are Not Obviously Malignant

The differential diagnosis of a papillary lung lesion is extensive and includes benign and malignant primary or metastatic neoplasms. In a situ-ation where the pathologist is uncertain whether the process in the lung is malignant, the diagnosis should be deferred, or perhaps simply descriptive. The most conservative procedure which completely encompasses the lesion should be carried out, with evaluation of the surgical margins. If, on the following morning, the permanent sections are found to contain a malignant neoplasm, the surgeon and pathologist can at least be reassured that the neoplasm was excised, preventing a possible second thoracotomy.

Frozen section diagnostic problems related to papillary lesions in the lung are discussed in a separate section (see p. 127).

Spindle Cell Lesions That Are Not Obviously Malignant

As with papillary lesions, spindle cell proliferations may represent re-active, benign or malignant primary or metastatic neoplasms. Spindle cell lesions of uncertain malignant potential should be handled in a manner similar to that for papillary lesions. Frozen section diagnostic problems related to spindled cell lesions in the lung are discussed in a separate section of this chapter (see p. 130).

Pleural Mesothelial Proliferations Which Cannot Be Definitively Classified (see Mesothelial Proliferations, p. 138).

REFERENCES

1. Naruke T, Suemasu K, Ishikama S: Lymph node mapping and curability at various levels of metastasis in resected lung cancer. *J Thorac Cardiovasc Surg* 76:832–839, 1978.
2. Mountain CF, McMurtrey MJ, Frazier OH: Regional extension of lung cancer. *Rad Oncol Biol Phys* 6:1013–1020, 1980.
3. Smith SR, Beechler CR, Whitcomb MF: Indications for mediastinal lymph node evaluation. *Chest* 5:599–604, 1982.
4. Kirschner PA: Surgical significance of mediastinal lymph node metastasis. *NY State J Med* 79:2036–2041, 1979.
5. Jolly PC, Li W, Anderson RP: Anterior and cervical mediastinoscopy for determining operability and predicting resectability in lung cancer. *J Thorac Cardiovasc Surg* 79:366–371, 1980.
6. McNeil TM, Chamberlain JM: Diagnostic anterior mediastinotomy. *Ann Thorac Surg* 2:532–539, 1966.
7. Kirsch MM, Kahn DR, Gago O, Lampe I, Fayos J, Prio M, Moores WY, Haight C, Sloan H: Treatment of bronchogenic carcinoma with mediastinal metastasis. *Ann Thorac Surg* 12:11–21, 1971.
8. Pearson FG, Nelems JM, Henderson RD, Delarue NC: The role of mediastinoscopy in the selection of treatment for bronchial carcinoma with involvement of superior mediastinal lymph nodes. *J Thorac Cardiovasc Surg* 64:382–390, 1972.
9. Frazier OH, McMurtrey MJ, Mountain CF: Cancer of the lung. In Edward Copeland, III (ed): *Surgical Oncology.* New York, Wiley & Sons, 1983, p 264.
10. Rubinstein I, Baum GL, Pauzner Y, Lieberman Y, Bubis JJ: Resectional surgery in the treatment of primary carcinoma of the lung with mediastinal lymph node metastases. *Thorax* 34:33–35, 1979.
11. Rabinovitch M, Castaneda A, Reid L: Lung biopsy with frozen section as a diagnostic aid in patients with congenital heart defects. *Am J Cardiol* 47:77–84, 1981.
12. Heath D, Edwards JE: The pathology of hypertensive heart disease. A description of six grades of structural changes in the pulmonary arterioles with special references to congenital cardiac septal defects. *Circulation* 18:533–547, 1958.
13. Wagenvoort CA: Lung biopsy specimens in the evaluation of pulmonary vascular disease. *Chest* 77:614–625, 1980.
14. American Joint Committee for Cancer Staging and End-Results Reporting Task Force on Lung: *Staging of Lung Cancer.* Chicago American Joint Committee, 1979.
15. Nohl HC: An investigation into the lymphatic and vascular spread of carcinoma of the bronchus. *Thorax* 11:172–185, 1956.
16. Carlens E: Mediastinoscopy: a method for inspection and tissue biopsy in the superior mediastinum. *Dis Chest* 36:343–352, 1959.
17. Schechter DC, Acinapura AJ: Pulmonary diagnostic invasive procedures (Part II). *NY State J Med* 80:1702–1711, 1980.
18. Steiger Z, Chaudhry S, Wilson RF: The use of anterior mediastinoscopy to assess intrathoracic lesions. *Am Surg* 47:251–253, 1981.
19. Bowen TE, Rajtchuk R, Green DC, Brott LNH: Value of anterior mediastinoscopy in bronchogenic carcinoma of the left upper lobe. *J Thorac Cardiovasc Surg* 76:269–271, 1978.
20. Schatzlein MH, McAuliffe S, Orringer MB, Kirsch MM: Scalene node biopsy in pulmonary carcinoma: When is it indicated? *Ann Thorac Surg* 31:322–324, 1981.
21. Schmidt FE, Kahle HR: Biopsy of apical pulmonary tumors: An open technique with needle biopsy. *Surgery* 70:614–615, 1971.
22. Wise WS, Read RC: Apical lung biopsy. *Ann Thorac Surg* 12:139–145, 1971.
23. DeCaro LF, Pak, HY, Yokota S, Teplitz RL, Benfield JR: Intraoperative cytodiagnosis of lung tumors by needle aspiration. *J Thorac Cardiovasc Surg* 85:404–408, 1983.
24. Pak HY, Yokota S, Teplitz RL, Shaw SL, Werner TL: Rapid staining techniques employed in fine needle aspirations of the lung. *Acta Cytol* 25:178–184, 1981.

25. Gottlieb MS, Schroff R, Schanker HM, Weisman J, Fan PT, Saxon A: Pneumocystis carinii pneumonia and mucosal candidiasis in previously healthy homosexual men. Evidence of a new acquired cellular immunodeficiency. *N Engl J Med* 305:1425–1431, 1981.
26. Gottlieb MS: Pulmonary disease in the acquired immune deficiency syndrome. *Chest* (*Suppl*) 86:29–31, 1984.
27. Murray JE, Felton CP, Garay S, Gottlieb M, Hopewell PC, Stover DE: Special Report: Report of a National Heart, Lung, and Blood Institute Workshop. *N Engl J Med* 310:1682–1688, 1984.
28. Hopewell PC, Luce JM: Pulmonary involvement in the acquired immunodeficiency syndrome. *Chest* 87:104–112, 1985.
29. Burt ME, Flye MW, Webber BL, Wesley RA: Prospective evaluation of aspiration needle, cutting needle, transbronchial, and open lung biopsy in patients with pulmonary infiltrates. *Ann Thorac Surg* 32:146–153, 1981.
30. Bennett WF, Smith RA: Segmental resection for bronchogenic carcinoma: A surgical alternative for the compromised patient. *Ann Thorac Surg* 27:169–172, 1979.
31. Jensik RJ, Faber P, Milloy FJ, Amato JJ: Sleeve lobectomy for carcinoma. A ten year experience. *J Thorac Cardiovasc Surg* 64:400–412, 1972.
32. Weisel R, Cooper JD, Delarue NC, Theman TE, Todd TRJ, Pearson FG: Sleeve lobectomy for carcinoma of the lung. *J Thorac Cardiovasc Surg* 78:839–849, 1979.
33. Paulson DL, Urschel HC, McNamara JJ, Shaw RR: Bronchoplastic procedures for bronchogenic carcinoma. *J Thorac Cardiovasc Surg* 59:38–48, 1970.
34. Deslauriers J, Beaulieu M, Benazera A, McClish A: Sleeve pneumonectomy for bronchogenic carcinoma. *Ann Thorac Surg* 28:465–474, 1979.
35. Von Hoff DD, LiVolsi VA: Diagnostic reliability of needle biopsy of the parietal pleura. A review of 272 biopsies. *Am J Clin Pathol* 64:200–203, 1973.
36. Ryckman FC, Rodgers BM: Thoracoscopy for intrathoracic neoplasms in children. *J Ped Surg* 17:521–524, 1982.
37. Carter D: Small cell carcinoma of the lung. *Am J Surg Pathol* 7:787–793, 1983.
38. Azzopardi JG: Oat cell carcinoma of the bronchus. *J Pathol Bacteriol* 78:513–519, 1959.
39. Hansen HH: Management of small-cell anaplastic carcinoma, 1980–1982. In Ishikana S, Hayata Y (eds): *Lung Cancer.* Amsterdam-Oxford, Excerpta Medica, 1982, p 31–54.
40. Mark EJ: Carcinomas. In: *Lung Biopsy Interpretation.* Baltimore, William & Wilkins, 1984, p 211.
41. Ihde D: Current status of therapy for small cell carcinoma of the lung. *Cancer* 54:2722–2728, 1984.
42. Mills SE, Cooper PH, Walker AN, Kron IL: Atypical carcinoid of the lung. A clinicopathologic study of 17 cases. *Am J Surg Pathol* 6:643–654, 1982.
43. Arrigoni MG, Woolner CB, Bernatz PE: Atypical carcinoid tumors of the lung. *J Thorac Cardiovasc Surg* 64:413–421, 1972.
44. Ranchod M, Levine GD: Spindle-cell carcinoid tumors of the lung. *Am J Surg Pathol* 4:315–331, 1980.
45. Scharifker D, Kaneko M: Localized fibrous mesothelioma of pleura (submesothelial fibroma). A clinicopathologic study of 18 cases. *Cancer* 43:627–635, 1979.
46. Hernandez FJ, Fernandez BB: Localized fibrous tumors of pleura: A light and electron microscopic study. *Cancer* 34:1667–1674, 1974.
47. Briselli M, Mark EJ, Dickerson GR: Solitary fibrous tumors of the pleura: Eight new cases and review of 360 cases in the literature. *Cancer* 47:2678–2689, 1981.
48. Mark EJ, Quay SC, Dickerson GR: Papillary carcinoid tumor of the lung. *Cancer* 48:316–324, 1981.
49. Mark EJ: Benign and borderline neoplasms. In: *Lung Biopsy Interpretation.* Baltimore, Williams & Wilkins, 1984, p 186–188.
50. Churg A, Warnock ML: Pulmonary tumorlet. A form of peripheral carcinoid. *Cancer* 37:1469–1477, 1976.
51. Mark EJ: Benign and borderline neoplasms. In: *Lung Biopsy Interpretation.* Baltimore, Williams & Wilkins, 1984, p 187.
52. Katzenstein ALA, Gmelich JT, Carrington CB: Sclerosing hemangioma of the lung. A clinicopathologic study of 51 cases. *Am J Surg Pathol* 4:343–356, 1980.
53. Mark EJ: Carcinomas. In: *Lung Biopsy Interpretation.* Baltimore, Williams & Wilkins, 1984, p 214–215.

54. Liebow AA: Bronchiolo-alveolar carcinoma. *Adv Int Med* 10:329–358, 1960.
55. Manning JT, Spjut HJ, Tschen JA: Bronchioloalveolar carcinoma: The significance of two histopathologic types. *Cancer* 54:525–534, 1984.
56. Donaldson JC, Kaminsky DB, Elliott RC: Bronchiolar carcinoma. Report of 11 cases and review of the literature. *Cancer* 41:250–258, 1978.
57. Miller WT, Husted J, Freiman P, Atkinson B, Pietra GG: Bronchioloalverolar carcinoma: Two clinical entities with one pathologic diagnosis. *Am J Roentgenol* 130:905–912, 1978.
58. Rosenblatt MB, Lisa JR, Collier F: Primary and metastatic bronchiolo-alveolar carcinoma. *Dis Chest* 52:147–152, 1967.
59. Kirschner RH, Esterly JR: Pulmonary lesions association with Busulfan therapy of chronic myelogenous leukemia. *Cancer* 27:1074–1080, 1971.
60. Pearl M: Busulfan lung. *Am J Dis Child* 131:650–652, 1977.
61. Holoye PY, Luna MA, Mackay B, Bedrossian CWM: Bleomycin hypersensitivity pneumonitis. *Ann Intern Med* 88:47–49, 1978.
62. Samuels ML, Johnson DE, Holoye PY, Lanzotti, VJ: Large dose bleomycin therapy and pulmonary toxicity: A possible role of prior radiotherapy. *JAMA* 235:1117–1120, 1976.
63. Weiss RB, Muggia FM: Cytotoxic drug-induced pulmonary disease: Update 1980. *Am J Med* 68:259–264, 1980.
64. Sostman HD, Matthay RA, Putman CE: Cytotoxic drug-induced lung disease. *Am J Med* 62:608–615, 1977.
65. Fajardo LF, Berthrong M: Radiation injury in surgical pathology (Part I). *Am J Surg Pathol* 2:159–199, 1978.
66. Katzenstein ALA, Purvis R, Gmelich J, Askin FB: Pulmonary resection for metastatic renal cell carcinoma. Pathologic findings and therapeutic value. *Cancer* 41:712–723, 1978.
67. Middleton RG: Surgery for metastatic renal cell carcinoma. *J Urol* 97:973–977, 1967.
68. Tannenbaum M: Ultrastructural pathology of human renal cell tumors. *Pathol Annu* 6:249–277, 1971.
69. Katzenstein ALA, Prioleau PG, Askin FB: The histologic spectrum and significance of clear-cell change in lung carcinoma. *Cancer* 45:943–947, 1980.
70. Liebow AA, Castleman B: Benign clear cell ("sugar") tumors of the lung. *Yale J Biol Med* 43:213–222, 1971.
71. Harbin WP, Mark GJ, Greene RE: Benign clear-cell tumor ("sugar tumor") of the lung: A case report and review of the literature. *Radiology* 129:595–596, 1978.
72. Azumi N, Churg A: Intravascular and sclerosing bronchioloalveolar tumor. A pulmonary sarcoma of probable vascular origin. *Am J Surg Pathol* 5:587–596, 1981.
73. Dail DH, Liebow AA, Gmelich JT, Friedman PJ, Mijai K, Meyer W, Patterson SD, Hammar SP: Intravascular, bronchiolar, and alveolar tumor of the lung (IVBAT). An analysis of twenty cases of a peculiar, sclerosing endothelial tumor. *Cancer* 51:452–464, 1983.
74. Bhagavan BS, Dorfman HD, Murthy MSN, Eggleston JC: Intravascular bronchiolo-alveolar tumor (IVBAT). A low-grade sclerosing epithelioid angiosarcoma of lung. *Am J Surg Pathol* 6:41–52, 1982.
75. Corrin B, Manners B, Millard M, Weaver L: Histogenesis of the so-called "intravascular bronchioloalveolar tumor". *J Pathol* 128:163–167, 1979.
76. Weldon-Linne CM, Victor TA, Christ ML, Fry WA: Angiogenic nature of the "intravascular bronchioloalveolar tumor" of the lung. *Arch Pathol Lab Med* 105:174–179, 1981.
77. Bahadori M, Liebow AA: Plasma cell granulomas of the lung. *Cancer* 31:191–208, 1973.
78. Spyker MA, Kay S: Plasma cell granuloma of a mediastinal lymph node with extension to right lung. *J Thorac Cardiovasc Surg* 31:211–216, 1956.
79. Tomita T, Dixon A, Watanabe I, Mantz F, Richany S: Sclerosing vascular variant of plasma cell granuloma. *Hum Pathol* 11:197–202, 1980.
80. Butler C, Kleinerman J: Pulmonary hamartoma. *Arch Pathol* 88:584–592, 1969.
81. Bateson EM: So called hamartoma of the lung—a true neoplasm of fibrous connective tissue of the bronchi. *Cancer* 31:1458–1467, 1973.
82. Bateson EM: Relationship between intrapulmonary and endobronchial cartilage-containing tumors (so-called hamartomata). *Thorax* 20:447–461, 1963.
83. Ramchand S, Baskerville L: Multiple hamartomas of the lung. *Am Rev Respir Dis* 99:932–935, 1969
84. Bateson EM, Hayes JA, Woo-Ming M: Endobronchial teratoma associated with bronchiectasis and bronchiolectasis. *Thorax* 23:69–76, 1968.

85. Trapnell DH: Recognition and incidence of intrapulmonary lymph nodes. *Thorax* 19:44–50, 1964.

86. Blakely RW, Blumenthal BJ, Fred HL: Benign intrapulmonary lymph node presenting as a coin lesion. *South Med J* 67:1216–1218, 1974.

87. McKenna RJ, Mountain CF, McMurtrey MJ: Open lung biopsy in immunocompromised patients. *Chest* 86:671–674, 1984.

88. Smith MJ, Naylor B: A method for extracting ferruginous bodies from sputum and pulmonary tissue. *Am J Clin Pathol* 58:250–254, 1972.

89. Churg A, Warnock ML: Analysis of the cores of ferruginous (asbestos) bodies from the general population. I. Patients with and without lung cancer. *Lab Invest* 37:280–286, 1977.

90. Churg A, Warnock ML, Green N: Analysis of the cores of ferruginous (asbestos) bodies from the general population. II. True asbestos bodies and pseudoasbestos bodies. *Lab Invest* 40:31–38, 1979.

91. Rosen PP, Martini N, Armstrong D: Pneumocystis carinii pneumonia. Diagnosis by lung biopsy. *Am J Med* 58:794–802, 1975.

92. Rosen PP: Frozen section management of a lung biopsy for suspected Pneumocystis pneumonia. *Am J Surg Pathol* 1:79–82, 1977.

93. Weber WR, Askin FB, Dehner LP: Lung biopsy in Pneumocystis carinii pneumonia. A histopathologic study of typical and atypical features. *Am J Clin Pathol* 67:11–19, 1977.

94. Mark EJ: Bacteria and Protozoa. In: *Lung Biopsy Interpretation,* Baltimore, Williams & Wilkins, 1984, p 39.

95. Campbell WG: Ultrastructure of Pneumocystis in human lung. *Arch Pathol Lab Med* 93:312–324, 1972.

96. Mark EJ: Bacteria and Protozoa. In: *Lung Biopsy Interpretation.* Baltimore, Williams & Wilkins, 1984, p 39.

97. Sale GE, Shulman HM, Hackman RC, Meyers JD: Frozen section diagnosis of Cytomegalovirus infections. *Diag Obstet Gynecol* 4:389–396, 1982.

98. Shulman HM, Hackman RC, Sale GE, Meyers JD: Rapid cytologic diagnosis of Cytomegalovirus interstitial pneumonia on touch imprints from open lung biopsy. *Am J Clin Pathol* 77:90–94, 1982.

99. Blumenfeld W, Wagar E, Hadley WK: Use of the transbronchial biopsy for diagnosis of opportunistic pulmonary infections in acquired immunodeficiency syndrome (AIDS). *Am J Clin Pathol* 81:1–5, 1984.

100. Zakowski P, Fligiel S, Berlin BW, Johnson BL: Disseminated Mycobacterium avium intracellulare infection in homosexual men dying of acquired immunodeficiency. *JAMA* 248:2980–2982, 1982.

101. Osborne BM, Guarda LA, Butler JJ: Bone marrow biopsies in patients with the acquired immunodeficiency syndrome. *Hum Pathol* 15:1048–1053, 1984.

102. Chalvardjian AM, Grawe LA: A new procedure for the identification of Pneumocystis carinii cysts in tissue sections and smears. *J Clin Pathol* 16:383–384, 1963.

103. Musto L, Flanigan M, Elbadawi A: Ten minute silver stain for Pneumocystis carinii and fungi in tissue sections. *Arch Pathol Lab Med* 106:292–294, 1982.

104. Bowling MC, Smith IM, Wescott SL: A rapid staining procedure for Pneumocystis carinii. *Am J Med Technol* 39:267–268, 1973.

105. Mahan C, Sale G: Rapid methenamine silver stain for Pneumocystis and fungi. *Arch Pathol Lab Med* 102:351–352, 1978.

106. Pintozzi R: Modified Grocott's methenamine silver nitrate method for quick staining of Pneumocystis carinii. *J Clin Pathol* 31:803–805, 1978.

107. Ohali VS, Garcia RL, Skolon J: Fluorescence of Pneumocystis carinii in Papanicolaou smears. *Hum Pathol* 15:907–909, 1984.

108. Brinn N, Bossen E, and Szpak C: Rapid silver impregnations using the microwave oven. *Lab Invest* 50:6–7(Abstract), 1984.

109. Soorae HS, Stevenson HM: Survival with residual tumor on the bronchial margin after resection for bronchogenic carcinoma. *J Thorac Cardiovasc Surg* 78:175–180, 1979.

110. Carter D: Pathology of early squamous carcinoma of the lung. *Pathol Annu* 13 (*Part 1*):131–147, 1978.

111. Marsh BR, Frost JK, Erozan YS, Carter D: The role of fiberoptic bronchoscopy in lung cancer. *Semin Oncol* 1:199–203, 1974.

112. Marsh BR, Frost JK, Erozan YS, Carter D: Occult bronchogenic carcinoma. Endoscopic localization and television documentation. *Cancer* 30:1348–1352, 1972.

113. Marsh BR, Frost JR, Carter D, Proctor DF: Flexible fiberoptic bronchoscope—its place in the search for lung cancer. *Trans Am Bronchoesophagol Assoc* 53:101–110, 1973.

114. Shields TW: The fate of patients after incomplete resection of bronchial carcinoma. *Surg Gynecol Obstet* 139:569–572, 1974.

115. Jarvi OH, Kunnas RJ, Laitio MT, Tyrkko JES: The accuracy and significance of cytologic cancer diagnosis of pleural effusions. *Acta Cytol* 16:152–158, 1972.

116. Bolen JW, Thorning D: Mesotheliomas. A light and electron microscopical study concerning histogenetic relationships between the epithelial and mesenchymal variants. *Am J Surg Pathol* 4:451–464, 1980.

117. Klima M, Gyorkey F: Benign pleural lesions and malignant mesothelioma. *Virch Arch A Pathol Anat Histol* 376:181–193, 1977.

118. Wagner JC, Mundray DE, Harrington JS: Histochemical demonstration of hyaluronic acid in pleural mesotheliomas. *J Pathol Bacteriol* 84:73–78, 1962.

119. Peterson H, Snider HL, Yam LT, Bowlds CF, Arnn EH, Li CY: Primary pulmonary lymphoma. A clinical and immunohistochemical study of six cases. *Cancer* 56:805-813, 1985.

7

Gastrointestinal Tract, Pancreas, and Liver

Luis Guarda, M.D.

The percentage of frozen sections taken from the gastrointestinal tract, including the esophagus, pancreas, and liver, varies from 8.2 to 18.7% depending on the series and the hospital setting (1–4). Some frozen sections are submitted for intraoperative histologic evaluation to assess nodal spread or local invasion and dissemination. Most commonly, these specimens are lymph nodes, pleural or peritoneal implants, and liver or other visceral nodules. Touch imprints for rapid intraoperative cytologic study may be of help in the frozen section diagnosis of these specimens. Confirmation of tumor spread beyond the confines of the organ in which the neoplasm originated will often determine nonresectability.

ESOPHAGUS

Frozen sections from the esophagus are rarely necessary. The one indication for frozen section during esophageal surgical procedures is to determine the status of resection margins when an esophageal neoplasm is removed. The neoplasm itself does not need to be examined by frozen section if the diagnosis has been established by endoscopic biopsy before the operation. A tumor-free margin cannot be determined by gross inspection or palpation because esophageal cancer can spread submucosally through lymphatic channels far beyond the gross extension of the tumor (Fig. 7.1); some are known to have spread up to 7 cm beyond the gross limits of the neoplasm (5). The specimen(s) submitted will be a resected segment of esophagus containing the margins, or short ring-shaped segments separate from the main portion of the tumor. Transverse sections must be taken from the specimen's proximal and distal ends to assure the adequacy of the operative procedure.

Histologic interpretation of these frozen sections is generally not difficult. Most patients undergoing esophageal surgery receive preoperative irradiation, but radiation change is rarely a problem in frozen section. The esophageal epithelium is only moderately sensitive to radiation and usually regenerates rapidly. Subacute and chronic ulceration may occur. The epi-

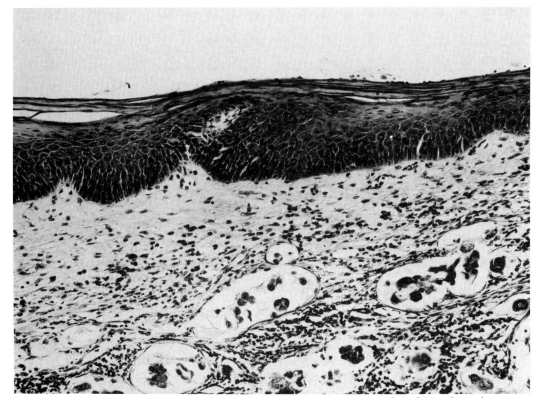

Figure 7.1. Esophageal submucosal spread of adenocarcinoma; tumor in lymphatic channels.

thelium is thickened and parakeratotic, with homogenized collagen, small-vessel telangiectasia, and atypical fibroblasts underlying the epithelium. Mucous esophageal glands show changes similar to those of radiation sialadenitis, and their ductal elements may become lined with squamous metaplastic epithelium. The latter must not be confused with submucosal nests of squamous carcinoma (6).

STOMACH

Fewer than 5% of gastrointestinal tract frozen sections are from the stomach (1–4). Indications for frozen section include the following: a) to help in the diagnosis of gastric lesions that on the basis of clinical, radiologic, or endoscopic examinations are believed to be malignant, but in which the preoperative histopathologic diagnosis has not been established. This category of lesions includes carcinomas, Ménétrier's disease, ulcers, and polyps; b) to help diagnose perforated ulcers which must be differentiated as benign or malignant; and c) to determine the status of the resection margins during the course of gastrectomy for gastric carcinoma. The specimen available for evaluation will be either a partial or a total gastrectomy.

We have encountered several problems in interpretation and diagnosis, the most common and difficult one being evaluation of margins in the course of gastrectomy for signet-ring carcinoma. The tumor cells are small and

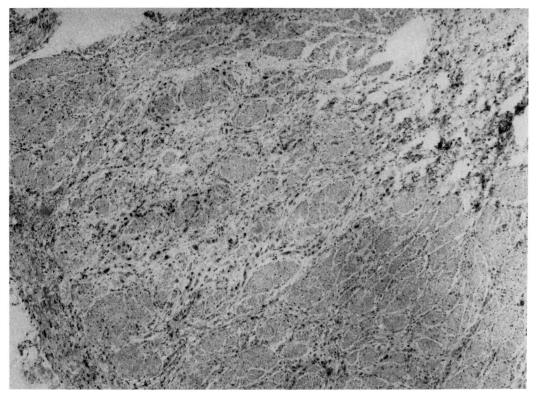

Figure 7.2. Frozen section of signet-ring carcinoma of stomach infiltrating a resection margin transmurally. The low power view gives the mistaken impression of inflammatory cells.

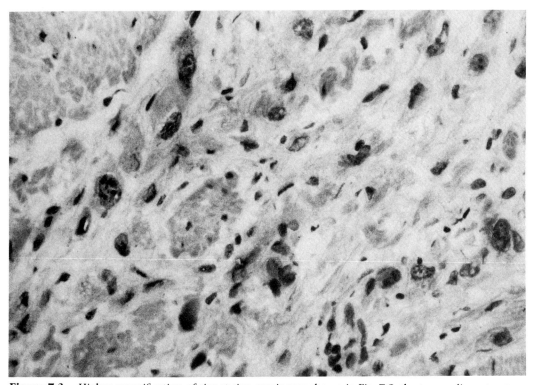

Figure 7.3. Higher magnification of signet-ring carcinoma shown in Fig. 7.2; the true malignant nature of the infiltrate is evident.

frequently isolated; they do not form glandular lumina, and marked fibroblastic and inflammatory reaction accompanies the infiltration of the stomach wall (Figs. 7.2 and 7.3). Close attention to the morphology of the individual tumor cells in the infiltrate often helps to establish the diagnosis. The most difficult cases may be resolved by the use of special stains, for example, ethanol fixed frozen sections stained with 1% alcian blue at pH 2.5 for 1 min and then counterstained with nuclear fast red. Neoplastic signet-ring cells must be differentiated from mast cells, the granules of which also stain positively with this technique (7).

In evaluating margins, one must be aware of the existence of a small mucosal lesion called gastric xanthelasma, which might be confused with a focus of signet-ring cells, especially in frozen section slides of poor quality. Gastric xanthelasma, also known as lipid island, is a yellow mucosal plaque, usually smaller than 2 mm, formed by a collection of foamy macrophages containing neutral fats (Fig. 7.4).

In patients with chronic gastric ulcers, the mucosal proliferation at the margins may grow downward, giving rise to deep epithelial penetration with distorted mucosa trapped in the fibrous and granulation tissue of the ulcer. This process may reach as deep as the muscularis propria. These entrapped islands of mucosa may be mistaken for invasive carcinoma (Fig.

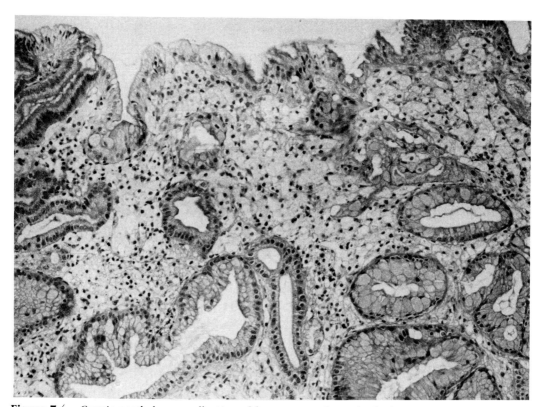

Figure 7.4. Gastric xanthelasma; collection of foamy macrophages in the lamina propria.

7.5). Regenerative atypia at the edge of the ulcer may make diagnosis of the lesion even more difficult. Close scrutiny of cellular detail, especially pleomorphism and mitotic activity, and low power scanning of the lesion's architectural features will often resolve the problem. In addition, if the ulcer is located in the gastric body mucosa, the presence of acid or pepsinogen secreting cells in the mucosal islands argues for the lesion's benign nature (Fig. 7.6).

Other conditions that may display benign glandular invaginations within the submucosa and the muscularis propria of the stomach are Ménétrier's disease (8, 9) and gastritis cystica profunda.

SMALL AND LARGE INTESTINES—INDICATIONS FOR FROZEN SECTION

There are few indications for frozen sections of small and large intestines, the two most important being assessment of resection margins during surgical procedures for inflammatory and malignant bowel diseases and the identification of ganglion cells during operations for Hirschsprung's disease. Occasionally, the nature of an intestinal mass requires frozen section diagnosis before a therapeutic decision can be made. Endoscopically resected specimens, especially polyps, should be evaluated with the use of permanent

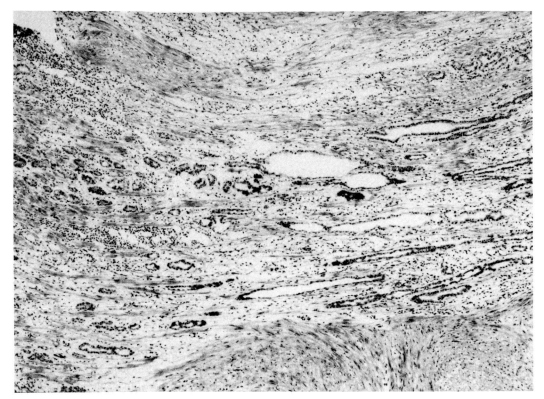

Figure 7.5. Penetration of gastric glands at the edge of a benign ulcer.

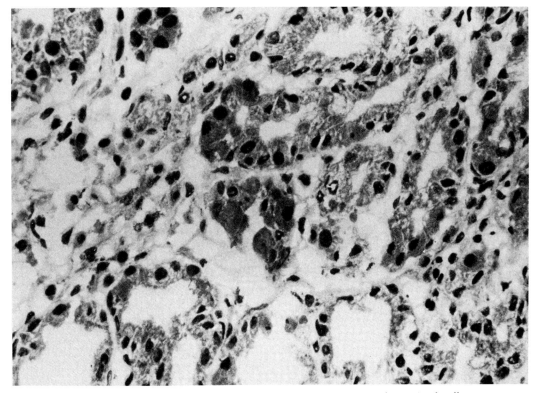

Figure 7.6. Higher magnification of the gastric glands in Fig. 7.5. Note the parietal cells.

sections. Adequate fixation and quality sections are needed for classification of the lesion, presence or absence of neoplasia, the status of the stalk, and its resection margin.

FROZEN SECTION DIAGNOSIS

Margins of Resection

Frozen section evaluation of resection margins for intestinal neoplasms is rarely necessary. Pathologists do not even agree that margins should be submitted routinely as permanent sections. In most cases, the resected segments proximal and distal to the tumor are such that macroscopic inspection alone confirms the absence of neoplastic involvement. The current trend seems to be toward more conservative extirpations, and it is possible that as the segments proximal and distal to the resected tumor become shorter, intraoperative histopathologic margin evaluation will be required.

Pathologists must be aware of the special problems presented by resection margins obtained in patients undergoing low anterior resection and low anastomosis for rectal carcinoma (10–13). The development of circular stapling devices has made it possible to remove low rectal tumors in patients who formerly would have needed an abdominoperineal resection with a permanent colostomy. In this operation, the margin of resection distal to the rectal tumor is quite close to the neoplasm. Yet this type of resection, with a short distal margin, is safe because the lymphatic spread of rectal carcinomas is mainly upward, thus allowing adequate clearance with a shorter distal margin (11). The stapler permits approximation of the colorectal ends to be anastomosed, after which the instrument is used to place a double, staggered circular row of stainless steel staples that join the two ends of bowel, while two rings of tissue are cut with a circular knife inside the staple line. The two rings, commonly called "doughnuts" (12–13), must be identified by the surgeon as proximal and distal, and they must be inspected to ensure that they are intact, indicating a complete and safe anastomosis. Evidence of discontinuity may indicate a defect in the anastomosis (13). The entire distal ring must be submitted for frozen section evaluation to establish whether it is tumor free.

Signet-Ring Carcinoma Compared With Mucinophages

Some situations may prove misleading in the pathologic interpretation of a frozen section from the bowel. Signet-ring carcinoma, although rare, may also occur in this location, and the diagnosis must be approached as described for the stomach. Mucinophages found in the lamina propria are macrophages that have engulfed mucin and which stain positively with alcian blue and mucicarmine. Close evaluation of their cytomorphologic character and their recognition as macrophages will lead to correct identification and avoid confusion with poorly differentiated carcinoma or signet-ring carcinoma. These mucinophages constitute a diagnostic pitfall analogous to that of gastric xanthelasma.

Colitis Cystica Profunda

Colonic glands, often accompanied by their surrounding lamina propria, may be found deep in the submucosa or muscularis propria of the colonic and rectal walls. Such findings are often secondary to radiation. These abnormally located glands should not be mistaken for invasive malignant disease. Colitis cystica profunda is an acquired condition related to radiation, solitary ulcer syndrome of the rectum, or to inflammation like that of ulcerative colitis and dysentery. Histologically, mucus filled cysts are lined with normal colonic epithelium and are associated with inflammatory changes. In these instances serial sections sometimes show luminal connections through narrow channels. Colitis cystica profunda may be localized, segmental, or diffuse, the first condition being by far the most common. It usually presents anteriorly or anterolaterally in the midrectum (14, 15).

Radiation Colitis

Chronic, healed radiation proctocolitis may have striking similarities to colitis cystica profunda except for the absence of inflammation. In radiation colitis, benign colonic glands may be seen as islands deep in the muscularis propria, and they must not be confused with invasive carcinoma (Fig. 7.7). Radiation may alter ganglionic cells so that they display distorted and bizarre nuclei that may superficially simulate malignancy (6).

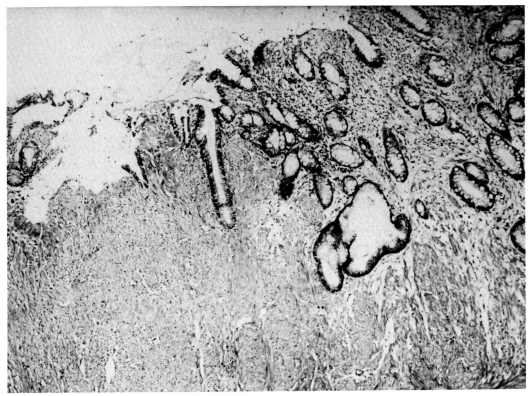

Figure 7.7. Benign colonic glands penetrating the colonic muscularis propria in a case of radiation colitis.

Endometriosis

Endometriosis within the bowel wall may also be confused with invasive adenocarcinoma. The diagnostic clue is the identification of endometrial stroma around the endometrial glands.

Crohn's Disease

The use of frozen section examination to ensure disease-free resection margins in patients with inflammatory bowel disease, especially Crohn's disease, and to determine the site of an ileocolic anastomosis, has been recommended with the idea of reducing relapses. Traditionally, if a margin is inflamed, additional segments are resected until a histologically free margin is obtained. This strategy has led, in some cases, to the development of short bowel syndrome, especially when recurrences have required further segments of bowel to be resected. The idea of inflammation-free margins in Crohn's disease has been recently challenged by studies which claim that frozen section is a poor technique for detecting margin involvement and that outcomes or recurrence rates are not affected when surgical margins are selected by means of frozen section or visual inspection by the surgeon (16, 17).

Hirschsprung's Disease

Most cases of Hirschsprung's disease are diagnosed during the first few weeks of life. The histochemical acetylcholinesterase reaction, in addition to routine hematoxylin and eosin staining, applied to frozen sections of rectal mucosal suction biopsies, allows rapid diagnosis or exclusion of Hirschsprung's disease without exposing the child to general anesthesia or an operative procedure. The aim of the initial treatment is to relieve obstruction until a definitive operation can be performed safely, usually when the child has grown to 20 to 30 lb. A stoma site is selected with the help of frozen section via intraperitoneal biopsy (18), and a stoma proximal to the aganglionic segment is constructed. This specimen identifies the most distal portion of the ganglionated bowel where the colostomy can be placed. The specimen usually consists of an ellipse of bowel wall, about 1 × 0.5 cm, including serosa and muscularis propria. To avoid peritoneal contamination when the colonic lumen is entered, the mucosa is not included. The biopsy must be oriented so that sections are perpendicular to the muscular wall. Multiple frozen sections may be needed to identify ganglia. The identification of the normal myenteric plexus of Auerbach indicates normal ganglionated bowel. The absence of ganglion cells (aganglionic segment) or a significant reduction in their numbers (hypoganglionic segment) associated with hypertrophic nerves (19) indicates an abnormally innervated segment; a more proximal level must be selected for the colostomy.

There are several pitfalls in diagnosing Hirschsprung's disease. Tissue from the distal colon (1.0 to 1.5 cm from the pectinate line) is hypoganglionic. In neonates, especially premature babies, the ganglion cells are immature. They are smaller than the ganglionic cells in infants and have small, dark nuclei without nucleoli. They can be easily confused with stromal cells (20). A potential for error exists in the association of Hirschsprung's disease complicated by enterocolitis with cytomegalovirus infection. The characteristic histologic picture of the latter shows enlarged endothelial cells that have intranuclear and intracytoplasmic inclusion bodies. These cells must be correctly identified and not confused with ganglion cells (21).

The pathologist has an important role in determining the proximal resection line of an aganglionic segment during the course of definitive corrective surgery for Hirschsprung's disease (22). When the surgeon asks for frozen section evaluation of the resection margin, it is important to know the histologic features of the aganglionic and hypoganglionic segments. If any of the latter type is detected, the surgeon must resect more intestine. Multiple sections may be necessary for adequate evaluation. With experience, ganglion cells are easily identified in properly cut and stained frozen sections.

LIVER

Frozen section diagnosis of liver is frequently requested to evaluate hepatic nodules or masses in the course of intrabdominal surgery and to assess resection margins in patients undergoing segmental resections, lobectomies, or partial hepatectomies.

Frozen Section Diagnosis

Surgeons routinely explore the abdominal cavity, including the liver, during the course of abdominal operations. In a cancer operation, this exploration becomes more exhaustive. The presence of a hepatic nodule is often an ominous sign of metastatic spread to the liver, although certainly not all liver nodules represent metastatic or primary cancer. Such liver nodules must be evaluated by frozen section. If they are malignant, the surgical procedure originally planned will probably have to be changed. If the lesion is benign, the operation will proceed as planned. Liver specimens submitted for intraoperative histologic evaluation are needle and wedge biopsies and resection specimens.

The majority (40–60%) of liver frozen section examinations are to confirm the presence of metastatic disease (1–4). Bile duct hamartomas and adenomas may be confused with metastasic adenocarcinoma. Cases of liver cell adenomas, focal nodular hyperplasia, and hepatocellular pseudotumor in cirrhotic liver (23) may be misdiagnosed as hepatocellular carcinoma.

Bile duct hamartomas, also known as Meyenburg's complexes, are usually multiple, well-circumscribed lesions composed of a collagenous stroma that contain irregularly shaped ductal structures often filled with bile material (24). Most bile duct adenomas are single lesions less than 1 cm in diameter and located in a subcapsular distribution (25) (Figs. 7.8 and 7.9). Bile duct hamartomas and adenomas lack the histologic and cytologic features of malignancy (Fig. 7.10). Metastatic lesions frequently have associated necrosis, a feature not seen in benign bile duct nodules. The accurate classification of these lesions has a great influence on the surgical therapy. The differential diagnosis of liver cell adenoma, focal nodular hyperplasia, hepatocellular pseudotumor in the cirrhotic liver, and hepatocellular carcinoma may be difficult, especially on a small specimen that may not represent the entire lesion. Localized surgical resection of the involved liver area, if technically feasible, is the treatment of choice for all these lesions regardless of their histopathologic features. Correct classification can wait until the entire lesion can be examined both grossly and by permanent sections (26, 27). Resectability is determined by the surgeon with the help of preoperative scans, ultrasonography, computerized tomography, angiographic studies, and, most importantly, direct examination during the operation.

One curious finding we have encountered in frozen section evaluation of liver nodules is the so-called pseudolipoma of Glisson's capsule (28). This rare lesion is not a tumor, but an appendix epiploica that has lost its attachment to the bowel and has become engrafted to the liver capsule. Microscopically, a thick fibrous capsule surrounds poorly preserved, partly necrotic, semicalcified fibroadipose tissue (Fig. 7.11).

PANCREAS

Pancreatic frozen sections comprise between 1 and 5.3% of all frozen sections performed (1–4).

It is well known that pancreatic cancer is a neoplasm that carries a very high mortality rate. Pancreatoduodenectomy, also known as Whipple's operation, and total pancreatectomy are the only recommended surgical

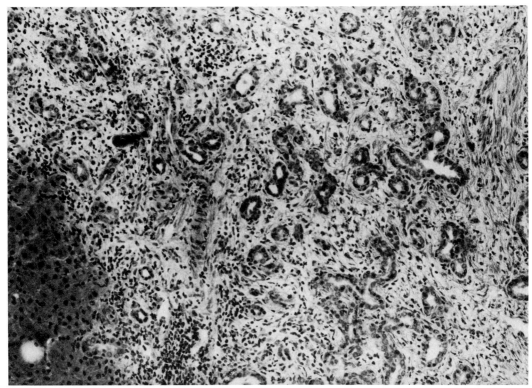

Figure 7.8. Bile duct adenoma. Benign ductal structures lie in a loose fibrous stroma.

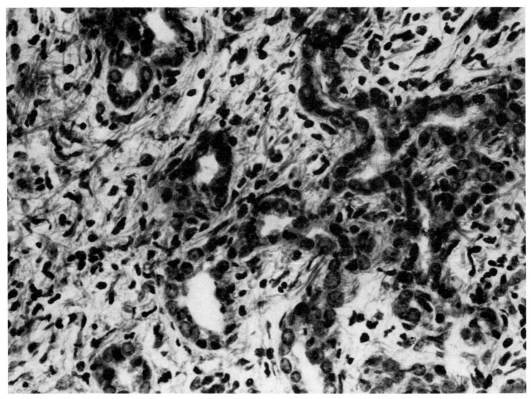

Figure 7.9. Higher magnification of Fig. 7.8.

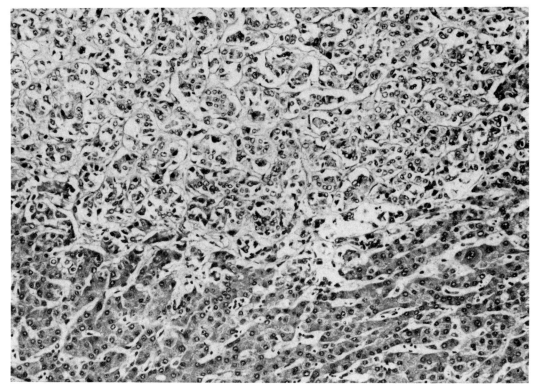

Figure 7.10. Metastatic breast carcinoma in liver. Well demarcated group of malignant epithelial cells.

therapies (29–36). Many patients diagnosed as having pancreatic cancer are found to be inoperable. Percutaneous fine needle aspiration cytologic examination is an excellent diagnostic tool when an experienced radiologist, using a modern imaging technique, can obtain an adequate sample to be interpreted by a skillful cytopathologist.

Extrapancreatic tissues are often submitted to evaluate extrapancreatic spread. The absence of spread to peripancreatic lymph nodes is one of the most significant determinants of long-term survival of pancreatic cancer. Patients with localized tumors have been cured by resection (29, 30, 33, 35). If the surgeon proceeds with a definitive operation, the resection margins must be evaluated. Although most errors are caused by incorrect sampling rather than errors in interpretation, false negative, false positive, and deferred diagnoses occur in almost all series, illustrating the interpretative difficulties of frozen sections from this area (1, 3, 4, 37).

False positive diagnoses are an obvious problem because of the potentially grave complications of a radical procedure, such as the Whipple's operation. False negative and deferred diagnoses are a problem because of the possible complications of a two-stage procedure and the likelihood of tumor dissemination during the first operation. Furthermore, patients who have small tumors and the best chance of a favorable outcome may never undergo resection because the histologic diagnosis was not rendered (33). Some surgeons prefer not to carry out a radical procedure without histologic evidence of carcinoma. Others believe that clinical evaluation at laparotomy

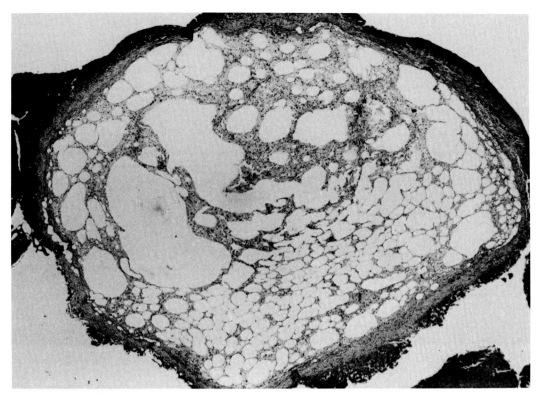

Figure 7.11. Pseudolipoma of Glisson's capsule, surrounded by a fibrous capsule and attached to hepatic tissue.

remains the most important factor in diagnosis and surgical decision-making (30, 32–34). The latter is controversial. Chronic pancreatitis may result in a mass that is indistinguishable from cancer by gross examination or palpation alone. Despite these arguments, experienced pancreatic surgeons believe that, in the majority of patients, they can differentiate benign from malignant lesions based on clinical examination at laparotomy; the margin of error given in the literature is between 3 and 25% (32, 34). In contrast, some surgeons believe that pancreatic biopsy at laparotomy may lead to seeding of cancer and other troublesome complications, and that some patients have been "biopsied to death" (32). Others believe that the complications of operative pancreatic biopsy have been overrated and that in the hands of an experienced surgeon, it is a safe procedure.

Indications for Frozen Section

The most common indication for frozen section is diagnosis of a pancreatic mass. If the neoplasm is malignant and a radical resection is carried out, the margins of resection should be checked by frozen section.

Types of Specimens

Several types of pancreatic specimens may be submitted for frozen section evaluation. A needle biopsy, obtained with a Tru-Cut or Vim-Silverman needle passed transduodenally or through the pancreatic capsule into the mass, provides an adequate core of tissue. Knife or shave biopsies are adequate for lesions that invade the pancreatic capsule (30, 37, 38). When the resected specimen of a radical operation is submitted for evaluation of margins, the most critical margins to examine are those of the common duct and pancreatic transection line (31, 35, 39). Local recurrences are the result of inadequate removal of all microscopic disease. Tumor extension up the common duct, intrapancreatic extension, and multicentricity of tumor account for the majority of failures (29, 35).

An acceptable alternative to intraoperative diagnostic frozen section is the use of fine needle aspiration technique for rapid cytologic diagnosis (30, 38). The procedure is less traumatic than needle biopsy, and several punctures and aspirations can be done. After a smear is prepared from the aspirated material, a rapid stain of the type commonly used for cytologic diagnosis can be done. The result is available as soon as or sooner than the frozen section report.

Frozen Section Diagnosis

Carcinoma of Pancreas

The most common type of primary pancreatic neoplasm, accounting for 80% to 95% of all pancreatic tumors of epithelial origin (40–43), is nonendocrine carcinoma originating in the duct cells. Microscopically, pancreatic duct carcinoma is often well differentiated, which may make histologic diagnosis difficult. The best frozen section criteria for diagnosing pancreatic cancer were outlined in 1981 in a landmark article by Hyland and associates (43). These criteria are: nuclear size variation of 4 : 1 or more between tumorous ductal cells, presence of incomplete ductal lumina, disorganized duct distribution, large irregular eosinophilic nucleoli, glands unaccompanied by connective tissue infiltrating duodenal smooth muscle, and vascular and perineural invasion (Figs. 7.12–7.15).

Other distinct morphologic variants of ductal carcinoma are giant cell carcinoma (epulis-osteoid and pleomorphic types) adenosquamous carcinoma, microadenocarcinoma, signet-ring carcinoma, mucinous adenocarcinoma, and anaplastic carcinoma (41). The malignant character of these variants is, in general, not difficult to determine in frozen section.

Carcinoma Versus Pancreatitis

In examining a frozen section from the pancreas, the pathologist must be wary of several problems and pitfalls. For pathologist and surgeon, chronic pancreatitis is the source of most problems. About 10% of patients with carcinoma have an associated chronic pancreatitis (44, 45). Ductal obstruction by the tumor induces acinar rupture with secondary inflammation, fibrosis, and distortion of ducts. The biopsies submitted for frozen section evaluation may not be representative of the underlying neoplasm, especially if the tumor is small and surrounded by a thick mantle of chronic pancreatitis. On occasion, the tumor will become evident only after the entire specimen has been removed by the surgeon. Multiple levels of the specimen submitted should be sectioned to maximize the chances of arriving at the correct diagnosis.

Histologically, chronic pancreatitis can also be difficult to separate from ductal carcinoma. In cases of pancreatitis, there is exaggerated lobulation due to increased amounts of connective tissue. The ducts appear more prominent because the caliber of the lumina, which often contain protein plugs, is enlarged. The larger interlobular ducts are surrounded by fibrosis, and the epithelial lining may show some infoldings and papillations. The islets of Langerhans are often unchanged, but in severe cases of pancreatitis they can be quite distorted.

In advanced stages of chronic pancreatitis, there is extensive loss of acinar epithelium. There is also marked fibrosis, which is pan- and intralobular, and peripancreatic. The interlobular ducts frequently contain coagulated protein and calculi. The ductal epithelium may show papillary or squamous features, and duct ectasia with cystic dilatation may be present. The distortion of the pancreatic anatomy may cause dramatic architectural disarray of ductal elements. Distorted islets of Langerhans and loss of pancreatic acini may cause great difficulties in interpretation. The distortion of the islets of Langerhans can be severe enough to result in their close apposition to nerves, a phenomenon that should not be confused with perineural invasion. Finally, simulation of incomplete lumina by atrophic acini and ductules may exacerbate the problem (Fig. 7.16). Close attention to the histologic criteria of carcinoma is the only way of resolving the problem.

Carcinoma Versus Proliferation of Ducts

Numerous small accessory pancreatic ducts may mimic invasive carcinoma. These ducts are normal anatomic variants of the ampullary region.

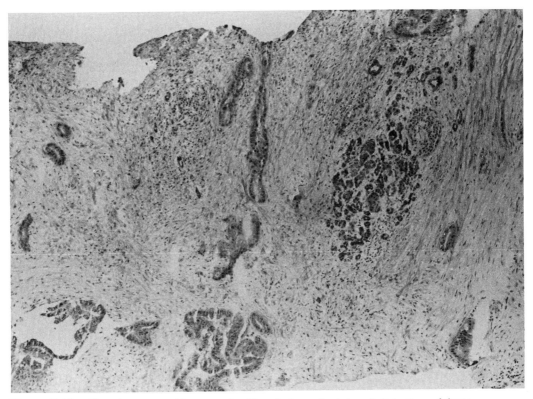

Figure 7.16. Chronic pancreatitis: extensive fibrosis, loss of acini, and distortion of ducts.

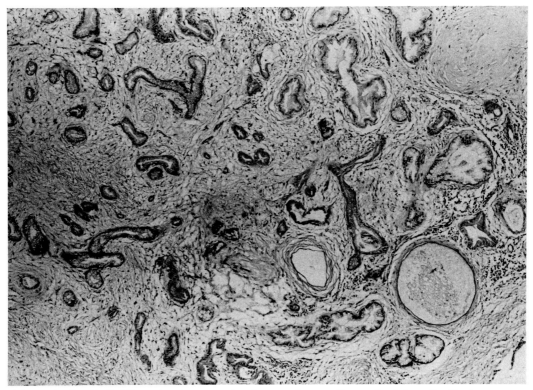

Figure 7.12. Well differentiated pancreatic adenocarcinoma; disorganized duct distribution.

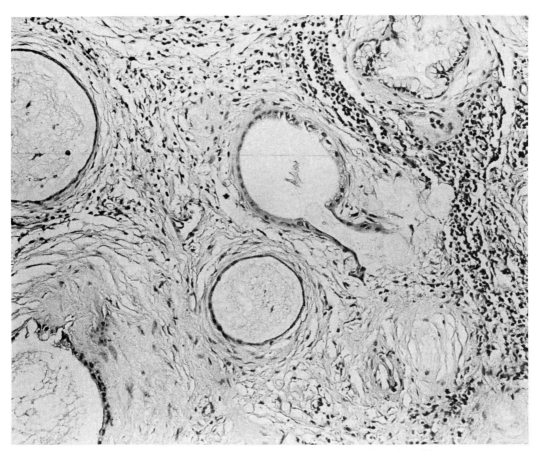

Figure 7.13. Well differentiated pancreatic adenocarcinoma: incomplete ductal lumina.

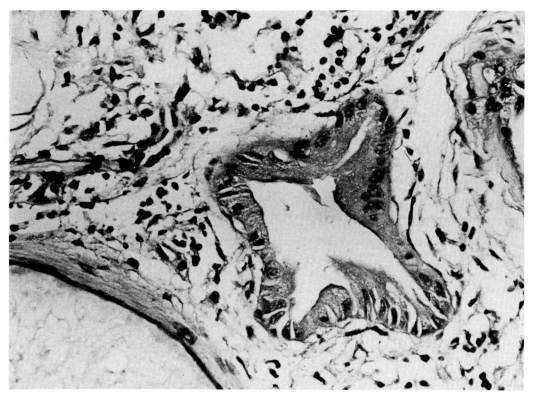

Figure 7.14. Well differentiated pancreatic adenocarcinoma: tumor cell nuclear size variation of more than 4 :1.

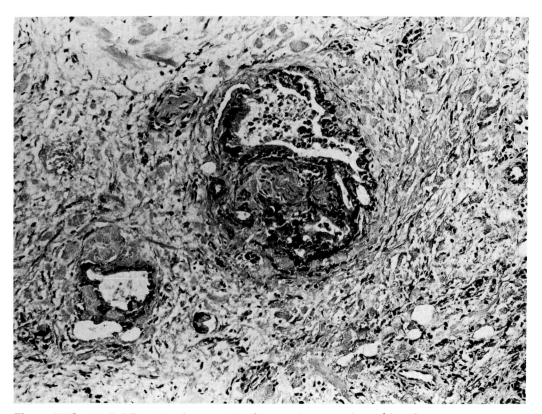

Figure 7.15. Well differentiated pancreatic adenocarcinoma: perineural invasion.

They are usually arranged in groups and surrounded by loose connective tissue stroma. They penetrate between duodenal smooth muscle without eliciting a desmoplastic reaction (43, 45).

Pancreatic ductal hyperplasia may mimic carcinoma, especially if it displays atypical characteristics. Ductal hyperplasia accompanies pancreatic cancer in many cases, but it may also be a feature of non-neoplastic conditions (46–48).

Strict adherence to the diagnostic criteria outlined above will avoid mistaking such lesions as malignancies.

Perineural invasion is a finding that strongly favors a malignant process in the pancreas and classically has been one of the most reliable criteria for such a diagnosis. It is not an absolute criterion, however, because benign intraneural and perineural epithelial inclusions have been reported in pancreases showing no evidence of malignancy (49), a situation similar to what has been described in the breast (50).

Carcinoma Versus Islet Cell Tumor—(see Chapter 13)

Microcystic Adenoma Versus Mucinous Tumor

Two cystic neoplasms easily recognized on frozen section include microcystic adenoma and the mucinous cystic tumor. Each has a totally different biologic behavior. Microcystic or glycogen-rich adenoma is a lesion often found in the head of the pancreas of elderly patients. These tumors are large (mean diameter of 10 cm) with a grossly spongy appearance, secondary to numerous cystic structures divided by trabeculae. Some trabeculae may be calcified. In the center there is often a stellate calcified scar, an important gross characteristic feature. The microscopic appearance is diagnostic and reflects the macroscopic appearance. Many cysts lined by small, flat or cuboidal cells have regular and central nuclei without pleomorphism and clear cytoplasm (Figs. 7.17 and 7.18) (51, 52).

The mucinous cystic tumor is formed by large, multilocular or rarely unilocular cysts lined by columnar mucin producing epithelium, which often form papillae. The underlying stroma is quite cellular. The gross and histologic appearance is similar to the ovarian mucinous counterpart. The most common location is the body and tail of the pancreas. There are both benign and malignant forms, but this distinction is not always easy. The diagnosis of the malignant form is based on the presence of invasion of the wall or frank anaplasia of the epithelial component. Malignant foci can be small and very localized, which makes adequate sampling of utmost importance. These tumors have been given the generic name of mucinous cystic neoplasms of the pancreas with overt and latent malignancy (53, 54).

Other Forms of Pancreatic Cancer

A rare form of pancreatic cancer that occurs most often in young women is the papillary and cystic neoplasm (55, 56) which should not be difficult to recognize on frozen section.

Acinar cell carcinomas are rare tumors comprising 1 to 2% of all pancreatic cancers. Microscopically, they are made up of solid nests of cells

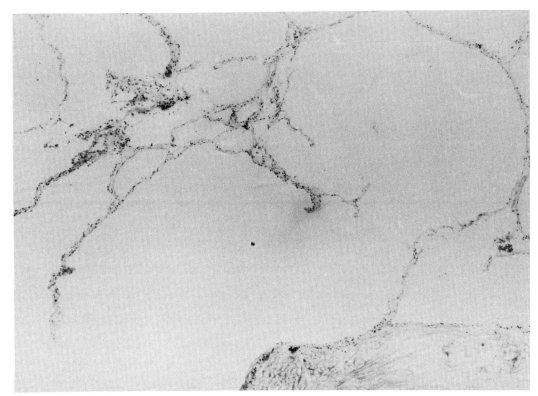

Figure 7.17. Microcystic adenoma of pancreas. Multiple cysts are divided by thin septae.

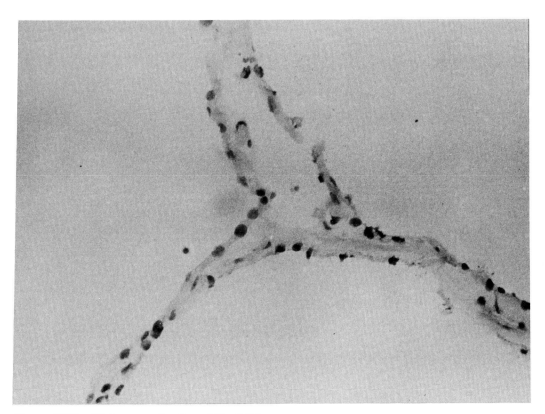

Figure 7.18. Higher magnification of Fig. 7.17.

that resemble the appearance of normal acini. The abundant cytoplasm is distinctly granular (41, 57). They can sometimes be difficult to distinguish from islet cell tumors.

REFERENCES

1. Ackerman LV, Ramirez GA: The indications for and limitations of frozen section diagnosis. A review of 1269 consecutive frozen section diagnoses. *Br J Surg* 46:336–350, 1959.
2. Dehner LP, Rosai J: Frozen section examination in surgical pathology. A retrospective study of one year experience, comprising 778 cases. *Minn Med* 60:83–94, 1977.
3. Elsner B: La biopsia por congelacion: su valor asistencial y en la educacion medica del patologo. *Pren Med Argent* 55:1741–1749, 1968.
4. Nakazawa H, Rosen P, Lane N, Lattes R: Frozen section experience in 3000 cases. Accuracy, limitations, and value in residency training. *Am J Clin Pathol* 49:41–52, 1968.
5. Rosai J: *Ackerman's Surgical Pathology,* ed. 6, St. Louis, C. V. Mosby, 1981, p 408.
6. Berthrong M, Fajardo LF: Radiation injury in surgical pathology. Part II. Alimentary tract. *Am J Surg Pathol* 5:153–178, 1981.
7. Rosai J: *Ackerman's Surgical Pathology,* ed. 6. St. Louis, C. V. Mosby, 1981, p 417.
8. Rosai J: *Ackerman's Surgical Pathology,* ed. 6. St. Louis, C. V. Mosby, 1981, p 423–424.
9. Kenney FD, Dockerty MB, Waugh JM: Giant hypertrophy of gastric mucosa. A clinical and pathological study. *Cancer* 7:671–681, 1954.
10. Heald RJ, Leicester RJ: The low stapled anastomosis. *Br J Surg* 68:333–337, 1981.
11. Hurst PA, Prout WG, Kelly JM, Bannister JJ, Walker RT: Local recurrence after low anterior resection using the staple gun. *Br J Surg* 69:275–276, 1982.
12. Gordon PH, Vasilevsky CA: Experience with stapling in rectal surgery. *Surg Clin North Am* 64:555–566, 1984.
13. Vezeridis M, Evans JT, Mittelman A, Ledesma EJ: EEA stapler in low anterior anastomosis. *Dis Colon Rectum* 25:364–367, 1982.
14. Herman AH, Nabseth DC: Colitis cystica profunda: localized, segmental, and diffuse. *Arch Surg* 106:337–341, 1973.
15. Saul SH, Sollenberger LC: Solitary rectal ulcer syndrome. Its clinical and pathological underdiagnosis. *Am J Surg Pathol* 9:411–421, 1985.
16. Fazio VW: Regional enteritis (Crohn's disease): Indications for surgery and operative strategy. *Surg Clin North Am* 63:27, 1983.
17. Hamilton SR, Reese J, Pennington L, Boitnott JK, Bayless TM, Cameron JL: The role of resection margin frozen section in the surgical management of Crohn's disease. *Surg Gyn Obstet* 160:57–62, 1985.
18. Lavery IC: The surgery of Hirschsprung's disease. *Surg Clin North Am* 63:161–175, 1983.
19. Corkery JJ: Hirschsprung's disease. *Clin Gastroenterol* 4:531–544, 1975.
20. Yunis EJ, Dibbins AW, Sherman FE: Rectal suction biopsy in the diagnosis of Hirschsprung's disease in infants. *Arch Pathol Lab Med* 10:329–333, 1976.
21. Ariel I, Vinograd I, Lernau OZ, Nissan S, Rosenmann E: Rectal mucosal biopsy in aganglionosis and allied conditions. *Hum Pathol* 14:991–995, 1983.
22. Preston HS, Bale PM: Rapid frozen section in pediatric pathology. *Am J Surg Pathol* 9:570–576, 1985.
23. Nagasue N, Akamizu H, Yukaya H, Yuuki I: Hepatocellular pseudotumor in the cirrhotic liver. Report of three cases. *Cancer* 54:2487–2494, 1984.
24. Chung EB: Multiple bile-duct hamartomas. *Cancer* 26:287–296, 1970.
25. Rosai J: *Ackerman's Surgical Pathology,* ed. 6. St. Louis, C. V. Mosby, 1981, p. 623.
26. Adson MA: Diagnosis and surgical treatment of primary and secondary solid hepatic tumors in the adult. *Surg Clin North Am* 61:181–196, 1981.
27. Fortner JG: Current management of tumors of the liver. *Surg Clin North Am* 57:465–472, 1977.
28. Edmondson HA: Tumors of the liver and intrahepatic bile ducts. In: *Atlas of Tumor Pathology,* section VII, fasc 25. Washington DC, Armed Forces Institute of Pathology, 1958, p 216.
29. Barton RM, Copeland EM: Carcinoma of the ampulla of Vater. *Surg Gynecol Obstet* 156:297–301, 1983.

30. Cooperman AM: Cancer of the pancreas: A dilemma in treatment. *Surg Clin North Am* 61:107–115, 1981.

31. Edis AJ, Kiernan PD, Taylor WF: Attempted curative resection of ductal carcinoma of the pancreas. Review of Mayo Clinic experience, 1951–1975. *Mayo Clin Proc* 55:531–536, 1980.

32. Fortner JG: Recent advances in pancreatic cancer. *Surg Clin North Am* 54:859–863, 1974.

33. Hermann RE, Cooperman AM: Current concepts in cancer. Cancer of the pancreas. *N Engl J Med* 301:482–486, 1979.

34. Malt RA: Treatment of pancreatic cancer. *JAMA* 250:1433–1437, 1983.

35. Tryka AF, Brooks JR: Histopathology in the evaluation of total pancreatectomy for ductal carcinoma. *Ann Surg* 190:373–381, 1979.

36. Whipple AO, Parsons WB, Mullins CR: Treatment of carcinoma of the ampulla of Vater. *Ann Surg* 102:763–779, 1935.

37. Wise L, Pizzimbono C, Dehner LP: Periampullary cancer. A clinicopathologic study of sixty-two patients. *Am J Surg* 131:141–148, 1976.

38. Moossa AR, Altorki N: Pancreatic biopsy. *Surg Clin North Am* 63:1205–1214, 1983.

39. Cubilla AL, Fitzgerald PJ: Tumors of the exocrine pancreas. In: *Atlas of Tumor Pathology,* second series, fasc 19. Washington DC, Armed Forces Institute of Pathology, 1984, p 269.

40. Cubilla AL, Fitzgerald PJ: Morphological patterns of primary nonendocrine human pancreas carcinoma. *Cancer Res* 35:2234–2248, 1975.

41. Cubilla AL, Fitzgerald PJ: Surgical pathology of tumors of the exocrine pancreas. In Moossa AB (ed): *Tumors of the Pancreas.* Baltimore, Williams & Wilkins, 1980, p 159.

42. Cubilla AL, Fitzgerald PJ: Tumors of the exocrine pancreas. In: *Atlas of Tumor Pathology,* second series, fasc 19. Washington DC, Armed Forces Institute of Pathology, 1984, p 111.

43. Hyland C, Kheir SM, Kashlan MB: Frozen section diagnosis of pancreatic carcinoma. A prospective study of 64 biopsies. *Am J Surg Pathol* 5:179–191, 1981.

44. Gambill EE: Pancreatitis associated with pancreatic carcinoma: a study of 26 cases. *Mayo Clin Proc* 46:174–177, 1971.

45. Loquvam GS, Russell WO: Accessory pancreatic ducts of the major duodenal papilla. Normal structures to be differentiated from cancer. *Am J Clin Pathol* 20:305–313, 1950.

46. Cubilla AL, Fitzgerald PJ: Morphological lesions associated with human primary invasive nonendocrine pancreas cancer. *Cancer Res* 36:2690–2698, 1976.

47. Kozuka S, Sassa R, Taki T, Masamoto K, Nagasawa S, Saga S, Hasegawa K, Takeuchi M: Relation of pancreatic duct hyperplasia to carcinoma. *Cancer* 43:1418–1428, 1979.

48. Cubilla AL, Fitzgerald PJ: Tumors of the exocrine pancreas. In: *Atlas of Tumor Pathology,* second series, fasc 19. Washington DC, Armed Forces Institute of Pathology, 1984, p 72.

49. Costa J: Benign epithelial inclusions in pancreatic nerves. *Am J Clin Pathol* 67:306–307, 1977.

50. Taylor HB, Norris HJ: Epithelial invasion of nerves in benign disease of the breast. *Cancer* 20:2245–2249, 1967.

51. Compagno J, Oertel JE: Microcystic adenomas of the pancreas (glycogen-rich cystadenomas). A clinicopathologic study of 34 cases. *Am J Clin Pathol* 69:289–298, 1978.

52. Cubilla AL, Fitzgerald PJ: Tumors of the exocrine pancreas. In: *Atlas of Tumor Pathology,* second series, fasc 19. Washington DC, Armed Forces Institute of Pathology, 1984, p 100.

53. Compagno J, Oertel JE: Mucinous cystic neoplasms of the pancreas with overt and latent malignancy (cystadenocarcinoma and cystadenoma). A clinicopathologic study of 41 cases. *Am J Clin Pathol* 69:573–580, 1978.

54. Cubilla AL, Fitzgerald PJ: Tumors of the exocrine pancreas. In: *Atlas of Tumor Pathology,* second series, fasc 19. Washington DC, Armed Forces Institute of Pathology, 1984, p 104.

55. Bombi JA, Milla A, Badal JM, Pinlachs J, Estape J, Cardesa A: Papillary-cystic neoplasm of the pancreas. Report of two cases and review of the literature. *Cancer* 54:780–784, 1984.

56. Cubilla AL, Fitzgerald PJ: Tumors of the exocrine pancreas. In: *Atlas of Tumor Pathology,* second series, fasc 19. Washington DC, Armed Forces Institute of Pathology, 1984, p 201.

57. Cubilla AL, Fitzgerald PJ: Tumors of the exocrine pancreas. In: *Atlas of Tumor Pathology,* second series, fasc 19. Washington DC, Armed Forces Institute of Pathology, 1984, p 208.

8

Central Nervous System and Pituitary

Bernd W. Scheithauer, M.D.

Frozen section technique, as applied to surgical neuropathology, frequently provides an immediate and final tissue diagnosis. However, in view of the wide spectrum of lesions affecting the various compartments of the nervous system, this technique often represents only the initial step in the diagnostic process. This is particularly true with respect to medical disorders such as infectious, demyelinative, and metabolic diseases. This discussion will limit itself largely to the application of frozen sections in the diagnosis of neoplasms.

The goal of the pathologist is to guide the neurosurgeon in making clinically relevant intraoperative decisions. Most often this consists of confirming that a neoplasm is present and determining whether it is benign or malignant, primary or secondary, or of a type that lends itself to total extirpation. The frozen section method also provides much needed information about the quality of the operative specimen and whether it is sufficient for further studies, including electron microscopy, immunocytochemistry, surface marker studies, and biochemical determinations, to name a few.

It must be understood by both the pathologist and neurosurgeon that the frozen section is the first step in establishing a morphologic diagnosis and that the method has its limitations. Latitude must remain for diagnostic refinement on permanent sections in diagnostically difficult cases. The pathologist, although guided by clinical and operative data, must be objective in interpreting frozen sections. The pressures applied by the plaintiff's attorney are invariably more unpleasant than the frustration expressed by surgical colleagues.

A diagnosis made without the benefit of clinical data and without consideration of radiographic data or gross anatomy is significantly compromised. Accurate identification of the process is based in part on such factors as patient age and sex, neurologic signs, tempo of symptom progression, and radiographic and gross operative features. More so than in other areas surgical pathology, it is important to know the precise location of a central nervous system lesion in differential diagnosis. Developments in comput-

Table 8.1.
Topographic Distribution of Tumors of the Central Nervous System and Sellar Region by Patient Age

	Children and Adolescents	Adults
Cerebral hemisphere	Astrocytoma (pilocytic/ fibrillary, etc.), anaplastic astrocytoma Ependymoma Oligodendroglioma "Primitive neuroectodermal tumor" Ganglioglioma	Astrocytoma, anaplastic astrocytoma, glioblastoma Metastatic carcinoma Oligodendroglioma Ependymoma Lymphoma "Primitive neuroectodermal tumor"
Corpus callosum	Astrocytoma, anaplastic astrocytoma Oligodendroglioma	Astrocytoma, anaplastic astrocytoma, glioblastoma
Lateral ventricle	Ependymoma Choroid plexus papilloma>> carcinoma Subependymal giant cell astrocytoma	Ependymoma Meningioma Subependymoma Choroid plexus papilloma
3rd Ventricle	Ependymoma Choroid plexus papilloma>> carcinoma	Colloid cyst Ependymoma
Region of 3rd ventricle	Astrocytoma (pilocytic) Oligodendroglioma	Astrocytoma, anaplastic astrocytoma, glioblastoma Oligodendroglioma Ependymoma
Optic nerve, chiasm, and sheath	Astrocytoma, pilocytic	Meningioma Astrocytoma (pilocytic or fibrillary)
Pineal region	Germ cell tumor Pineoblastoma	Germ cell tumors Pineocytoma Pineoblastoma
Cerebellum	Medulloblastoma Astrocytoma (pilocytic) Dermoid cyst	Hemangioblastoma Metastatic carcinoma Astrocytoma (fibrillary or pilocytic) Medulloblastoma
4th Ventricle	Ependymoma Choroid plexus papilloma>> carcinoma	Ependymoma Choroid plexus papilloma Subependymoma
CP angle	Ependymoma Choroid plexus papilloma	Neurilemmoma Meningioma Epidermoid cyst Choroid plexus papilloma Glomus jugulare tumor
Brainstem	Astrocytoma, anaplastic astrocytoma, glioblastoma	Astrocytoma, anaplastic astrocytoma, glioblastoma

Table 8.1.
**Topographic Distribution of Tumors of the Central Nervous System
and Sellar Region by Patient Age (*Continued*)**

	Children and Adolescents	Adults
Spinal region	Ependymoma Astrocytoma	Ependymoma Astrocytoma Hemangioblastoma Meningioma Neurilemmoma Neurofibroma Paraganglioma
Pituitary-sellar region	Craniopharyngioma Germ cell tumor Pituitary adenoma	Pituitary adenoma Meningioma Germ cell tumors Chordoma/chondroid chordoma Metastasis

erized axial tomography (CT) have greatly contributed to the assessment of pathologic processes within the nervous system. The pathologist whose practice includes a sizable neurosurgical load should become acquainted with the technique and recognize its utility in differential diagnosis. Needless to say, there is no substitute for personal communication between pathologist and neurosurgeon.

Included in this chapter are summary lists correlating age, lesion location, and differential diagnosis (Table 8.1) as well as pertinent epidemiologic, gross, and microscopic features of commonly occurring lesions according to their site (Table 8.2). Additional information on the subject of frozen section interpretation in neuropathology includes the excellent two-part work of Burger and Vogel (1, 2). The technique is of particular use in the pediatric setting (3).

APPROACH TO THE SPECIMEN

In that the frozen section is an intraoperative diagnostic guide and not necessarily the final step in the evaluation of the specimen, care must be taken to insure that sufficient tissues remain for routine histology, special stains, immunocytochemistry, and, when necessary, electron microscopy. Indiscriminate freezing of entire specimens is to be avoided.

When the specimen is scant, one should consider diagnosis by touch preparation or smear (4). Air-dried touch preparations permit histochemical studies as well as detection of cell surface markers. Tissue conservation is also achieved by cutting consecutive unstained microsections at the time of permanent section preparation; the latter obviates the need for block recutting and the resultant waste.

For practical purposes, there is never so little tissue that material cannot be set aside for ultrastructural study. A single 1-mm tissue fragment fixed in glutaraldehyde often suffices. Such tissue may remain in fixative for days; if not needed, the specimen may be discarded. Fixation in formaldehyde solution, although less effective in preserving ultrastructural details, is adequate.

Table 8.2.
Compartments of Nervous System Differential Diagnosis
and Clinicopathologic Features

	Extraparenchymal	
	Supratentorial	Meningioma Metastasis
	Infratentorial	Schwannoma Meningioma Metastasis
	Foramen Magnum and Spinal Canal	Meningioma Schwannoma Neurofibroma
	Clivus	Chordoma Meningioma

Meningioma		
	Gross	Discrete, globoid Tan and/or gritty Compression and displacement of nervous tissue Dural attachment (not invariable) ± Hyperostosis of bone
	Locations (classic)	Parasagittal Convexity Olfactory groove Sphenoid ridge Suprasellar Cerebellopontine Angle Foramen magnum Intraventricular Spinal Optic sheath
	Micro	Oval nuclei ± cytoplasmic inclusions Epithelioid to spindle cells Whorls, psammoma bodies, xanthomatous change Collagenized vessels Cellular touch prep, variable cytology
	DDX	Metastatic carcinoma, eg melanoma or squamous carcinoma (more anaplastic) Hemangioblastoma (abundant cytoplasmic lipid, complex uniform microvascular pattern) Hemangiopericytoma, i.e. "angioblastic meningioma," (staghorn vasculature, mitoses, abscence of whorls, psammoma bodies and nuclear cytoplasmic inclusions)

Schwannoma		
	Clinical	Tinnitus, deafness Unilateral, bilateral (neurofibromatosis)
	Gross	Encapsulated Solid/cystic Tan, yellow
	Location	Cerebellopontine angle 8th nerve, (occasionally nn 5, 9, or 10) Spinal (see below)

Table 8.2.
Compartments of Nervous System Differential Diagnosis
and Clinicopathologic Features (*Continued*)

Micro	Spindle cells Benign elongate nuclei (bizarre nuclei in old lesions) Collagenous vessels with hemosiderin deposition ± Xanthoma cells Antoni A and B pattern (frequent in spinal but infrequent in acoustic tumors)
DDX (CP angle)	Glomus jugulare (Zellballen pattern, vascular) Meningioma Brainstem glioma
Miscellaneous Neoplasms	Metastatic carcinoma Myeloma Olfactory neuroblastoma Histiocytosis X Fibrous dysplasia Aneurysmal bone cyst Chondroma Chondrosarcoma Chordoma/chondroid chordoma
Inflammatory	Sarcoidosis (basal leptomeninges, hypothalamus-infundibulum) Tuberculosis

Intraparenchymal

Supratentorial
   Astrocytoma

Gross	Ill-defined (fibrillary or gemistocytic types) Fairly defined (pilocytic, or protoplasmic types) ± Cysts Rubbery or gelatinous
Micro	Irregularly distributed hypercellularity (as compared to gliosis) Cytologic atypia ± Microcysts ± Secondary structures (perineuronal, subpial, subependymal or perivascular aggregation of tumor cells)

Anaplastic
astrocytoma

Gross	Hyperemia ± friability
Micro	*Cytologic malignancy, mitoses* Early vessel proliferation Absence of palisading necrosis

Glioblastoma
multiforme

Clin	Short duration of symptoms A-V shunting on angiogram Central hypodensity and peripheral enhancement on CT scan
Gross	Necrosis, friability, hemorrhage ± Apparent circumscription
Micro	Variable cytology (small cell/spindle cell/ gemistocytic/pleomorphic/giant cell) *Necrosis with pseudopalisading* *Glomeruloid microvascular* *proliferation*

Table 8.2.
**Compartments of Nervous System Differential Diagnosis
and Clinicopathologic Features (*Continued*)**

Oligodendroglioma

        Clin   Long term symptoms, eg seizures

        Gross   Variable circumscription on gross examination and CT
                  ± Calcification, gross or x-ray (50%)

        Micro   *Uniform cytology;* round nuclei, evenly-spaced cells; perinuclear
                  haloes are seen on permanent sections only
                  Intersecting "chickenwire" vasculature
                  Calcospherites, ± vascular calcification
                  Nuclear pleomorphism and mitoses as well as variable
                  microvascular proliferation and necrosis in anaplastic forms

Ependymoma [see Infratentorial (Posterior Fossa), below]

Lymphoma
(reticulum cell
sarcoma-
microglioma)

        Clin   ± Association with immunosuppression

        Gross   Simulates glioblastoma or infarct

        Micro   Lymphocyte cytology (small cell ± plasmacytoid differentiation,
                  mixed, *large cell, immunoblastic*)
                  Multicellular infiltrate includes reactive astrocytes and
                  macrophages
                  Intramural and circumferential perivascular infiltrates

Metastases

        Gross   ± Multiple
                  Discreet, subject to enucleation
                  Associated edema (extensive on CT)

        Micro   Microscopic circumscription
                  High nuclear cytoplasmic ratio, coarse chromatin, prominent
                  nucleoli
                  High mitotic index
                  Variable necrosis
                  Little vascular proliferation. Note: some metastases, particularly
                  renal cell carcinoma, may induce marked vessel proliferation
                  ± Fibrosis

Infarct

        Clin   Subacute clinical course
                  A-V shunting on angio
                  Expanding lesion on CT, enhancement only in early phase

        Gross   Necrosis (glioblastoma-like grossly)
        Micro   Early infarction
                      Neuronal necrosis
                      Hypocellular, edematous
                      Early capillary proliferation with prominent endothelial cells
                  Organizing infarct
                      Necrosis (not serpiginous or palisading)
                      Cellular process (reactive astrocytes; macrophages with
                          defined borders, foamy cytoplasm and uniform benign nuclei;
                        variable chronic inflammation)
                      Microvascular proliferation
                      (*not* glomeruloid)

Table 8.2.
Compartments of Nervous System Differential Diagnosis
and Clinicopathologic Features (*Continued*)

	DDX	Demyelination (loss of myelin but retention of neurons and their processes)

Abscess

	Early	Ill-defined, soft Necrotic vessels, acute inflammation
	Organizing	Circumscription Central liquefaction Peripheral fibrosis, gliosis and chronic inflammation

Infratentorial (Posterior Fossa)

Brainstem (Pontine)
Glioma

	Clin	First two decades of life Diagnosis largely clinical, radiographic and gross. Note: These biopsies are small; spare tissues for permanent sections
	Micro	Two types (1) Similar to supratentorial astrocytoma (2) Similar to pilocytic astrocytoma of cerebellum or 3rd ventricle (see below)

Cerebellar Pilocytic
Astrocytoma

	Clin	Young patients Indolent, slow evolution of symptoms
	Gross	Discreet, solid or cystic with mural nodule
	Micro	Biphasic microscopic pattern: *Loose* with microcysts; *compact* with Rosenthal fibers Cytology—benign or mild atypia *No mitoses* Mild vessel proliferation ± Microcalcification
	DDX	Hemangioblastoma (adults, grossly yellow, lipid-rich, highly vascular) Gliosis eg. around AVM Fibrillary astrocytoma (adults)

Medulloblastoma

	Clin	Childhood—vermis, roof of 4th ventricle Young adults—hemispheric Short clinical course Hydrocephalus and cerebellar signs
	Gross	Soft ill-defined (classic) to firm localized (desmoplastic variant)
	Micro	Highly cellular "Indian file" and "follicular" patterns in desmoplastic variant High nuclear-cytoplasmic ratio Oval to carrot-shaped nuclei Variable mitotic activity and necrosis ± Homer Wright rosettes (neuroblastic differentiation) Variable desmoplasia (leptomeningeal infiltration)

Table 8.2.
Compartments of Nervous System Differential Diagnosis
and Clinicopathologic Features (*Continued*)

DDX	Normal cerebellar cortical granular cells (benign cytology, uniformly distributed cells with small round nuclei, high nuclear cytoplasmic ratio, no mitoses, associated Purkinje cells)
	Ependymoma (originates from floor of 4th ventricle; pseudorosettes, true rosettes, lower nuclear cytoplasmic ratio, few mitoses)
	Anaplastic "small cell" carcinoma (adults)
Ependymoma	
Gross	Related to ventricular system
	Soft, grey, lobulated, circumscribed
	May fill or exit ventricular system via foramina
Micro	Variable microscopic patterns (cellular, papillary, etc.)
	Perivascular pseudorosettes
	± True rosettes
	± Mild atypia
	Few mitoses (grades I and II); numerous mitoses (grade III)
	± Focal necrosis
DDX	Medulloblastoma (see above)
	Choroid plexus papilloma (connective tissue stroma in papillae, cuboidal to columnar cells)
Hemangioblastoma	
Clin	Adults
Gloss	± von Hippel-Lindau syndrome
	Cerebellum, brainstem, spinal cord; (dura, rare)
	Solid or cyst-associated, discreet yellow-red, circumscribed from parenchyma
	Leptomeningeal attachment
Micro	Lipid-rich cells in nests separated by intersecting vascular network (distinction of vasculature from tumor cells may be obscured on frozen section)
DDX	Metastatic renal cell carcinoma (IVP may be needed)
	Xanthomatous meningioma (whorls, psammoma bodies, dural attachment)
	Cerebellar astrocytoma (gliosis surrounding hemangioblastoma may simulate glioma)
Metastatic Neoplasms	Common primary sites:
	Lung > melanoma > kidney > GI
	Cerebral:cerebellum (8:1)
	Brainstem (uncommon)

	Optic Nerve and Sheath

Astrocytoma	
Clin	Young patients
	Unilateral/bilateral (neurofibromatosis)
	Tendency to proximal extension with optic foramen enlargement
Gross	Fusiform nerve enlargement
Micro	Pilocytic astrocytoma
	Leptomeningeal involvement induces desmoplasia

Table 8.2.
Compartments of Nervous System Differential Diagnosis
and Clinicopathologic Features (*Continued*)

	DDX	Meningioma of optic nerve sheath (see below, reactive meningothelial cells of optic nerve sheath may mimick meningioma)
Meningioma		Adults Tumor surrounds optic nerve ± Hyperostoses of involved orbital bones Usual morphology

Spinal Region Lesions

INTRAMEDULLARY
(SPINAL CORD)
  Astrocytoma

	Clin	Young patients
	Gross	Fusiform cord enlargement Ill-defined, ± cystic, ± associated syrinx
	Micro	Fibrillary or pilocytic pattern
	NOTE	Don't freeze entire specimen; artifacts may preclude diagnosis on permanent section
	DDX	Syrinx (thick hypocellular glial lining, benign cytology or "degenerative atypia")

  Ependymoma

	Clin	Adults
	Gross	Intraparenchymal Variably circumscribed. NOTE: Ependymomas are potentially resectable; intraoperative distinction from astrocytoma is of importance
	Micro	Cellular Papillary
Hemangioblastoma		± Associated cyst or syrinx Highly vascular (see above)

Filum Terminale
  Ependymoma

	Gross	Encapsulated (sausage-shaped mass) or nonencapsulated. NOTE: The prognosis of encapsulated tumors is related to their intact total removal Perivascular myxoid change
	Micro	Myxopapillary (most common variant) Cellular Papillary
	DDX	Schwannoma (see above) Paraganglioma (filum or cauda equina origin, argyrophilic) ± Zellballen pattern)

INTRADURAL—
EXTRAMEDULLARY
  Meningioma
    Cervicothoracic > lumbosacral
    Laterally situated, sessile, dural origin
    Frequently psammomatous variety

Table 8.2.
Compartments of Nervous System Differential Diagnosis
and Clinicopathologic Features (*Continued*)

Neurilemmoma		
	Clin	Benign course, slow growing
	Gross	Posterior > anterior root Eccentric to nerve of origin Globular, ± "dumbell" configuration with extradural component, ± ganglion involvement Solid-cystic, yellow
	Micro	Antoni A and B pattern, palisading, Verocay bodies Thick hyalinized vessels, hemosiderin deposition
Neurofibroma		
	Clin	Neurofibromatosis
	Gross	Fusiform, diffusely enlarged nerve Translucent, mucoid
	Micro	Bundles of wavy cells in mucoid matrix
	NOTE	Potential malignant transformation Examine nerve margins for tumor extension
Cysts		Dermoid cyst Epidermoid cyst Arachnoid cyst Enteric cyst
"Lipoma" Metastases SPINE AND EPIDURAL SPACE		
		Abscess Aneurysmal bone cyst Chordoma Giant cell tumor Hemangioma Lymphoma Lipoma Metastatic carcinoma Myeloma Tuberculosis

Pituitary and Sellar Region

Craniopharyngioma		
	Clin	Childhood > adulthood Suprasellar, 3rd ventricle, intrasellar component (20%) Calcification (gross/x-ray)
	Gross	Cystic or solid "Machine oil" content of cyst
	Micro	Adamantinomatous epithelium. NOTE: fibrous tissue, keratinized "ghost cells" or "wet keratin" cholesterol and foreign body cells qualify for *presumptive diagnosis*)
	DDX	Rathke's cleft cyst (rarely symptomatic, simple glandular epithelium and occasional pituitary secretory cells). Epidermoid cyst (simple stratified epithelium, older age group) Dermoid cyst (adnexal structures)

Table 8.2.
Compartments of Nervous System Differential Diagnosis
and Clinicopathologic Features (*Continued*)

	Arachnoidal diverticulum (empty sella syndrome) Glioma. NOTE: Peritumoral gliosis with Rosenthal fibers is characteristic of craniopharyngioma and may mimick pilocytic astrocytoma
Pituitary Adenoma	Adulthood, Fancommon in children Sellar abnormality (tomography)
Surgical/radiographic classification	Macroadenoma < 1 cm Microadenoma (diffuse) > 1 cm Invasive
Endocrinologic classification	Functional—often intrasellar microadenomas Nonfunctional—often diffuse with sellar expansion or destruction, suprasellar extension or invasion
Pathologic classification	Based on immunocytochemistry; terms such as "acidophilic, basophilic and chromophobic" are of no clinical significance
Micro	Highly variable histologic pattern Uniform cytology Mild atypia Few mitoses Variable cytoplasmic granularity Microcalcifiation (20% of prolactinomas)
DDX	Plasmacytoma (clockface nuclei, paranuclear hoff) Metastatic carcinoma (anaplasia) Olfactory neuroblastoma (cribriform plate involvement, nasal presentation)
Germinoma ("ectopic pinealoma")	
Clin	1st and 2nd decade (rare in aged); male predominance Associated diabetes insipidus, visual disturbance, hypopituitarism Pineal region and suprasellar optic chiasm, 3rd ventricle, pituitary stalk involvement; infrequently intrasellar); one third of patients have region both suprasellar and pineal involvement
Micro	Large tumor cells with indistinct cytoplasm, vesicular nuclei, prominent nucleoli, and mitoses Lymphocytes, granulomatous infiltrate (uncommon). Other associated germ cell elements
DDX	Lymphoma (Continuous morphologic spectrum of cells, i.e., no "two cell population") NOTE: germinoma may occur in pure form or in combination with other germ cell tumors
Inflammatory Lesions	Lymphocytic hypophysitis (females, frequently pregnancy associated)
	Giant cell granuloma Sarcoidosis Histiocytosis X Cultures for fungi and tubercle bacilli are negative

Pathologic features of common lesions are shown. These are considered in context of regional differential diagnosis.

PITFALLS IN DIAGNOSIS

In most instances, the operative, as well as the pathologic diagnosis of an intracranial neoplasm is readily evident. The principal function of the frozen section is to determine its primary or secondary nature and to assess its malignancy and degree. Nonetheless, numerous "lookalikes" do occur among tumors of the nervous system. Even non-neoplastic conditions may simulate glioma. What follows is a discussion of major diagnostic problems or pitfalls in frozen section diagnosis. Attention is given primarily to differential diagnostic issues that affect intraoperative decision making.

Gliosis or Glioma?

The response of astrocytic cells to irritation may mimic glioma, particularly in tissues surrounding processes such as arteriovenous malformation, craniopharyngioma, hemangioblastoma, organizing abscess, subacute infarction, or demyelination.

Subacute gliosis in tissue sections, and particularly in smear preparations, is characterized by evenly spaced astrocytes of uniform size with somewhat gemistocytic features and long processes (Fig. 8.1*A* and *B*). Mitotic figures are morphologically normal and usually sparse. Gemistocytic astrocytomas are more cellular, cytologically atypical, and show distinctly different features on smear preparation (Fig. 8.2). With time, reactive astrocytes become more densely fibrillated; such chronic gliosis (Fig. 8.3)

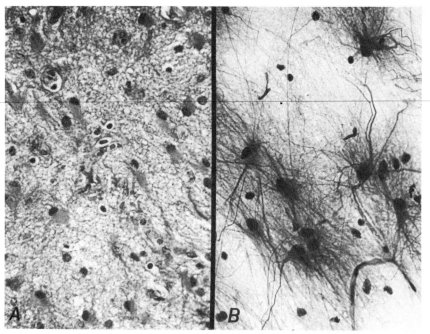

Figure 8.1. Subacute gliosis. The reactive astrocytes are regularly distributed in tissue sections (*A*) and possess relatively abundant cytoplasm. Their tapering processes are best seen on smear (*B*). *A* and *B*, hematoxylin and eosin, ×400.

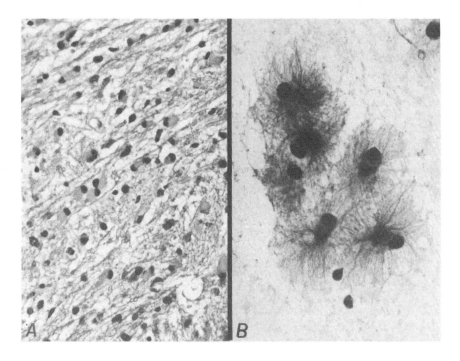

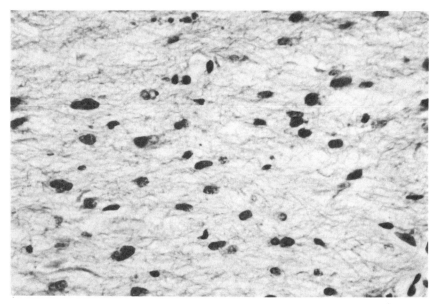

Figure 8.3. Fibrillary astrogliosis exemplified by long-standing gliosis within a demyelinative plaque. Note nuclear variation and narrow, stiff, fibrilrich processes. Hematoxylin and eosin, × 400.

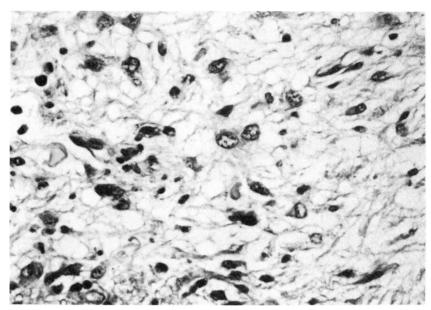

Figure 8.4. "Degenerative atypia" and multinucleation may be observed in long-standing, slow-growing gliomas such as this cerebellar astrocytoma of childhood as well as in juvenile pilocytic astrocytoma, ependymoma, and subependymoma, to name a few. Lack of mitoses and attention to clinical and radiographic data should prevent an erroneous diagnosis of malignancy. Hematoxylin and eosin, × 400.

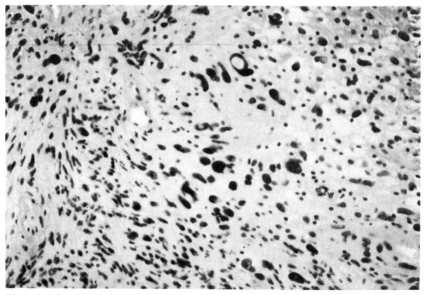

Figure 8.5. Neurilemmomas of the central as well as peripheral nervous system not infrequently display "degenerative nuclear atypia". Hematoxylin and eosin, × 250.

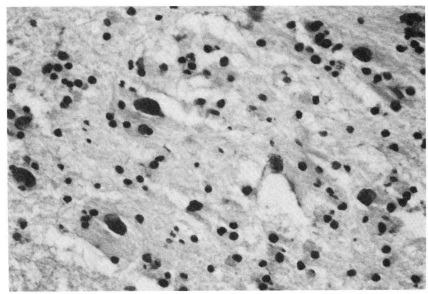

Figure 8.6. Radiation-induced atypia in non-neoplastic astrocytes. Such nuclear alterations may prompt a mistaken diagnosis of residual or recurrent astrocytoma. Relative lack of mitotic activity and degenerative, rather than proliferative, vasculature aids in the identification of radiation reaction. Hematoxylin and eosin, × 320.

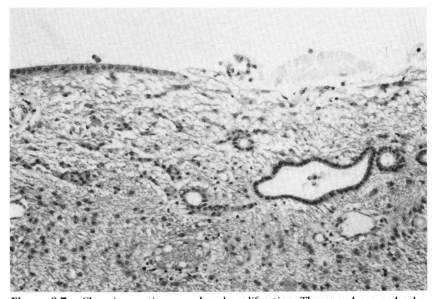

Figure 8.7. Chronic reactive ependymal proliferation. The ependyma and subependymal glial cells react to chronic irritation by proliferation and the formation of ependymal rosettes and canals. Such changes are rarely biopsied or mistaken for neoplasia. Hematoxylin and eosin, × 250.

may simulate fibrillary astrocytoma. Reactive astrocytes do not engage in the formation of secondary structures (i.e., dense subpial, subependymal, perivascular, and perineuronal aggregation) and are unassociated with complex neovascularity. In summary, there is a disparity between cytologic appearance and other features usually associated with malignancy.

Chronic gliosis may also be accompanied by "degenerative atypia," i.e., nuclear enlargement and hyperchromasia unaccompanied by mitotic activity. Similar nuclear changes may also be noted in benign tumors of long duration, both glial (cerebellar astrocytoma, ependymoma, subependymoma, etc.) and nonglial (nuerilemmoma, meningioma) (Figs. 8.4 and 8.5). Cytologic atypia, usually mild in degree, may be observed, particularly in irradiated tissues (Fig. 8.6).

Both tumors and non-neoplastic processes adjacent to the ventricular cavity may prompt reactive subependymal gliosis and ependymal proliferation. The latter often takes the form of scattered rosettes or canals, either attached to or lying immediately beneath the ependyma (Fig. 8.7). Confusion with ependymoma is unlikely.

Non-Neoplastic Conditions Simulating Glioma

Frozen sections obtained from normal cerebellar cortex contain sheetlike arrays of granular neurons, which may mimic medulloblastoma. The error is avoided by noting their uniform distribution, round rather than

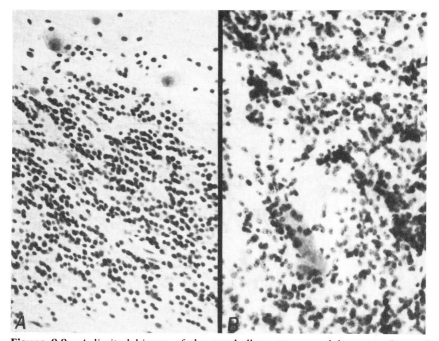

Figure 8.8. A limited biopsy of the cerebellum may reveal large numbers of granular neurons (*A*). Attention to their uniform round nuclei, central nucleoli, total lack of mitoses and association with Purkinje cells should prevent an erroneous diagnosis of medulloblastoma (*B*), *A,* hematoxylin and eosin, ×400; *B* (smear), ×400.

oval-or carrot-shaped nuclei, delicate solitary nucleoli, association with Pur-kinje cells, and, most importantly, their total lack of mitotic activity (Fig. 8.8). For comparison, the morphologic features of medulloblastoma are illustrated in Figure 8.9.

Infarcts, particularly in their subacute and organizing phases, are mark-edly cellular and may be mistaken for glioma (Fig. 8.10). Both its CT ap-pearance and information regarding the clinical evolution of the process are diagnostically helpful. The symptoms of infarction, unlike gliomas, are rather abrupt in onset and, other than in their acute phase, infarcts are not contrast enhancing. Microscopically, the predominant cells are ovoid to polygonal lipid-rich histiocytes ("gitter" cells) with round nuclei and solitary uniform nucleoli (Fig. 8.10*B*). Mitoses may be observed, but are not atypical (Fig. 8.10*C*). Aggregation of histiocytes in cuffs about the vasculature is common and is often accompanied by small numbers of lymphocytes or polymorphonuclear leukocytes. The reactive astrocytes are characteristi-cally large with prominent cell bodies and, unlike the gemistocytic astro-cytes of glioma, possess long processes that are best visualized on smear preparations (Fig. 8.1). The microvasculature surrounding infarcts is pro-liferative (Fig. 8.10*A*), but in contrast to the neovascularity of high grade glioma, the capillaries in an infarct are not glomeruloid in architecture. Multilayer endothelial proliferation is not observed.

Demyelinative foci are rarely biopsied, particularly when they are mul-tiple or assume their typical periventricular distribution. When solitary,

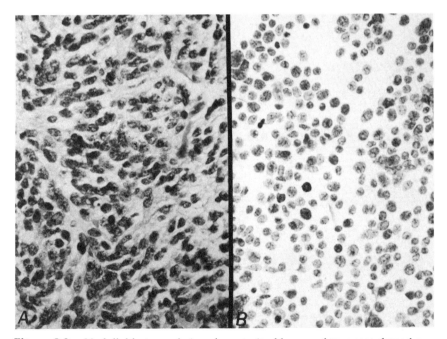

Figure 8.9. Medulloblastomas being characterized by round to carrot-shaped nu-clei, lack of prominent nucleoli, and relative abundance of mitotic figures should not be confused with a biopsy consisting of normal cerebellar granular neurons (Fig. 8.8). *A,* hematoxylin and eosin, × 400; *B,* smear preparation, hematoxylin and eosin, × 400.

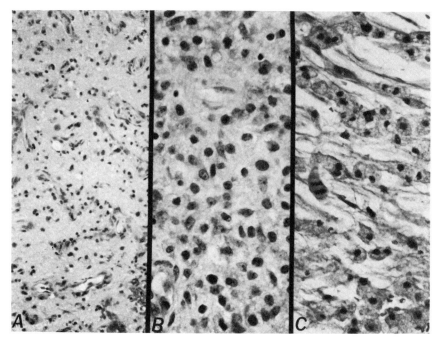

Figure 8.10. During their subacute phase, infarcts are cellular processes and may show enhancement on CT scan. Foamy histiocytes (*B,C*) and microvascular proliferation are characteristic of ischemia (*A*) and should not prompt a diagnosis of glioma. Clinical data regarding abrupt onset is also helpful. *A–C,* hematoxylin and eosin; *A,* × 250; *B,* × 320; *C,* × 400.

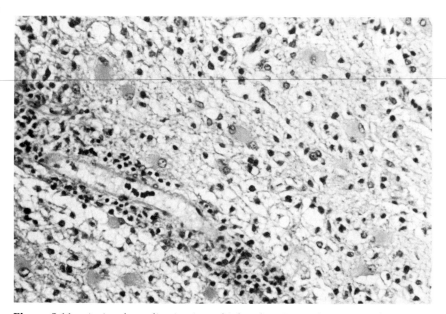

Figure 8.11. Active demyelination in multiple sclerosis may be mistaken for glioma. Cellular polymorphism, e.g., the presence of subacute gliosis, histiocytes disposed about vessels, and lymphoplasmacytoid cells should, in addition to clinical and CT data, suggest the correct diagnosis. Hematoxylin and eosin, × 250.

however, the radiographic features may simulate glioma. A biopsy from such an active focus (Fig. 8.11) is occasionally mistaken for low grade mixed oligoastrocytoma. Perivascular histiocytes are present in varying number, as are lymphocytes. Special stains show these lesions to be devoid of myelin, but unlike in infarcts, neurons and their processes are seen to be intact. Necrosis is rare in demyelination, but may be observed particularly in spinal lesions, where it is likely due to ischemia secondary to tissue swelling within the nonyielding leptomeninges.

Fragments of subacute abscess tissue may grossly and microscopically resemble glioma. If removed intact, the somewhat circumscribed lesion with a liquefied center is more easily recognized (Fig. 8.12). The polymorphous nature of the infiltrate, which includes polymorphonuclear leukocytes, lymphocytes, plasma cells and histiocytes, as well as broad areas of necrosis, plump reactive astrocytes, and fibrocapillary proliferation, assist greatly in making the correct diagnosis. Characteristically, the lesion is laminated, progressing from *a*) a center of polymorphonuclear leukocytes to *b*) layers of necrotic tissue and *c*) foamy macrophages among reactive capillaries, mononuclear leukocytes, and proliferating fibroblasts (Fig. 8.13*A–C*). The surrounding brain shows intense reactive gliosis (Fig. 8.13*D*).

Progressive multifocal leukoencephalopathy (PML), an infectious disease due to papova viruses, is the only viral infection that may be mistaken for glioma. A history of immunosuppression and the presence of multifocal lesions on CT are helpful diagnostic features. In a minority of cases, the essentially demyelinating lesions may be large or accompanied by limited necrosis. Histiocytes and reactive astrocytes may be numerous. Although the astrocytes are markedly atypical (Fig. 8.14*A*) and may show abnormal mitotic figures, the overall cellularity falls short of that seen in high grade astrocytomas. A helpful feature is the presence of eosinophilic inclusions,

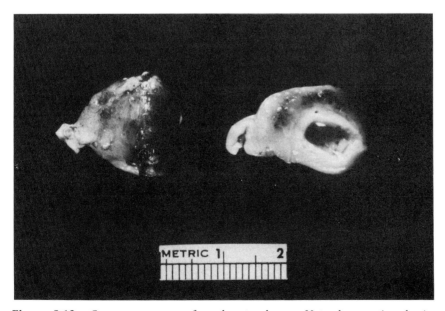

Figure 8.12. Gross appearance of a subacute abscess. Note demarcation, lamination, and central necrosis.

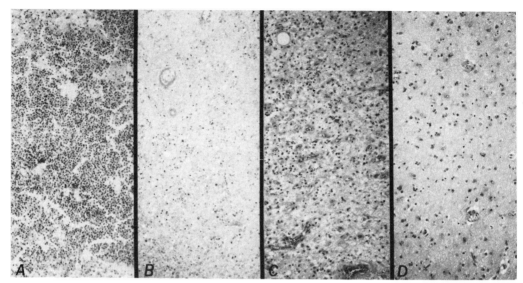

Figure 8.13. Attention to the zonation of abscesses will prevent an erroneous diagnosis of glioma. Note the central to peripheral zonation of purulent exudate (*A*), necrosis (*B*), capillary proliferation, and histiocytic reaction (*C*) as well as gliosis (*D*). *A–D*, hematoxylin and eosin, × 160.

most apparent in oligodendroglial cells (Fig. 8.14*B*). Features of glioma such as microvascular proliferation, palisading necrosis, and secondary structures are not noted. Electron microscopy is diagnostic.

Tumors Simulating Glioma

Neurilemmomas of the cerebellopontine angle, when deeply indenting the pons, may grossly or radiographically appear to arise from the brainstem

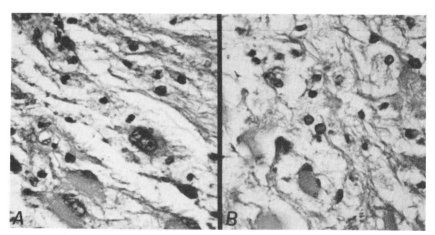

Figure 8.14. Progressive multifocal leukoencephalopathy is characterized by astrocytic atypia (*A*) and has, on rare occasion, been associated with the development of glioma. Its occurrence in the setting of immunosuppression, multifocal changes on CT scan, and the recognition of nuclear inclusions (*B*) in oligodendroglial cells (*arrows*) should preclude a mistaken diagnosis of glioma. *A* and *B*, hematoxylin and eosin, × 400.

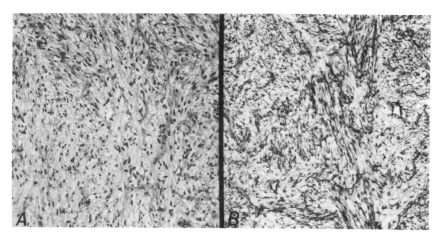

Figure 8.15. Brainstem gliomas are often composed of aligned elongate astrocytes and may, on a limited biopsy, resemble neurilemmoma (*A*) of the cerebellopontine angle. The latter is the most common tumor of the posterior fossa. Astrocytomas at this site are usually mitotically active and, unlike neurilemmoma (*B*), are devoid of intercellular reticulin. A modified reticulin method applicable to frozen sections has been described (13). *A* and *B*, hematoxylin and eosin, × 160.

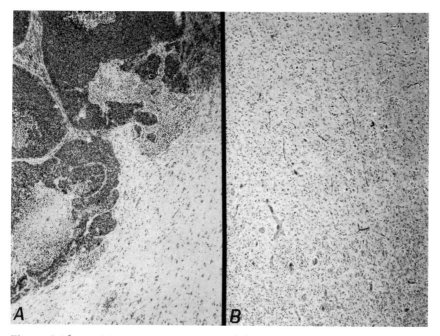

Figure 8.16. Unlike metastatic carcinoma (*A*) which is usually multifocal, sharply circumscribed, and devoid of glomeruloid vasculature, malignant gliomas, such as this glioblastoma (*B*), are characteristically solitary, merge imperceptibly with normal brain parenchyma, and show the formation of complex neovasculature. *A* and *B*, hematoxylin and eosin, × 160.

and thus mimic astrocytoma. The reverse, extension of brainstem glioma into the angle, is rare. The error is promoted by their microscopic similarity, both tumors being composed of elongate bipolar cells. Helpful diagnostic features of neurilemmoma include encapsulation, vascular hyalinization, hemosiderin deposition, and a biphasic growth pattern (Antoni A and B). Verocay bodies, a diagnostic feature of neurilemmoma consisting of focal exaggerated palisading of Schwann cells, are regularly seen in spinal neurilemmomas but are an infrequent finding in cerebellopontine angle tumors. The reticulin stain method adapted for frozen sections (5) may be helpful in distinguishing small fragments of a reticulin-free spindle cell glioma from neurilemmoma (Fig. 8.15), which characteristically shows dense pericellular reactivity.

Few tumors demonstrate as broad a spectrum of histologic appearances as do meningiomas (6). They may simulate a variety of gliomas, including fibrillary and gemistocytic astrocytomas, oligodendroglioma, and ependymoma (see below; Figs. 8.48–8.53).

Metastatic neoplasms are characteristically circumscribed, multiple, and frequently occur in the setting of known extracranial malignancy. Metastatic carcinomas far outnumber sarcomas. Nonetheless, when a solitary lesion presents in a patient not known to harbor a primary tumor at another site, diagnostic confusion may occur. Several tumors mimic glioblastoma, the most frequent being amelanotic malignant melanoma, poorly differentiated

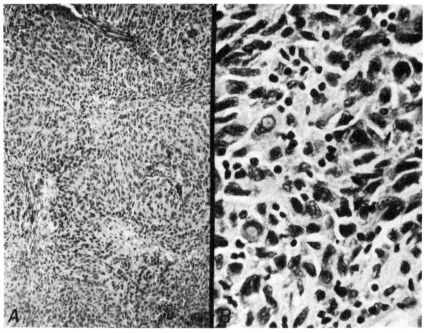

Figure 8.17. Metastatic amelanotic melanoma, a neuroectodermal neoplasm, may mimic glioblastoma. Melanomas frequently show pseudopapillae formation resulting from cuffs of viable perivascular cells separated by zones of necrosis. Glomeruloid endothelial proliferation is noticeably absent. Nuclear pseudoinclusions are often seen in melanoma (*B*). *A,* hematoxylin and eosin, × 160; *B,* hematoxylin and eosin × 400.

carcinoma of the lung, and sarcomatoid renal cell carcinoma (Fig. 8.18). Abrupt tumor margins and relative lack of microvascular proliferation are characteristic of metastases (Fig. 8.16*A*), whereas glioblastomas frequently merge imperceptably with surrounding parenchyma and induce glomeruloid vessel proliferation (Fig. 8.16*B*). Palisading necrosis is not a specific feature of glioblastoma and may be observed in metastases. Metastatic carcinomas, unlike gliomas, are keratin and epithelial membrane antigen immunoreactive. Renal cell carcinomas, in contrast to gliomas, are glycogen rich and thus strongly PAS positive.

It is no surprise that the cells of melanoma, also a neuroectodermal tumor, may closely resemble those of glioblastoma. In addition to circumscription, tendency to hemorrhage, and frequent multiplicity of melanoma deposits, they show a tendency to pseudopapillae formation and lack glomeruloid vessel proliferation (Fig. 8.17*A*). Nuclear inclusions similar to those of meningioma are common (Fig 8.17*B*). In the absence of stainable melanin, the identification of melanoma may require performance of glial fibrillary acidic protein immunostains, the reaction being negative. Both tumors are S-100 protein immunoreactive. Electron microscopy may be required.

In that medulloblastoma, principally a tumor of childhood, does occur in adults, the differential diagnosis of metastatic small cell carcinoma must be considered. Unlike the former (Fig. 8.9), small cell carcinomas characteristically show extensive necrosis (Fig. 8.18*A*), lack the desmoplastic growth

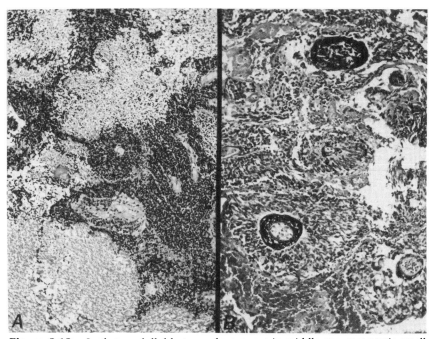

Figure 8.18. In that medulloblastoma does occur in middle age, metastatic small cell (oat cell) carcinoma may enter into the differential diagnosis. Deposits of the latter carcinoma are circumscribed, often show extensive necrosis (*A*), demonstrate no tendency to desmoplasia, less frequently form rosettes, are highly mitotically active, and may show vascular impregnation by nucleic acid (Azzopardi phenomenon) (*B*). *A,* hematoxylin and eosin, ×100; *B,* hematoxylin and eosin, ×160.

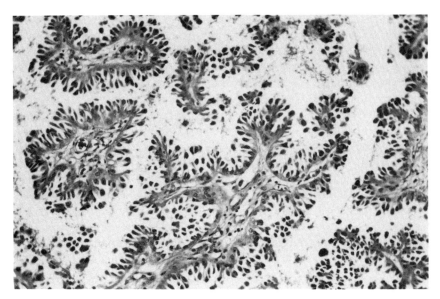

Figure 8.19. Metastatic papillary adenocarcinoma, such as this secondary deposit of pulmonary origin, may stimulate choroid plexus carcinoma. The rarity of the latter in adulthood, its largely intraventricular location and usual lack of cytoplasmic mucin should preclude misdiagnosis. Hematoxylin and eosin, × 250.

pattern often observed in medulloblastomas of adulthood, show less tendency to rosette formation, have a higher mitotic index, and may demonstrate nucleic acid impregnation of their vasculature (Azzopardi phenomenon; Fig. 8.18*B*).

Metastatic adenocarcinomas, particularly papillary forms involving the deep cerebrum or choroid plexus, may mimic papillary ependymoma or choroid plexus carcinoma (Fig. 8.19). Although both may occur in adults, the latter are clearly tumors of early life, most patients with choroid plexus carcinoma being less than 10 years of age. Fortunately, the distinction is not critical at the time of surgery. Choroid plexus carcinomas often show transition from atypical choroid plexus epithelium and are characteristically devoid of mucin. Glial fibrillary acidic protein immunoreactivity is regularly seen in ependymoma and is not uncommonly observed in tumors of choroid plexus origin as well.

BRAIN TUMORS SIMULATING NON-NEOPLASTIC PROCESSES

The distinction of gemistocytic astrocytoma from subacute gliosis has previously been discussed. The differences are illustrated in Figures 8.1 and 8.2.

On rare occasion, glioblastomas may be remarkably circumscribed. In such instances, central necrosis may result in a gross appearance resembling abscess (Fig. 8.20*A*). Unlike the zonation of abscesses, the viable periphery of such gliomas is composed entirely of tumor (Fig. 8.20*B*). Attention to cytologic features of malignancy avoids confusion.

Infection rarely supervenes on glioma. It may, however, be mimicked

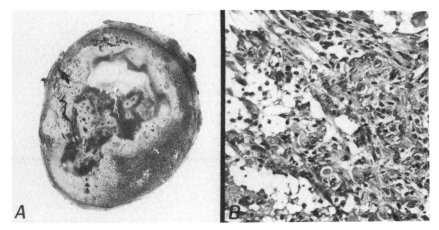

Figure 8.20. Glioblastomas may occasionally be circumscribed and centrally necrotic thus simulating abscess (*A*). Composed in part of fibroglial granulation tissue, abscesses lack both the nuclear anaplasia of glioma as well as glomeruloid proliferation (*B*). *A,* hematoxylin and eosin, × 3; *B,* hematoxylin and eosin, × 160.

by the occurrence of extensive acute inflammation in occasional high grade gliomas (Fig. 8.21). Such tumors are usually not infected, the inflammatory infiltrate being reaction to degenerating cell products. Cultures are negative.

Highly vascular, low grade gliomas may be encountered in the cerebrum or cerebellum. Such so-called "angiogliomas" may be mistaken for angioma or arteriovenous malformation (Fig. 8.22). Careful search for the monomorphous glial component usually resolves the problem.

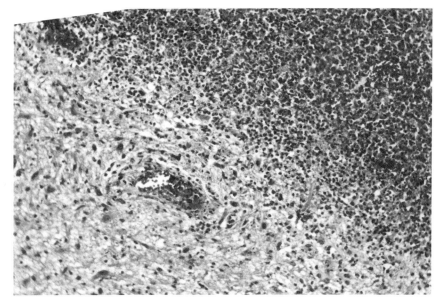

Figure 8.21. Necrosis in glioblastomas is sometimes accompanied by intense acute inflammation. The latter does not indicate infection but may simulate abscess. Cultures are negative. Hematoxylin and eosin, × 160.

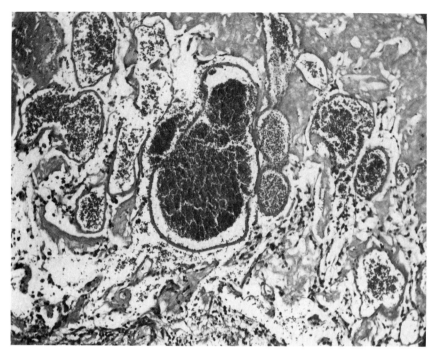

Figure 8.22. The so-called angioglioma, simply a highly vascular form of low-grade astrocytoma, may simulate hemangioma or arteriovenous malformation. A correct diagnosis depends upon a careful search for a monomorphous glial component (*bottom*). Hematoxylin and eosin, ×100.

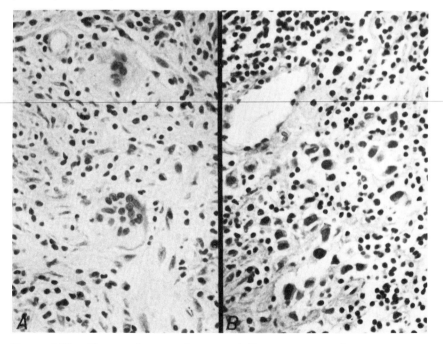

Figure 8.23. The reactive granulomatous infiltrate accompanying some germinomas (*A*), whether pineal or hypothalamic in origin, may mask the true nature of the process. The search for atypical cells (*B*) is facilitated by the PAS stain. *A* and *B,* hematoxylin and eosin, ×250.

Germinomas most frequently involve the pineal gland or the hypothalamus and suprasellar area. Granulomatous inflammation accompanying these tumors may obscure the neoplastic cells and result in an erroneous diagnosis of infectious granuloma or neurosarcoidosis (Fig. 8.23). Germinoma cells are strongly PAS-positive and are immunoreactive for placental alkaline phosphatase.

Gliomas Simulating Other Neoplasms

The vast majority of astrocytomas including glioblastoma are easily recognized, but the morphologic spectrum of astrocytic neoplasia is broad. Several variants mimic mesenchymal and even epithelial neoplasms. Although most high grade astrocytomas are composed of spindle and epithelioid cells, those gliomas consisting entirely of spindle cells may simulate fibrosarcoma (Fig. 8.24A). Gross, radiographic, and surgical circumscription as well as firm texture characterize true sarcomas of the nervous system. In contrast, glioblastomas are frequently ill defined and soft. The frozen section adapted reticulin stains will show dense intercellular staining in fibrosarcoma and its lack in glioma (Fig. 8.24B). It should be kept in mind that rare tumors composed of malignant glial and fibrous elements do occur, i.e., gliosarcoma.

Gliomas infiltrating the dura may, upon retraction, separate from brain substance in such a way as to mimic a dural deposit of metastatic carcinoma or a meningioma (Fig. 8.25). This is particularly true of astrocytomas inciting a dense fibroproliferative response. The latter may suggest a diagnosis of

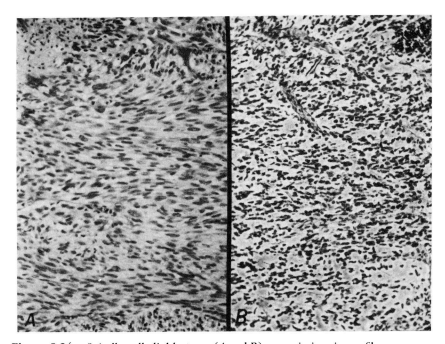

Figure 8.24. Spindle cell glioblastoma (*A* and *B*) may mimic primary fibrosarcoma of the brain. The latter, however, are sharply circumscribed, firm, devoid of glomeruloid vessel proliferation, and rich in intercellular reticulin. *A,* hematoxylin and eosin, × 160; *B,* Gomori's reticulin, × 160.

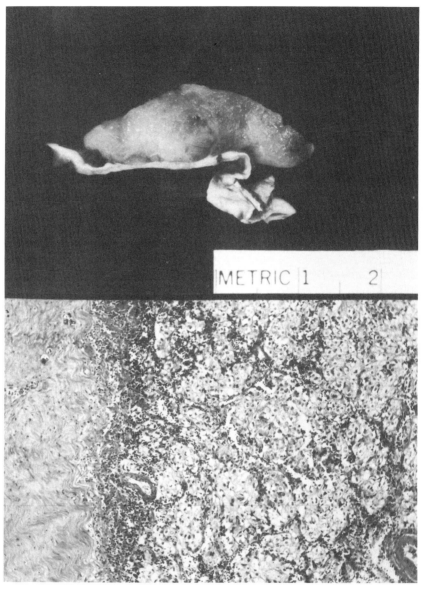

Figure 8.25. Oligodendroglioma showing dural attachment. Note its apparent circumscription (*above*) and epithelioid microscopic appearance (*below*). Such tumors may be mistaken for meningotheliomatous meningioma or metastatic carcinoma. *Below*, hematoxylin and eosin, ×100.

fibrous meningioma or of gliosarcoma. Confusion is avoided by attention to the benign appearance of the collagen rich reaction (Fig. 8.26*A*) and to the identification of classic glioma in its deeper portions (Fig. 8.26*B*). All elements of gliosarcoma appear cytologically malignant (Fig. 8.27).

Gliomas infiltrating the leptomeninges also incite desmoplasia, a feature which may suggest leptomeningeal sarcomatosis or carcinomatosis (Fig. 8.28*A* and *B*). Adequate sampling of the tumor usually permits diagnosis.

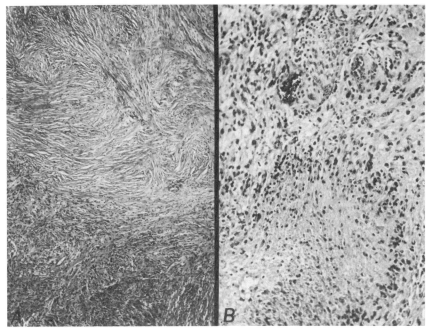

Figure 8.26. Glioblastoma with dural invasion showing intense fibroplasia (*A*). Deep portions of the process show the characteristic features of glioblastoma (*B*). *A,* hematoxylin and eosin, ×64; *B,* hematoxylin and eosin, ×160.

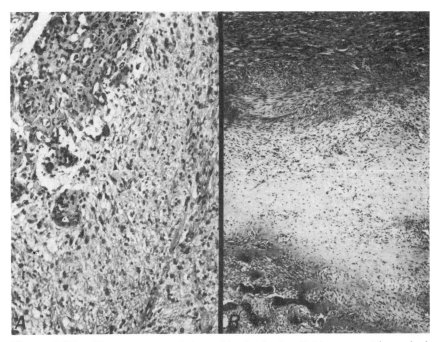

Figure 8.27. Gliosarcoma consisting of both classic glioblastoma with marked endothelial proliferation (*A*) and, in this unusual example, of malignant fibrous tissue, cartilage, and bone (*B, top to bottom*). *A,* hematoxylin and eosin, ×160; *B,* hematoxylin and eosin, ×64.

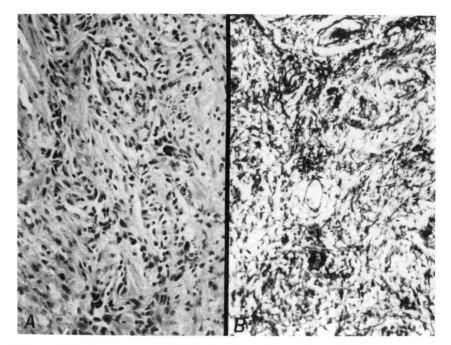

Figure 8.28. Leptomeningeal infiltration by malignant glioma (*A*) may prompt a desmoplastic reaction and thus simulate meningeal sarcomatosis. A sufficient biopsy of deep portions of the tumor as well as GFAP immunostains should serve to identify glioma, despite the abundance of intercellular reticulin (*B*) in meningeal portions of the lesion. *A*, hematoxylin and eosin, ×250; *B*, reticulin, ×250.

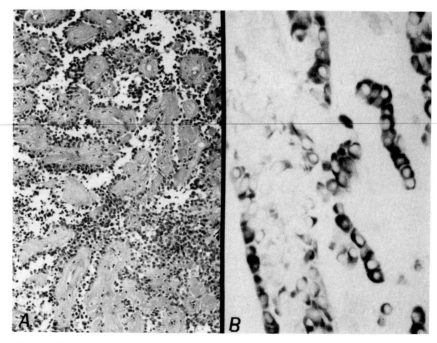

Figure 8.29. The perithelial cell arrangement of astroblastoma may mimic metastatic adenocarcinoma. Helpful cytologic features of this often circumscribed glioma are stout processes terminating upon vessels, lack of cytoplasmic vacuolation or mucin content, and a positive GFAP reaction (*B*). *A*, hematoxylin and eosin, ×160; *B*, peroxidase-antiperoxidase technique, ×400.

With minute biopsies, the most reliable method of identifying glial cells in such a setting is the glial fibrillary acidic protein immunostain performed on permanent sections.

The astroblastoma, an unusual form of astrocytoma with a striking tendency to circumscription and formation of papillary structures, may simulate adenocarcinoma (Fig. 8.29*A*). Fortunately, this pattern is rarely pure, and more characteristic features of astrocytoma are usually present in other portions of the tumor. Immunostains for glial fibrillary acidic protein are strongly positive (Fig. 8.29*B*).

Attention has recently been brought to adenoid cellular arrangements of astrocytic cells in gliosarcomas (7). Similar features may occasionally be seen in ordinary glioblastoma and may closely resemble metastatic carcinoma (Fig. 8.30). In small biopsies, the application of the glial fibrillary acidic protein immunostain on permanent sections may be required to identify these unusual gliomas.

Hemangioblastoma, a tumor of uncertain histogenesis limited to the cerebellum, brainstem and spinal cord, may simulate metastatic renal cell carcinoma based upon its circumscription, yellow color, and composition of foamy cells. Both tumors may be associated with von Hippel-Lindau disease; however, the renal cell carcinoma in this phakomatosis infrequently metastasizes. Hemangioblastomas characteristically abut the leptomeninges and may present as a mural nodule within a cyst. In the most common variant of hemangioblastoma, the vasculature is a dense interlacing network of capillaries surrounding small pockets of lipid rich stromal cells (Fig. 8.31*A*). More cellular forms of hemangioblastoma are composed of sheets of these cells with a less characteristic vascularity and greater similarity to

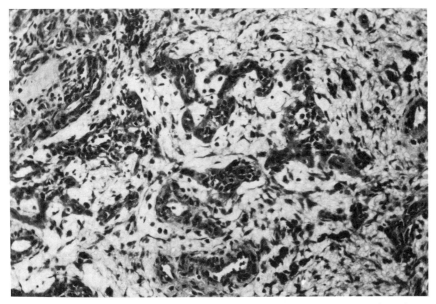

Figure 8.30. An "adenoid" pattern of glial cells may be observed in either gliosarcoma or glioblastoma. Astrocytic cells in clusters and pseudoglandular arrangements are best seen in the stroma-rich portions of such tumors. Hematoxylin and eosin, × 160.

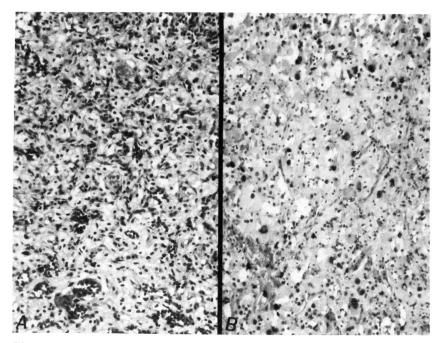

Figure 8.31. The classic hemangioblastoma (*A*), a tumor of the posterior fossa and spinal cord, is characterized by a rich vascular network of intersecting capillaries separating small groups of lipid-rich stromal cells. When the latter are more relatively abundant (*B*), the diagnosis of metastatic renal cell carcinoma may be entertained. Although hemangioblastomas of either pattern may contain cytologically atypical cells, they are largely devoid of mitoses. *A* and *B*, hematoxylin and eosin, × 250.

renal cell carcinoma (Fig. 8.31*B*). As in renal cell carcinoma, the cells of hemangioblastoma also contain considerable glycogen. Both may contain erythropoietin and show foci of extramedullary hemopoiesis. An intravenous pyelogram or abdominal CT scan may be required to exclude renal cell carcinoma in that by light microscopy the two tumors may be nearly indistinguishable.

Carcinoma Versus Lymphoma

There is an increasing tendency to resect solitary foci of metastatic carcinoma. In the setting of known carcinoma, the clinical and operative diagnosis is usually correct. In situations of no known extracranial primary, however, the distinction of carcinoma from lymphoma is of therapeutic importance.

In contrast to the highly radiosensitive infiltrative and less well-defined lymphoma, secondary deposits of carcinoma are characteristically sharply circumscribed, contain no functional brain parenchyma (Fig. 8.16) and respond only marginally to radiotherapy. As a result, gross total removal is a reasonable goal in carcinomas and is accompanied by little neurologic loss. In contrast, extensive resection of a lymphoma may leave the patient with considerable neurologic deficit due to loss of infiltrated functional parenchyma.

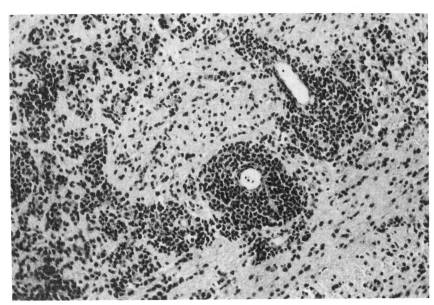

Figure 8.32. Cerebral lymphoma is characterized by dense infiltration of the peri-vascular spaces and, to a lesser extent, the intervening parenchyma, by atypical lymphocytes. Most are large cell or immunoblastic lymphomas. The parenchymal infiltrate may appear polymorphous in that it usually contains reactive astrocytes and macrophages. Hematoxylin and eosin, × 160.

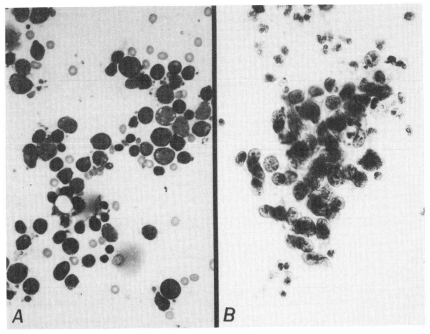

Figure 8.33. Touch preparations or smears of metastatic carcinoma (*A*) are char-acterized by cellular cohesion and nuclear molding, whereas such cytologic features are absent in lymphoma (*B*). *A,* hematoxylin and eosin, × 400; *B,* Giemsa, × 400.

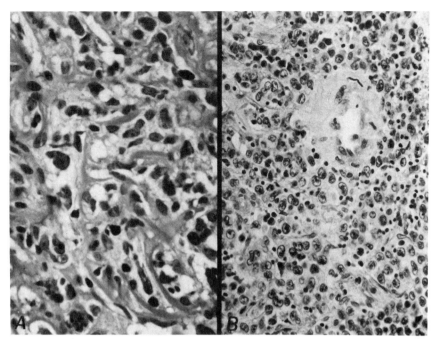

Figure 8.34. Confusion may arise in the identification of lymphoma in the spinal epidural space in that sclerosis may be extensive (*A*) and may produce a compartmentalizing pattern reminiscent of invasive carcinoma (*B*). *A*, hematoxylin and eosin, ×400; *B*, hematoxylin and eosin, ×250.

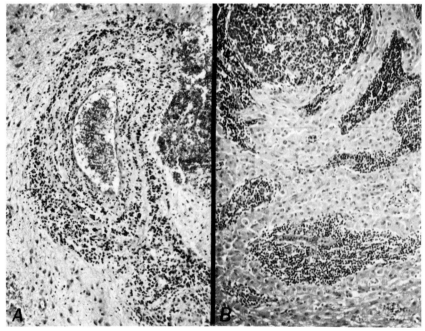

Figure 8.35. Abscesses (*A*) as well as gliomas, particularly gemistocytic astrocytomas (*B*), may show perivascular lymphocytic infiltrates which should not be mistaken for lymphomas. The infiltrates are composed primarily of small lymphocytes lacking atypia and may be accompanied by germinal center formation (*B*). *A*, hematoxylin and eosin, ×160; *B*, hematoxylin and eosin, ×160.

In most instances, the diagnosis of lymphoma is relatively straightforward, the cells having a distinct tendency to perivascular infiltration (Fig. 8.32). Histiocytes, reactive astrocytes, and nonspecific inflammatory cells may be numerous. Touch preparations usually show the characteristic cytology of lymphoma, most often large cell type (Fig. 8.33*A*). Carcinoma cells, on the other hand, are cytologically more monomorphous and tend to be cohesive (Fig. 8.33*B*). On occasion, however, the distinction may be difficult. A small proportion of lymphomas, particularly in the epidural space, show distinct desmoplasia or compartmentalization of lymphoma cells; the resulting pattern may be mistaken for carcinoma (Fig. 8.34). A careful search for perivascular infiltration, gradual blending of cells with brain parenchyma, and attention to cytologic features on smear are usually sufficient to make the distinction.

Both abscesses and some gliomas, particularly gemistocytic astrocytomas, may possess dense perivascular lymphoid infiltrates which may be mistaken for lymphoma (Fig. 8.35). Errors are avoided by attention to clinical and radiographic information and by noting the cytologic polymorphism of the lymphoid infiltrate.

The Spinal Cord

Astrocytoma or Ependymoma

The majority of astrocytomas of the spinal cord differ significantly from ependymomas in their gross relationship to surrounding cord parenchyma, astrocytomas being diffuse and ill defined (Fig. 8.16). Such tumors often incorporate surrounding tissue and usually do not lend themselves to resection without significant neurologic deficit. In contrast, ependymomas are characteristically demarcated, permitting a plane of dissection and gross total removal. Thus, the pathologist is frequently asked to intraoperatively classify spinal cord gliomas in order to guide the surgical approach. Ependymomas will be grossly resected, whereas astrocytomas may only be biopsied. Thus, in the case of an astrocytoma, the first specimen may be the last; tissue conservation is in order.

Although the epithelial and cellular forms of ependymoma pose no diagnostic problems, the tanycytic variant, composed of elongate bipolar and fibrillated cells (Fig. 8.36), may be mistaken for pilocytic astrocytoma.

Astrocytoma or Syrinx

A variety of slow growing spinal cord neoplasms may be associated with the formation of an intramedullary fluid filled cystic space or syrinx; such tumors include astrocytoma, ependymoma, and capillary hemangioblastoma (Fig. 8.37*A*). In that such a syrinx may be much larger than the tumor responsible for its development, the latter may be undetected. Syrinx formation may also be idiopathic or may be caused by non-neoplastic processes, particularly trauma. Biopsies from the wall of a syrinx of any origin consist of a mat of nondiagnostic gliotic tissue (Fig. 8.37*B*). The cyst fluid content is protein rich. Cytologic examination of syrinx fluid is of little or no diagnostic assistance. Preoperative clinical and radiographic studies are of primary importance in localizing a coexisting neoplasm. In summary, the

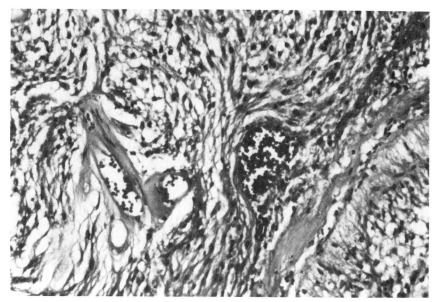

Figure 8.36. This so-called "tanycytic variant" of ependymoma may be micro-scopically mistaken for an astrocytoma, thus precluding attempts at total resection. Hematoxylin and eosin, ×250.

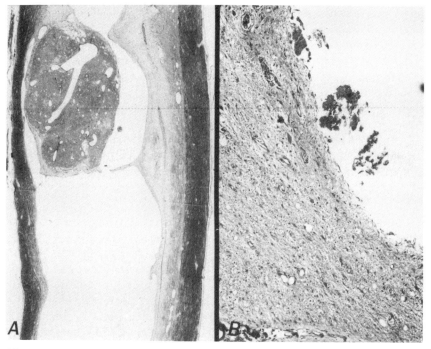

Figure 8.37. Syrinx accompanying a hemangioblastoma (_A_). Biopsies of such a secondary syrinx wall are nondiagnostic and demonstrate only reactive gliosis or degenerating glial cells (_B_). _A_, LFB-PAS, ×4; _B_, hematoxylin and eosin, ×100.

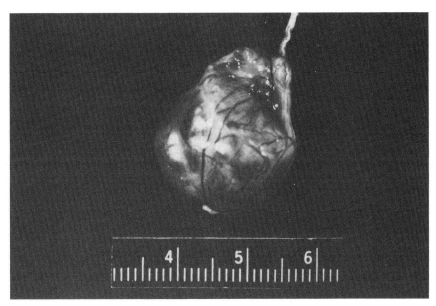

Figure 8.38. Schwannomas of the cauda equina region arise from nerve roots, not uncommonly show cyst formation, possess a thick fibrous capsule, and are yellow in color. Cellular pattern variation (Antoni A and B patterns) is characteristic of neurilemmoma (*A;* see Fig. 8.15*A*). As previously illustrated, reticulin stains show dense intercellular staining (*B;* see Fig. 8.15*B*), a feature lacking in myxopapillary ependymoma.

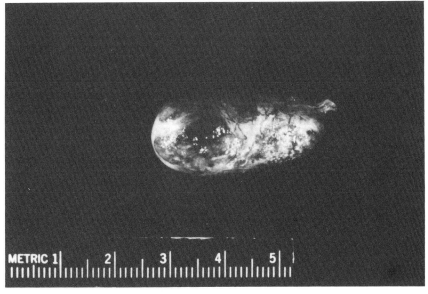

Figure 8.39. Ependymomas of the cauda equina region arise from the filum terminale, are solid, delicately encapsulated or unencapsulated, and are highly vascular.

diagnosis of tumor must be made on biopsy of the mass—not of the associated syrinx.

"Encapsulated Tumors" of the Cauda Equina Region

Three lesions of the cauda equina region, inclusive of the filum terminale, the fibroglial termination of the spinal cord, may present as sausage-shaped intradural tumors. These include nerve sheath tumors, most commonly the neurilemmoma, myxopapillary ependymoma of the filum terminale, and paraganglioma. In view of their gross similarities, the proper diagnosis is dependent on microscopy.

The neurilemmoma, a benign tumor of dorsal nerve root origin, is composed entirely of Schwann cells, is focally yellow, and occasionally partially cystic (Fig. 8.38). It may be opened in situ and "gutted" to facilitate removal. Neurilemmomas can be subtotally resected with no danger to the patient short of slow local recurrence. As previously described, they are characterized by the presence of a fibrous capsule, vascular hyalinization accompanied by hemosiderin deposition, and a biphasic pattern of cellular growth. Dense parallel arrangements of bipolar cells, occasionally in register, lie side by side with loosely arranged multipolar cells, the patterns being referred to as Antoni A and B, respectively. Degenerative cytologic atypia may be striking, but mitotic figures are not seen (Fig. 8.5). The reticulin stain pattern is dense and intercellular (Fig. 8.15).

Myxopapillary ependymomas, when intact, are solid, highly vascular tumors of the filum terminale surrounded by an attenuated delicate fibrous membrane (Fig. 8.39). They may show intimate attachment to surrounding cauda nerve roots. The cytologic appearance of such ependymomas varies greatly, the ependymal cells ranging from epithelial in appearance to ones in which their glial nature is more notable (i.e., elongate, sweeping, bipolar cells which may be confused with Schwann cells) (Fig. 8.40). Attention to the origin of the tumor from the filum terminale serves to distinguish ependymoma from neurilemmoma. Myxopapillary ependymomas must be entirely excised, intact if possible, to avoid local tumor seeding. Attention must be paid to documenting the integrity of the capsule, in that disrupted or subtotally excised lesions will require radiotherapy.

Paragangliomas of the cauda equina region are only one-fifth as frequent in occurrence as myxopapillary ependymoma, and they are grossly indistinguishable from the latter. They may arise either from the filum or, less commonly, from caudal nerve roots. The characteristic Zellballen pattern is frequently observed, as are ganglion cells (Fig. 8.41*A* and *B*).

TUMORS SIMULATING MENINGIOMA

Solitary deposits of metastatic carcinoma or melanoma are occasionally misdiagnosed as meningioma. The confusion is based largely upon their similar gross appearance as a globular dural-based mass (Fig. 8.42). At the microscopic level, the proper diagnosis may be further confounded in that whorl formation, the most obvious microscopic feature of meningioma, is seen in a variety of secondary neoplasms, notably melanoma and squamous, as well as mammary carcinoma (8) (Fig. 8.43). Whorl formation may also

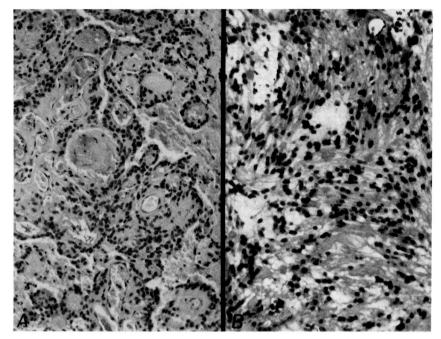

Figure 8.40. Ependymomas of the cauda equina microscopically show a spectrum of cytologic appearances ranging from epithelial (*A*) to glial (*B*). *A,* hematoxylin and eosin, × 160; *B,* hematoxylin and eosin, × 250.

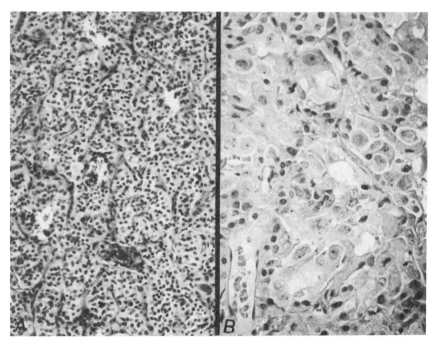

Figure 8.41. The Zellballen pattern characterizes paragangliomas of the filum terminale (*A*). Nearly half of such tumors at this location show gangliocytic elements (*B*). Unlike myxopapillary ependymoma, perivascular myxoid changes are absent or minimal and the cells show exclusively an epithelioid appearance. Grimelius stains are positive, whereas glial fibrillary acidic protein immunostains are negative. *A,* hematoxylin and eosin, × 160; *B,* hematoxylin and eosin, × 250.

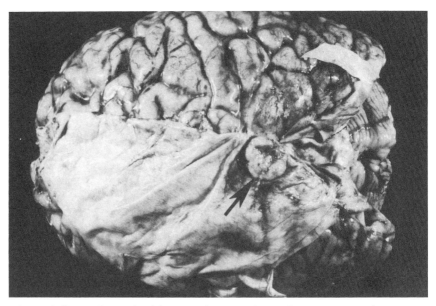

Figure 8.42. Solitary dural lesions of metastatic carcinoma may simulate meningioma (*arrow*).

be produced by cautery artifact. Cytologic atypia is of limited utility in the differential diagnosis, but metastases should be suspect in tumors showing conspicuous brain invasion, obvious anaplasia, significant necrosis, mitotic activity, and lack of psammoma bodies as well as of hyalinized vessels.

Neurilemmoma (schwannoma) may be mistaken for fibrous meningioma, particularly in the cerebellopontine angle. Both tumors are circum-

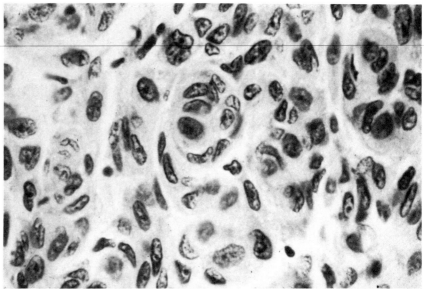

Figure 8.43. Whorl formation in this dural deposit of bronchogenic squamous carcinoma simulates meningioma. Hematoxylin and eosin, ×400.

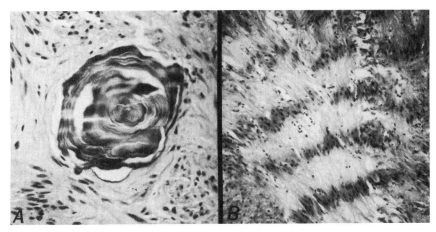

Figure 8.44. Psammoma bodies (*A*) are an unusual feature in otherwise ordinary schwannoma (*B*), but may prompt a mistaken diagnosis of meningioma. *A*, hematoxylin and eosin, × 250; *B*, hematoxylin and eosin, × 160.

scribed, composed of elongate bipolar cells, and may show whorl formation and nuclear intrusions (4). Psammoma bodies are uncommonly encountered in neurilemmoma (Fig. 8.44). The proper identification of neurilemmoma rests upon its gross attachment to a nerve rather than to the dura, the presence of a fibrous capsule, a biphasic (Antoni A and B) histologic pattern, the formation of Verocay Bodies; lack of psammoma bodies, and the presence of perivascular hemosiderin deposits. Both neurilemmomas and meningiomas show vascular hyalinization.

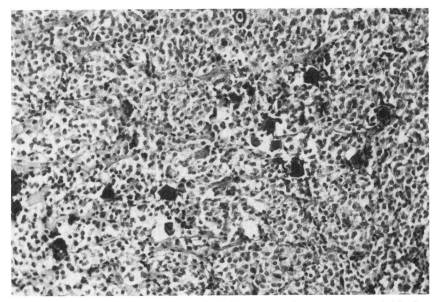

Figure 8.45. Approximately 20% of prolactinomas show psammoma body formation. Such tumors should not be mistaken for meningioma. Immunostains for prolactin are strongly reactive. Hematoxylin and eosin, × 100.

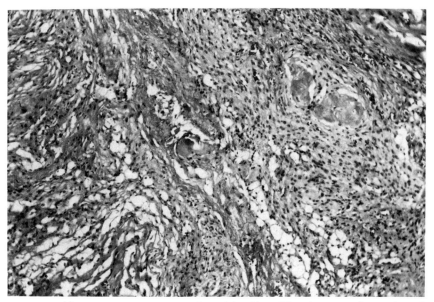

Figure 8.46. Chronic reactive arachnoidal cell proliferation may, due to its cellularity, suggest a diagnosis of meningioma. Hematoxylin and eosin, × 100.

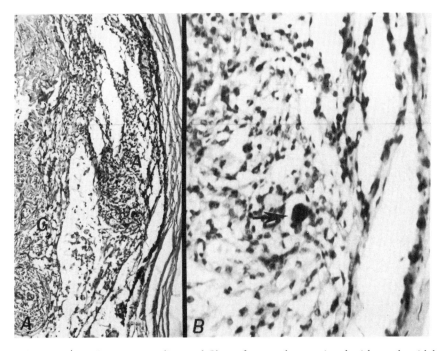

Figure 8.47. Optic nerve gliomas (*G*) are frequently associated with arachnoidal cell proliferation (*A*) in the surrounding leptomeninges. Scanty biopsies may suggest an erroneous diagnosis of optic nerve sheath meningioma. Note the psammoma body (*arrow*). Hematoxylin and eosin, × 60.

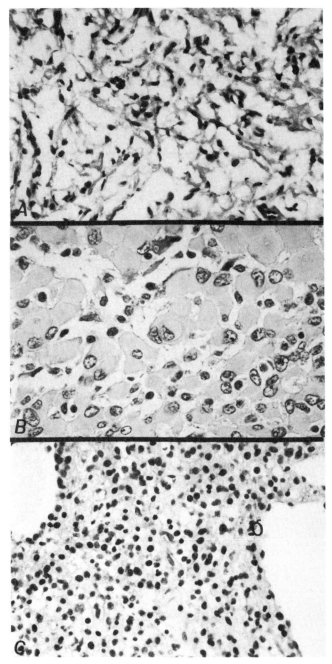

Figure 8.48. The morphologic spectrum of meningiomas includes patterns simulating glial neoplasms, e.g., fibrillary astrocytoma (*A*), gemistocytic astrocytoma (*B*) and oligodendroglioma (*C*). *A–C,* hematoxylin and eosin; *A,* ×250; *B,* ×400; *C,* ×250.

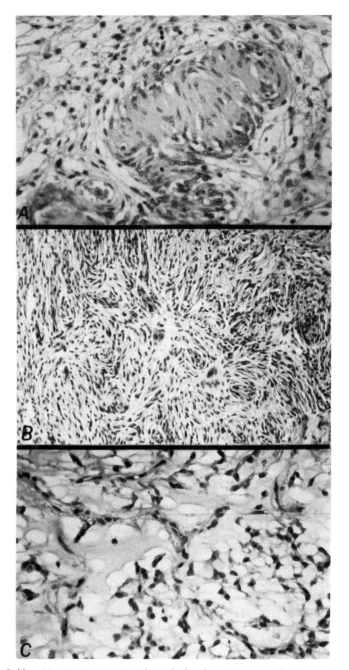

Figure 8.49. Meningiomas mimicking (*A*) schwannoma with Verocay body formation, (*B*) storiform fibrous histiocytoma, and (*C*) myxoma or myxoid sarcoma. *A–C,* hematoxylin and eosin; *A,* ×250; *B,* ×160; *C,* ×320.

Prolactin-producing pituitary adenomas, particularly when extending outside the sella, may be mistaken for meningioma in that this form of adenoma is prone to the formation of psammoma bodies (Fig. 8.45). Immunostains for prolactin are strongly positive.

Although rarely a point of confusion, a mistaken diagnosis of meningioma may be made if biopsies are obtained from a focus of reactive menigothelial cells (Fig. 8.46) or from a Paccionian granulation. Reactive meningothelial cells are regularly seen at the periphery of cystic astrocytomas involving the meningeal sheath of the optic nerve and may, on limited biopsy, prompt a mistaken diagnosis of meningioma (Fig. 8.47).

Meningioma—"The Chameleon"

Of all tumors affecting the nervous system, none assume such a broad range of morphology as do meningiomas (7). Most are solitary globular dural-based tumors, but meningiomas may be grossly diffuse, entirely intraparenchymal, or rarely extradural in location. Thus, the pathologist must be acquainted with the many faces of this common tumor. Communication with the surgeon, attention to radiographic studies and thorough tissue sampling usually assist in diagnosis, but the application of immunocytochemistry or electron microscopy may be required. The broad range of morphology of meningiomas is illustrated in Figures 8.48 through 8.53.

Meningiomas are prone to recurrence, particularly cellular tumors with brisk mitotic activity and foci of necrosis. Not infrequently, such aggressive meningiomas show the formation of pseudopapillae due to loss of cellular cohesion (Fig. 8.54). This "papillary meningioma" pattern is ominous in that it suggests malignant transformation.

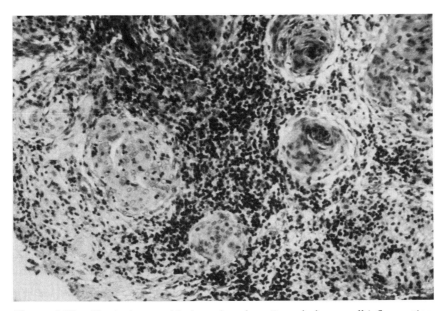

Figure 8.50. Meningiomas with dense lymphocytic and plasma cell inflammation may be mistaken for plasma cell granuloma or lymphoplasmacytic lymphoma. Hematoxylin and eosin, ×160.

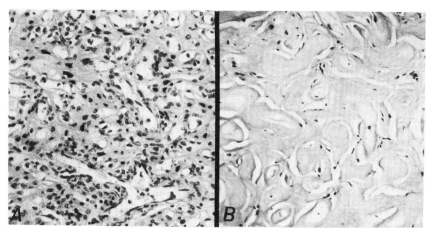

Figure 8.51. Vascular meningiomas (*A*) may resemble hemangioblastoma. Some undergo extensive sclerosis and simulate angioma (*B*). *A* and *B,* hematoxylin and eosin, × 160.

Although the angioblastic meningioma or "dural hemangiopericytoma" usually poses no diagnostic problem, spindle cell areas resembling fibrous meningioma as well as gland-like cellular arrangements mimicking adeno-carcinoma may be seen (Fig. 8.55).

SPECIAL CONSIDERATIONS IN TISSUE HANDLING

Pituitary Adenomas

The most common tumor of the sellar region is the pituitary adenoma. Its identification is assisted by information regarding endocrinopathy and by radiographic data suggesting a primary intrasellar lesion. Expansion and

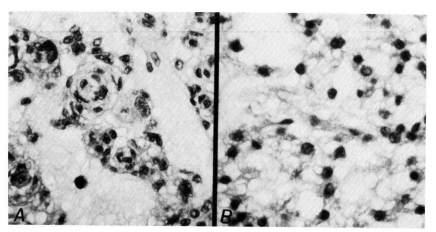

Figure 8.52. Meningiomas with mucosubstance accumulation (*A* and *B*) may mimic chordoma. The finding of cellular whorls (*A*) and the absence, on x-rays, of midline bone destruction is of assistance in diagnosis. *A* and *B,* hematoxylin and eosin, × 250.

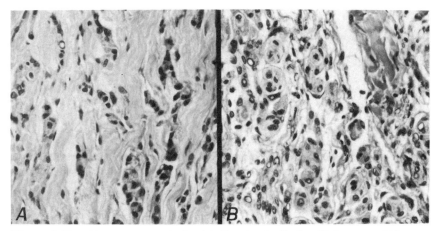

Figure 8.53. Meningioma with dural infiltration in "Indian file" pattern (*A*) mimicking metastatic carcinoma. Other portions of the tumor showed classic meningioma (*B*). *A,* hematoxylin and eosin, × 250; *B,* hematoxylin and eosin, × 160.

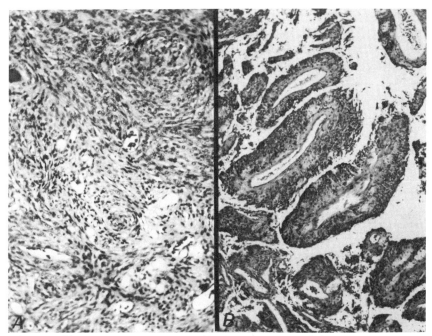

Figure 8.54. The formation of papillae in meningioma (*A*) is an ominous sign suggesting malignant transformation. When intraparenchymal, such tumors may be mistaken for ependymoma. Careful sampling shows the presence of more recognizable cellular mitotically active meningioma (*B*). *A,* hematoxylin and eosin, × 100; *B,* hematoxylin and eosin, × 160.

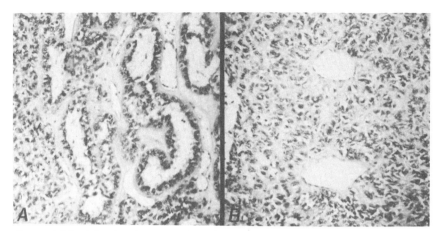

Figure 8.55. The development of an adenoid pattern (*A*) in an otherwise ordinary angioblastic meningioma (hemangiopericytoma of the dura) (*B*). *A* and *B,* hematoxylin and eosin, × 160.

destruction of the sella is common, as are visual field defects due to chiasmal compression. Clinical data regarding sellar lesions are of particular importance in view of the spectrum of histologic appearances of pituitary adenomas (9, 10) (Figs. 8.56 and 8.57) and the wide variety of other tumors occuring in this region (11). As with other endocrine neoplasms, the finding of cytologic atypia (Fig. 8.58) is of no prognostic significance.

Because the functional characterization of adenomas requires application of the immunoperoxidase technique, conservation of tissue again becomes a significant consideration. A methodologic scheme of tissue handling is shown in Table 8.3. When tissue is abundant, a frozen section serves to identify the process; however, more often than not, the specimen is small. This is particularly the case in prolactinomas in young females as well as in Cushing's disease. In such instances, smears, or preferably touch preparations, are a quick and economical means by which adenomas can be identified with little tissue loss. The making of touch preparations is both simple and rapid. Small portions of tissue are touched to dry, clean slides, which are then fixed in absolute alcohol for 30 sec and stained by the hematoxylin and eosin method. The cytologic features of the cells as well as their quantity and distribution in the touch preparation serve to distinguish adenoma from normal adenohypophysis (Fig. 8.59) (Table 8.4).

Once an adenoma has been identified and appropriate tissues are set aside for further study, frozen sections or smears may be further employed in the assessment of tissue margins or of dural infiltration. Special stains for the identification of pituitary adenomas on frozen section have, in our experience, been of little use (12, 13).

When despite a thorough search, no adenoma is identified at surgery, the pathologist may be asked to confirm the presence of hyperplasia. Adenohypophyseal hyperplasia is rare and is seen most frequently in the setting of Cushing's disease (9, 11). The diagnosis is suggested by expansion of

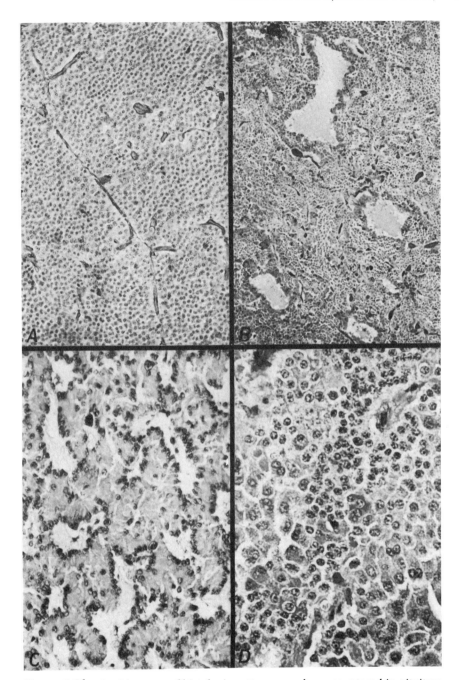

Figure 8.56. A wide range of histologic patterns may be encountered in pituitary adenomas. Knowledge of the clinical history and radiographic as well as operative findings precludes such erroneous diagnoses as carcinoma, glioma, or meningioma. Some adenomas are patternless (*A*), whereas others show microcyst formation (*B*), a carcinoid like appearance (*C*), or are composed of a bimorphic cell population (*D*). *A–D,* hematoxylin and eosin; *A,* ×160; *B,* ×64; *C,* ×250; *D,* ×400.

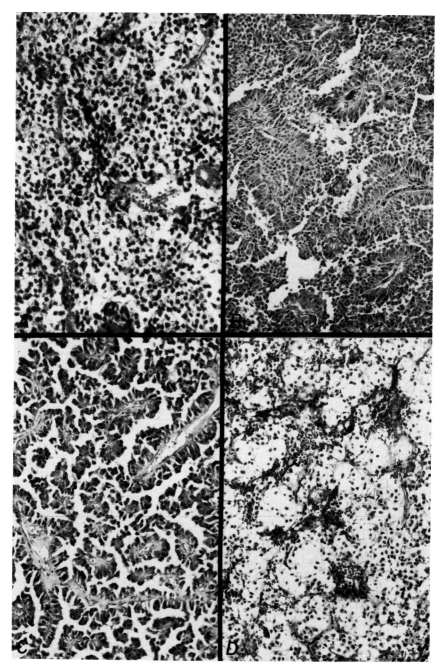

Figure 8.57.   Pituitary adenomas (*A–D*) simulating a variety of neoplasms including oligodendroglioma (*A*), papillary ependymoma (*B*), metastatic adenocarcinoma (*C*), and metastatic renal cell carcinoma (*D*). *A–D*, hematoxylin and eosin: *A*, ×250; *B–D*, ×160.

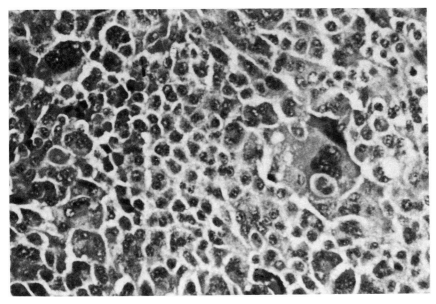

Figure 8.58. Cytologic atypia as well as modest mitotic activity are of no prognostic significance in pituitary adenomas. Hematoxylin and eosin, ×640.

Table 8.3.
Pituitary Tissue Evaluation[a]

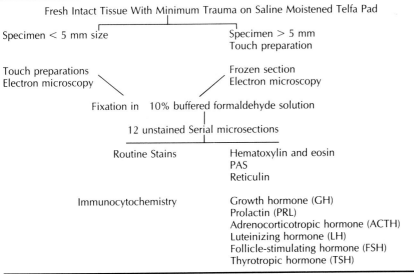

[a]Based on Scheithauer BW: Surgical Pathology of the Pituitary: The Adenomas, Part I. In Sommers SC, Rosen PP (eds): *Pathology Annual.* Connecticut, Appleton-Century-Crofts, 1984, p 317–374; and Scheithauer BW: Surgical Pathology of the Pituitary: The Adenomas, Part II. In Sommers SC, Rosen PP (eds): *Pathology Annual.* Connecticut, Appleton-Century-Crofts, 1984, p 269–329.

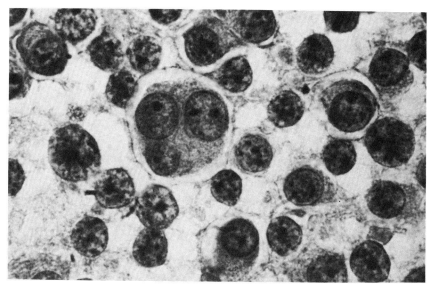

Figure 8.59. Touch preparations of pituitary adenoma show cytologic features distinct from those of the normal gland. These include abundance of cells, variation in nuclear size and number, prominent nucleoli, occasional mitoses and uniformity of cytoplasmic staining. Hematoxylin and eosin, ×640.

pituitary cords, a feature best seen on reticulin stain. On immunostains, such cords are seen to consist in large part of a single cell type. In that hyperplasia may coexist with adenoma, the diagnosis of hyperplasia is not valid unless the entire gland is available for examination. In any event, a diagnosis of hyperplasia is never made on the basis of frozen section.

The Specimen in Medical Disorders

In the setting of non-neoplastic diseases such as dimentia, diffuse encephalopathy, metabolic and storage disease, viral infection, etc., optimal specimen assessment may require special attention to specimen processing. A biopsy is frequently taken from a neurologically "silent" site, such as the frontotemporal region or cerebellum. The surgeon should be encouraged

Table 8.4.
Pituitary Touch Preparation

Diagnostic Criteria	
Normal gland	Adenoma
Hypocellularity	High cellularity
Even cell dispersion	Cell clusters
Uniform nuclei with mild size variation	Nuclear pleomorphism or multinucleation
Delicate chromatin	Coarse chromatin pattern
Round, small nucleoli	Prominent or irregular nucleoli
No mitoses	Mitoses

to obtain a full thickness biopsy including leptomeninges, cortex, and white matter with as little cautery artifact as possible. Touch preparations are made (both air dried and alcohol fixed), cortical and white matter sites are sampled for electron microscopy, and a portion of the tissue is frozen and stored at $-70°C$ for future use. If a diagnosis of infection is suspected, microbiologic specimens must be obtained in a sterile environment, preferably the operating room rather than the pathology laboratory. Although assessment of medical disorders requires clinical correlation and considerable interpretative time, a "pilot" frozen section should be performed to exclude obvious disease, such as bacterial, fungal, or tuberculous infection, lymphoma, or meningeal carcinomatosis. In addition to routine microsections, accompanying sequential unstained slides are simultaneously cut for the performance of special stains.

Acknowledgments: The author expresses his appreciation to Dr. J. J. Kepes, University of Kansas Medical Center, Kansas City, KS, for providing illustrative materials for Figures 8.23, 8.30, 8.43, 8.44, 8.48–8.50, 8.51B, 8.52, 8.53, 8.55.

REFERENCES

1. Burger PC, Vogel F: Frozen section interpretation in surgical neuropathology. I. Intracranial lesions. *Am J Surg Pathol* 1:323–347, 1977.
2. Burger PC, Vogel F: Frozen section interpretation in neuropathology. II. Intraspinal lesions. *Am J Surg Pathol* 2:81–95, 1978.
3. Preston HS, Bale PM: Rapid frozen section in pediatric pathology. *Am J Surg Pathol* 9:570–576, 1985.
4. Burger PC: Use of cytological preparations in the frozen section diagnosis of central nervous system neoplasia. *Am J Surg Pathol* 9:344–354, 1985.
5. Kepes JJ: Reticulin stain in differentiating astrocytoma from neurilemmoma on frozen section. *J Neurosurg* 51:124, 1979.
6. Kepes JJ: In Sternberg SS (ed): *Meningiomas: Biology, Pathology and Differential Diagnosis.* Masson Publishing, 1982.
7. Kepes JJ, Fulling KH, Garcia JH: The clinical significance of "adenoid" formations of neoplastic astrocytes, imitating metastatic carcinoma, in gliosarcoma. *Clin Neuropathol* 1:139–150, 1982.
8. Kepes JJ: Cellular whorls in brain tumors other than meningiomas. *Cancer* 37:2232–2237, 1976.
9. Scheithauer BW: Surgical Pathology of the Pituitary: The Adenomas, Part I. In Sommers SC, Rosen PP (eds): *Pathology Annual.* Norwalk, Appleton-Century-Crofts, 1984, p 317–374.
10. Scheithauer BW: Surgical Pathology of the Pituitary: The Adenomas, Part II. In Sommers SC, Rosen PP (eds): *Pathology Annual.* Norwalk, Appleton-Century-Crofts, 1984, p 269–329.
11. Scheithauer BW: Pathology of the Pituitary and Sellar Region: Exclusive of Pituitary Adenoma. Part I. In Sommers SC, Rosen PP (eds): *Pathology Annual.* Norwalk, Appleton-Century-Crofts, 1985, p 67–155.
12. Adelman LS, Post KD: Intra-operative frozen section technique for pituitary adenomas. *Am J Surg Pathol* 3:173–175, 1979.
13. Velasco ME, Sindley SD, Roessman U: Reticulum stain for frozen-section diagnosis of pituitary adenomas. *J Neurosurg* 46:548–550, 1977.

Genitourinary System

Elvio G. Silva, M. D.

Frozen sections are rarely requested from genitourinary specimens. Most of these requested are for diagnosis of prostate disease and for evaluations of tumors of the bladder.

PROSTATE

Indications for Frozen Section

It is common practice at M. D. Anderson Hospital to perform frozen section analysis of material from a needle biopsy of the prostate. In this situation, there are two indications for making a frozen section: (*a*) The patient presents with a nodule in the prostate and no other evidence of disease. The purpose of the frozen section in this instance is to be certain that the material submitted for pathologic examination is representative. (*b*) A totally different situation occurs when a patient presents with disseminated metastatic disease from what may be a possible prostatic primary neoplasm. In this case, if a prostatic nodule is detected on physical examination, a needle biopsy of the prostate is performed under general anesthesia. If the frozen section diagnosis shows an adenocarcinoma of the prostate, a bilateral orchiectomy is performed while the patient is still under anesthesia.

Frozen Section Diagnosis

Adenocarcinoma of Prostate

The diagnosis of adenocarcinoma of the prostate is based on the presence of histologic features that include changes in gland architecture, cellular characteristics, and invasion (Figs. 9.1 and 9.2).

Table 9.1 shows the histologic features of adenocarcinoma of the prostate.

Table 9.1.
Prostate Adenocarcinoma: Histologic Features

Architecture of glands	Small, Disorganized, Closely packed
Anaplasia and prominent nucleoli	
Invasion of	Prostatic capsule, Perineural spaces, Seminal vesicles

Differential Diagnosis

Several benign and non-neoplastic conditions are easily confused with prostatic adenocarcinoma. The most common diagnostic pitfalls of prostatic carcinoma are described below.

Benign Glands in Perineural Spaces. As an isolated histologic feature, the presence of glands in perineural spaces is not diagnostic of carcinoma (1). This finding helps to support the diagnosis of prostatic carcinoma when areas suspected of being cancerous are also found in the biopsy(2).

Benign Glands Between Skeletal Muscle. The prostatic capsule is incomplete in the anterior part of the gland which is why biopsies from the anterior portion of the prostate may show the presence of glands between skeletal muscle fibers (3). The benign appearance of these glands and the absence of areas of carcinoma are clues to the benign nature of the condition (Fig. 9.3).

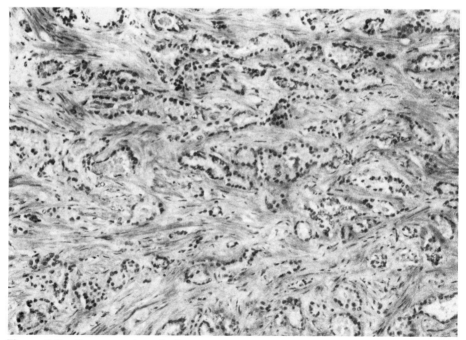

Figure 9.1. Frozen section of adenocarcinoma of prostate. Small glands with enlarged nuclei infiltrate the stroma.

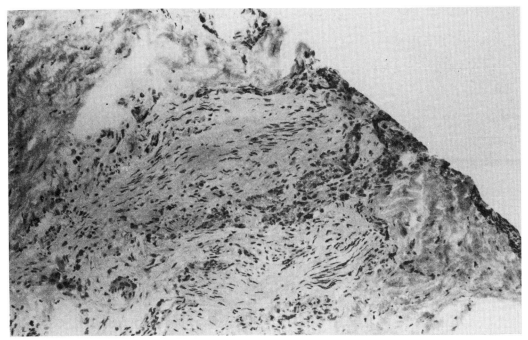

Figure 9.2. Frozen section of adenocarcinoma of prostate displaying perineural invasion.

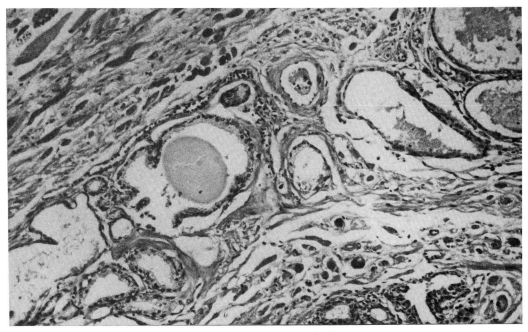

Figure 9.3. Benign prostatic glands between skeletal muscle fibers.

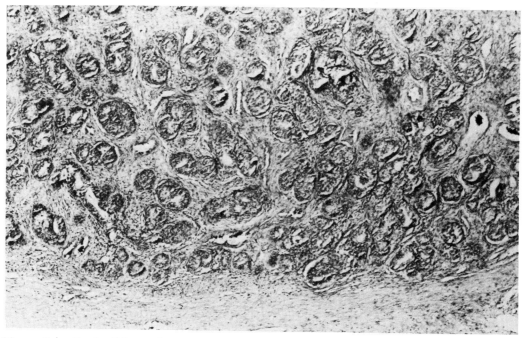

Figure 9.4. Basal cell hyperplasia of prostate. Nodular, well demarcated cellular proliferation.

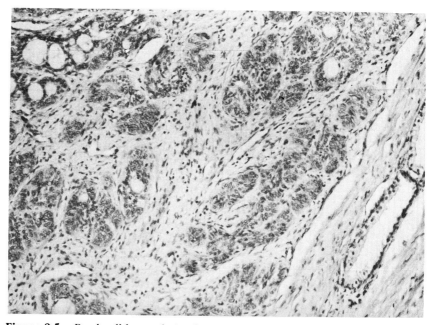

Figure 9.5. Basal cell hyperplasia of prostate. Proliferation of uniform basal cells without atypia.

Basal Cell Hyperplasia. The nodular lesion of basal cell hyperplasia is characterized by fibromuscular hyperplasia, sometimes clearly demarcated from the rest of the prostate, and by solid nests of basaloid cells with a high nucleocytoplasmic ratio and prominent peripheral palisading (4) (Figs. 9.4 and 9.5). The nuclei show evenly dispersed chromatin and rare nucleoli. This entity is also known as fetalization of the prostatic gland and as basal cell adenoma (5).

Seminal Vesicles with Atypical Epithelial Cells. Encountering portions of seminal vesicles in biopsies from the prostate is not unusual. To avoid misdiagnosing the condition as prostatic carcinoma (6,7), the pathologist must be aware of the histologic characteristics of seminal vesicles and the possibility of atypical cells in the epithelium. Seminal vesicles are characterized by irregular glandular structures that produce a large number of folds; they are connected to a central lumen and lined by columnar cells having lipochrome pigment (Fig. 9.6). When atypical cells with a high nucleocytoplasmic ratio, hyperchromatic nuclei, and prominent nucleoli are seen in the epithelium of seminal vesicles of middle-aged and elderly adults, they may be unrelated to any disease (Fig. 9.7). The clue to the reactive or non-neoplastic nature of these cells is that, of all the cells lining a given space, only one or two show the atypical features while the rest are unremarkable columnar cells.

Transitional Cell Metaplasia. Although recognizing transitional cell metaplasia in the prostate is not difficult, the presence of atypia in these

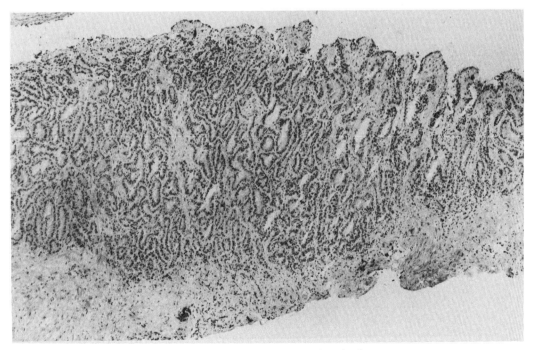

Figure 9.6. Frozen section of seminal vesicle. Small, irregular glands.

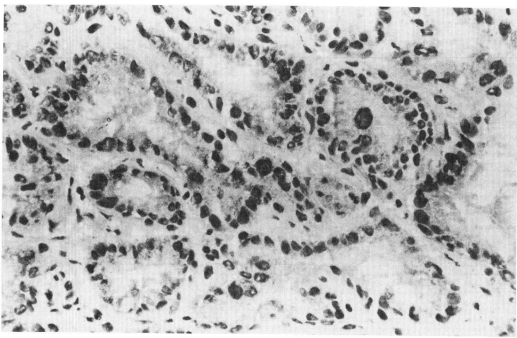

Figure 9.7. Seminal vesicle showing small dense granules of lipochrome pigment in the cytoplasm of the epithelial cells. A few enlarged, atypical cells are also seen. Compare with Fig. 9.1.

foci of metaplasia may cause confusion between simple metaplasia and poorly differentiated carcinoma of prostate. At our hospital, frozen section examination of 172 needle biopsies of the prostate resulted in false negative evaluations of six biopsied samples (3.5%) and a false positive evaluation of one (0.6%). The one false positive diagnosis was florid transitional cell metaplasia with atypia, which was misinterpreted as carcinoma (8).

In this situation, low power microscopic examination of the frozen section is of great value because, if some acini are involved by transitional cell metaplasia, the process is also evident in the prostatic ducts (Fig. 9.8). Usually transitional cell metaplasia in the prostate is accompanied by prostatic infarction, prostatitis, or both, without the cytologic features of carcinoma. When the frozen section contains atypical cells in areas of transitional cell metaplasia, we prefer to defer the diagnosis until we can examine permanent sections.

Fragments of Mucin. The pathologist must know what technique was employed in performing the needle biopsy of the prostate. If the biopsy results in penetration of the rectal wall (transrectal biopsy), fragments of mucin may be encountered between the prostatic tissue fragments and raises the possibility of mucinous prostatic carcinoma. Information about biopsy route coupled with the absence of other histologic features of carcinoma will indicate that the process is benign. A transperineal biopsy of the prostate avoids this potential frozen section problem.

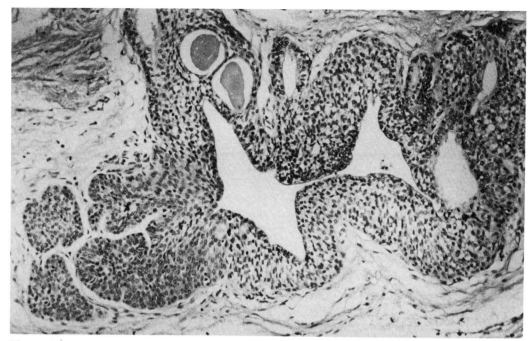

Figure 9.8. Transitional cell metaplasia of prostatic ducts.

Surgical Management and Implications of Frozen Section Diagnosis

Before performing a prostatectomy for prostatic carcinoma, the surgeon may request frozen section analysis of the patient's pelvic lymph nodes (9). In this situation, the lymph nodes are bisected, both halves are submitted on one slide, and sections from two different levels are microscopically examined. When metastatic prostatic carcinoma is identified in lymph nodes, even in cases where only a single micrometastasis is found, the surgeon does not perform the planned prostatectomy (see Chapter 12, **Lymph Nodes**).

Usually, when prostatic carcinoma is diagnosed from a needle biopsy of the prostate of a patient with disseminated disease, a bilateral orchiectomy is performed. This is not done, however, when the diagnosis is transitional cell carcinoma of the prostate, a prostatic carcinoma unresponsive to hormonal treatment (10,11). Failure to recognize transitional cell carcinoma in a prostatic biopsy will result in an unnecessary orchiectomy.

BLADDER

During a partial or total resection of a cancerous bladder, frozen section analysis of ureteral and urethral margins may be requested. Interpretation of these frozen sections usually is not difficult, even when the epithelium shows focal atypia. Only the diagnosis of carcinoma in situ or invasive carcinoma present at the margins justifies a new resection margin.

The presence of von Brunn's nests may create some difficulties in interpreting margins of resection. Von Brunn's nests are proliferations of transitional cell epithelium extending into the wall of different portions of the urinary tract. The absence of significant atypia in the area in question as well as in the overlying epithelium, the absence of stromal reaction, and the superficial location of the nests (usually involving only the lamina propria, and rarely, superficial muscularis) are indications of the benign nature of this process.

KIDNEY

We rarely evaluate frozen sections of the kidney because needle, incisional, and excisional biopsies of the kidney are not performed often at our institution. Although we often evaluate the specimens from a nephrectomy or radical nephrectomy, a frozen section is usually not necessary because it does not change the operative management. One exception, however, is the examination of partial nephrectomy specimens. In this situation the pathologist must evaluate the lesion and determine its benign or malignant nature, and assess the margin of resection.

Two lesions that must be differentiated from renal cell carcinoma in a partial nephrectomy specimen are benign multilocular cyst and renal oncocytoma.

Renal Cell Carcinoma versus Benign Multilocular Cyst

Benign multilocular cyst may be very difficult to differentiate from cystic renal cell carcinoma. An embarrassing situation is created when the pathologist, after opening the kidney, reports to the surgeon that the lesion

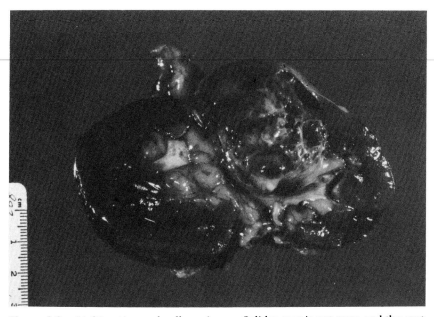

Figure 9.9. Multicystic renal cell carcinoma. Solid tumor is not seen, and the cyst walls are extremely thin.

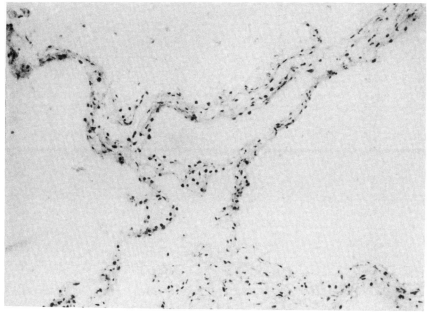

Figure 9.10. Multicystic renal cell carcinoma. Frozen section showing cells with uniform nuclei and poorly visualized cytoplasm.

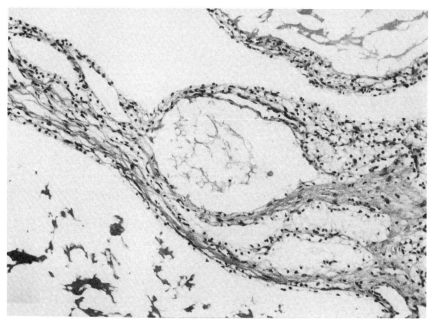

Figure 9.11. Multicystic renal cell carcinoma. Same case as Fig. 9.10. In this permanent section, the clear cytoplasm of the cells is easily appreciated. The stroma is hypocellular.

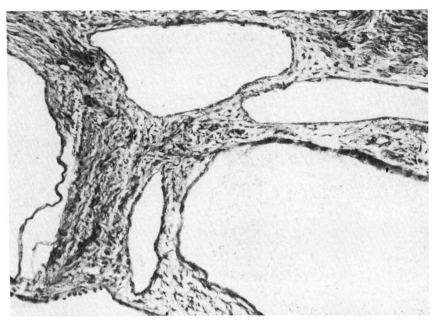

Figure 9.12. Benign multilocular cysts. The cystic spaces are lined by low cuboidal to flattened epithelial cells.

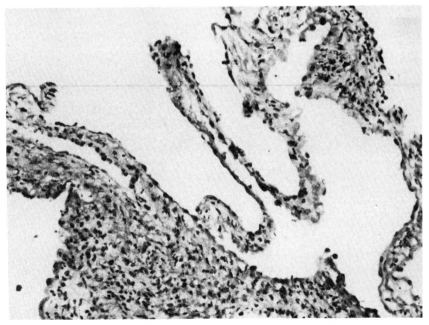

Figure 9.13. Benign multilocular cyst. Same case as Fig. 9.12. The stroma in this lesion is more cellular than the stroma in multicystic renal cell carcinoma. (Compare with Figs. 9.10 and 9.11).

in the kidney is only a multicystic structure—there is no evidence of renal cell carcinoma. The next day, after examining the permanent section, the pathologist finds a cystic renal cell carcinoma and has to reverse the diagnosis (Fig. 9.9). In the case of this differential diagnosis, if the pathologist decides to perform a frozen section analysis of a kidney, he should be aware of the difficulties inherent in diagnosing cystic renal cell carcinoma. Usually, the walls of cystic carcinoma are lined by low cuboidal or flattened epithelium. It is often difficult to identify these epithelial cells in frozen section, much less to render a diagnosis of carcinoma (Figs. 9.10 and 9.11). The stroma of cystic carcinoma is usually less cellular than that of multilobular benign cysts (Figs. 9.12 and 9.13). The pathologist must examine one or more frozen sections from any solid or papillary areas before reporting the lesion as a non-neoplastic renal cyst.

Renal Cell Carcinoma versus Oncocytoma

Differentiating renal oncocytoma from oncocytic renal cell carcinoma is also difficult, and whenever possible it should be reserved until permanent sections can be examined. Table 9.2 is a guide for separating these two entities (12–14).

Metastatic Renal Cell Carcinoma

The diagnosis of renal cell carcinoma in a nephrectomy specimen is fairly easy because of its primary location, but recognizing renal cell carcinoma in a metastasis can be extremely difficult. In our experience, the main problem is that the typical clear cell appearance of the metastatic tumor cells is not visualized as clearly in frozen section as in permanent section. In frozen section, the clear cytoplasm of these cells stained with hematoxylin and eosin appears light pink (Fig. 9.14). When this happens, and when we suspect the possibility of clear cell carcinoma, we prefer to fix the unstained frozen section slide in formalin for one minute and then overstain it with hematoxylin for more than 2 minutes (Fig. 9.15). The cells' classic clear cytoplasm can also be observed in cytologic preparations (Fig.

Table 9.2.
Comparison of Renal Oncocytoma and Renal Cell Carcinoma

	Diagnosis	
Examination	Renal Oncocytoma	Renal Cell Carcinoma
Gross	Well demarcated	Infiltrating
	Central scar	No central scar
	Tan-brown	Yellow
	Rare hemorrhage	Frequent hemorrhage
Microscopic	Pure oncocytes	Oncocytes and clear cells
Anaplasia	Absent	Present
Necrosis	Absent	Present
Mitoses	Absent	Present
Nucleoli	Absent	Frequently present
Clear cells	Absent	May be focally present
Papillary areas	Absent	Frequent

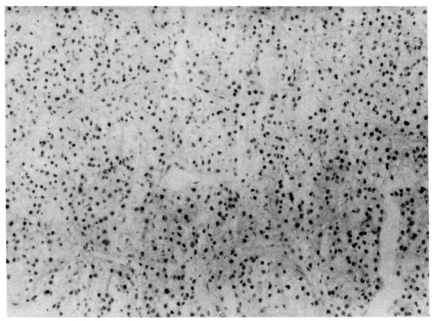

Figure 9.14. Renal cell carcinoma. Frozen section. The clear appearance of the cytoplasm is not well appreciated.

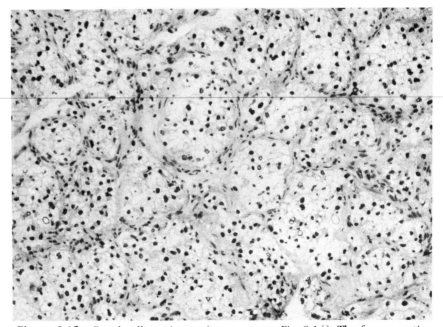

Figure 9.15. Renal cell carcinoma (same case as Fig. 9.14). The frozen section was fixed in formaldehyde solution for 1 min and overstained with hematoxylin for 2 min. The clear cytoplasm is now easily identified.

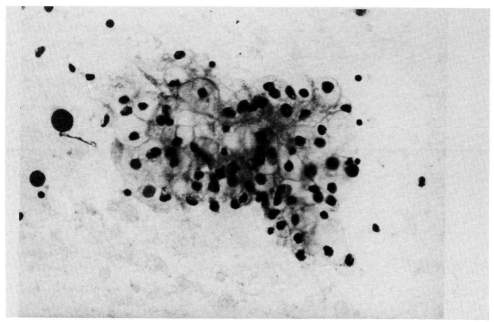

Figure 9.16. Touch imprint of renal cell carcinoma showing cells with clear cytoplasm.

9.16). With these minor variations in technique both the cytoplasm and cytoplasmic membrane of the clear cells can be identified better. We find these technical variations equally applicable to other neoplasms that have abundant clear cell cytoplasm.

REFERENCES

1. Carstens PHB: Perineural glands in normal and hyperplastic prostates. *J Urol* 123:686–688, 1980.
2. Byar PD, Mostofi FK, Veterans Administration Cooperative Urological Research Group: Carcinoma of the prostate: Prognostic evaluation of certain pathologic features in 208 radical prostatectomies examined by the step-section technique. *Cancer* 30:5–13, 1972.
3. Manley CB: The striated muscle of the prostate. *J Urol* 95:234–240, 1966.
4. Cleary KR, Choi HY, Ayala AG: Basal cell hyperplasia of the prostate. *Am J Clin Pathol* 80:850–854, 1983.
5. Lin JI, Cohen EL, Villacin AB, Garcia MB, Tseng CH: Basal cell adenoma of prostate. *Urology* 11:409–410, 1978.
6. Arias-Stella J, Takano-Moron J: Atypical epithelial changes in the seminal vesicles. *Arch Pathol* 66:761–766, 1958.
7. Kuo T, Gomez LG: Monstrous epithelial cells in human epididymis and seminal vesicles: A pseudomalignant change. *Am J Surg Pathol* 5:483–490, 1981.
8. Johnson DE: Cancer of the prostate: Overview. In Johnson DE, Boileau MA (eds): *Genitourinary Tumors: Fundamental Principles and Surgical Techniques.* New York, Grune & Stratton, 1982, p 1.
9. Kramolowsky EV, Narayana AS, Platz CE, Loening SA: The frozen section in lymphadenectomy for carcinoma of the prostate. *J Urol* 131:899–900, 1984.

10. Taylor G, Blom J: Transitional cell carcinoma of prostate. *Cancer* 51:1800–1802, 1982.
11. Johnson DE, Hogan JM, Ayala AG: Transitional cell carcinoma of the prostate. A clinical morphological study. *Cancer* 29:287–293, 1972.
12. Merino MJ, Livolsi VA: Oncocytomas of the kidney. *Cancer* 50:1852–1856, 1982.
13. Choi H, Almagro UA, McManus JT, Norback DH, Jacobs SC: Renal oncocytoma: A clinicopathologic study. *Cancer* 51:1887–1896, 1983.
14. Farrow GM, Melamed MR, Haggitt RC: Fall Anatomic Pathology Slide Seminar, Cases 2 and 3, Urologic Neoplasms. *American Society of Clinical Pathologists,* Nov. 1-2, 1984.

10

Mediastinum

B. Balfour Kraemer, M.D.

Frozen section interpretation of mediastinal masses is often difficult. Accuracy in diagnosis depends upon knowledge of the patient's clinical history, the anatomic site of the mass, the radiographic presentation, and representative tissue.

Resection is the preferred treatment for some mediastinal masses (1). The operative approach for a given mass is dependent on its anatomic location. For an anterior mediastinal mass, a median sternotomy is performed to allow full exposure of the entire anterior mediastinal compartment. Masses located within the middle or posterior compartments are explored via thoracotomy. If there is evidence of secondary extension of a posterior mediastinal mass into the spinal canal, a one-stage combined resection may be performed (2).

The most common primary mediastinal masses, according to age group, anatomic compartment, and expected frequency are listed in Table 10.1.

INDICATIONS FOR FROZEN SECTION

During mediastinal exploration, most surgeons request a frozen section diagnosis of a mediastinal mass to rapidly establish a tissue diagnosis. Frozen section evaluation of surgical margins may be requested at the time of surgery when complete excision is anticipated. The extent of mediastinal disease is sometimes greater than that predicted clinically or radiographically. In this situation, frozen section interpretation of involved tissues, such as lymph node or lung, aids in determining the feasibility of complete resection.

TYPES OF SPECIMENS

Needle, Flexible Bronchoscopic and Mediastinoscopic Biopsy

Tissue core and flexible bronchoscopic biopsies are not routinely employed in the frozen section evaluation of primary mediastinal masses, since these procedures are high risk and the small amount of material obtained

Table 10.1.
Mediastinal Masses According to Age Group, Site, and Frequency

	Anterior	Middle	Posterior
Child	Lymphoid hyperplasia or lymphoma (80%) Germ cell tumor (10%) Cyst (10%)	Lymphoid hyperplasia or lymphoma (90%) Cyst (10%)	Neoplasms of sympathetic origin (over 90%) Cyst (5%) Paraganglioma (5%)
Adult	Thymoma (50%) Lymphoma (20%) Germ cell tumor (10%) Cyst (10%) Paraganglioma, ectopia, sarcoma (10%)	Lymphoma (80%) Cyst (20%)	Neoplasms of nerve sheath origin (over 90%) Paraganglioma, cyst (10%)

is often inadequate for accurate tissue diagnosis (3-5). If a mediastinal mass appears widely invasive and unresectable by clinical evaluation, a needle biopsy may be performed in order to establish a tissue diagnosis for palliative therapy. Similarly, a tissue diagnosis may indicate the need for curative irradiation and/or chemotherapy rather than ablative surgical therapy. Cervical mediastinoscopy may be used to evaluate the middle compartment of the mediastinum (e.g., paratracheal and subcarinal lymph nodes), but is rarely used in conjunction with thoracotomy in evaluation of mediastinal masses. Anterior mediastinotomy (Chamberlain procedure) allows assessment and biopsy of lesions in the anterior compartment of the mediastinum (6).

Anterior Compartmental Dissection

An anterior mediastinal mass is usually explored via median sternotomy because it provides the best access to the entire thymus, anterior mediastinal lymph nodes, pericardium, and mediastinal fat. By opening the pleura, the surgeon can also perform most pulmonary resections.

Thoracotomy Tissue

Resection of an anterior mediastinal mass via thoracotomy is often more difficult. The surgeon may only submit biopsies. For posterior mediastinal masses that secondarily extend into the spinal canal, soft tissue from laminectomy may be submitted for frozen section to assess extent of disease.

FROZEN SECTION DIAGNOSIS OF MEDIASTINAL NEOPLASMS

Thymoma

Thymoma is the most common primary neoplasm of the anterior compartment and is one of the most common neoplasms arising from the mediastinum; treatment of choice is complete resection. Accurate frozen section interpretation is imperative (7–10).

The many different histologic appearances of thymoma along with the histologic variation present in any one thymoma can easily create diagnostic confusion at the time of frozen section, especially if only a small piece of the neoplasm is examined histologically.

The main histologic patterns of thymoma and their differential diagnoses are listed in Table 10.2.

Lymphocytic Thymoma

Lymphocytic thymoma presents special problems at the time of frozen section, primarily since it is so easily confused with malignant lymphoma. Accurate frozen section interpretation can be exceedingly difficult if the tissue sample is small and if the quality of the frozen section is less than adequate. The most common diagnostic errors are to misinterpret lymphocytic thymoma as lymphocytic lymphoma, or nodular sclerosing Hodgkin's disease. Since lymphocytic thymoma is, by definition, composed of predominantly lymphocytes (11), distinguishing it from a lymphoproliferative lesion can be difficult (Figs. 10.1 and 10.2). Approximately 20% of lymphocytic thymomas exhibit a "starry sky" pattern, a pattern usually ascribed to malignant lymphomas. To complicate the matter further, lymphocytic thymomas characteristically have fibrous trabeculae, which can be easily misinterpreted as the sclerotic bands of nodular sclerosing Hodgkin's disease.

Table 10.2.
Frozen Section Appearance of Thymoma

Predominant Pattern	Differential Diagnosis
Lymphocytic	Malignant lymphoma Hodgkin's disease
Epithelial	Malignant lymphoma Germinoma Angiofollicular hyperplasia Metastatic carcinoma
Cystic	Thymic cyst Endodermal sinus tumor
Spindled	Carcinoid Fibrous mesothelioma Nerve sheath neoplasm Paraganglioma Soft tissue sarcoma

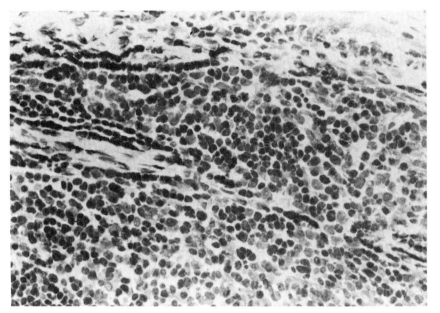

Figure 10.1. Frozen section of thymoma. Lymphocytes predominate.

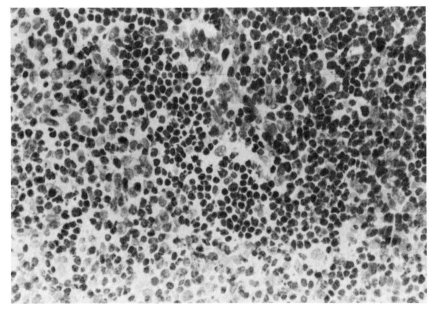

Figure 10.2. Frozen section of lymphocytic thymoma. Epithelial cell component is poorly visualized.

The Epithelial Component. Depending on the quality of the frozen section, the epithelial cell population may or may not be obvious. In hematoxylin and eosin stained frozen sections, the epithelial cells assume a faintly eosinophilic appearance. They may superficially resemble benign histiocytes or lacunar cells or nodular sclerosing Hodgkin's disease. To visualize this minor population of cells:

1.) Perform a touch preparation, sampling as much surface area as possible. The biphasic cell population is usually shown to better advantage on a touch imprint (Figs. 10.3 and 10.4). Cytologically, an epithelial cell is four to five times the size of a lymphocyte and has a vesicular nucleus with a tiny nucleolus. Lymphocytes in lymphocytic thymoma may appear slightly pleomorphic, and may have mitotic figures. The degree of pleomorphism or mitotic activity in a touch imprint should not cause alarm if an epithelial cell population is recognized.

2.) Overstain the frozen section with eosin, especially acidified eosin (12), which will accentuate the cytoplasm of the epithelial cells.

3.) Look for the epithelial cells adjacent to the fibrous trabeculae. The epithelial component of a lymphocytic thymoma always appears to be better visualized at the periphery of lobules (Fig. 10.5).

Arrangement of Fibrous Trabeculae. Architecturally, thymomas typically have a multilobulated appearance. The fibrous trabeculae are often thin and regular, serving to compartmentalize the thymoma into fairly uniform lobules. This is in contrast to the collagenous bands of sclerosis of nodular sclerosing Hodgkin's disease, in which there is no orderly arrangement of collagen deposition.

Perivascular Spacing. This is another characteristic feature of thymoma, and is usually easily identified in lymphocytic thymoma. Perivascular spacing is not a feature of malignant lymphoma. Expanded perivascular spaces may be empty, creating a halo-like effect around vessels, or they may be partially organized with hyalinized fibrous tissue. Occasionally, perivascular spaces are filled with proteinaceous material, lymphocytes, or foamy macrophages.

Medullary Differentiation. This key feature is apparently restricted to lymphocytic thymomas (13), and when present can be very helpful. Foci of medullary differentiation are defined as epithelial cells mixed with lymphocytes where the epithelial-lymphocytic ratio is higher than that in the surrounding thymoma. On frozen section these foci can easily be confused with germinal centers or nodules of follicular lymphoma. One distinguishing feature of medullary differentiation is the frequent associated presence of Hassall's corpuscles.

Lymphocytic thymoma is a common histologic type of thymoma associated with myasthenia gravis (14, 15). Syndrome-linked lymphocytic thymomas often have lymphoid follicles with germinal centers scattered within the thymoma. Residual thymus often has a prominent reactive follicular hyperplasia.

In contrast to thymoma, malignant lymphomas that involve the mediastinum may involve mediastinal lymph nodes, thymus, or both. When the thymus is involved, Hassall's corpuscles tend to resist lymphomatous

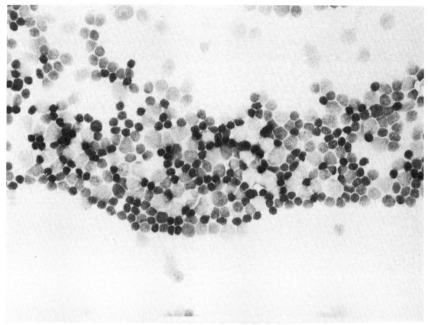

Figure 10.3. Touch imprint of lymphocytic thymoma. Both epithelial and lymphocytic cell populations are well visualized. Hematoxylin and eosin.

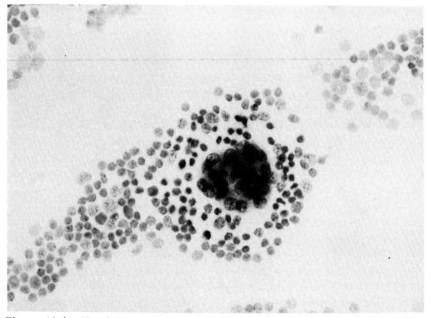

Figure 10.4. Touch imprint of lymphocytic thymoma. Epithelial cell cluster. Hematoxylin and eoxin.

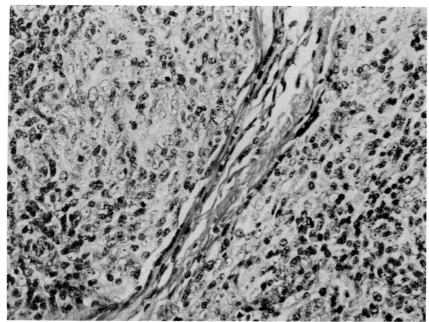

Figure 10.5. Thymoma. Epithelial component lies adjacent to fibrous trabeculum.

infiltrates. Lymphomatous involvement of lymph nodes may extend into mediastinal or pericardial fat, but usually preserves the fibroadipose network.

Epithelial Thymoma

In contrast to lymphocytic thymoma, this particular type of thymoma would be expected to pose fewer diagnostic problems since the epithelial component is so obvious. Unfortunately, this is not always the case. Thymomas having an epithelial cell predominance can be easily confused with a variety of other neoplasms on frozen section examination. Similar to lymphocytic thymoma, epithelial thymoma can be misinterpreted as malignant lymphoma, but for reasons different than those described for lymphocytic thymoma. The vesicular nuclei of epithelial thymoma can simulate the large transformed lymphocytes of diffuse large cell lymphoma. The important histologic distinction is made most easily by identification of other features common to thymoma, such as perivascular spaces and fibrous trabeculae. Germinoma is also easily confused with epithelial thymoma, since it has a minor lymphocytic cell population and fibrous septae, both of which are common morphologic features of epithelial thymoma. Again, the presence of other architectural features is helpful in distinguishing between these two neoplasms. Germinoma is typically monotonous in its pattern and may have an associated granulomatous component. Epithelial thymoma usually has a variety of patterns from one microscopic field to the next, and also has perivascular spaces, features absent in germinoma. Epithelial thymoma can also be confused with thymic carcinoid, since one of the common patterns in epithelial thymoma is a pseudorosette pattern. On frozen section, the distinction between a true rosette and a pseudorosette may be difficult, especially if hematoxylin staining is excessive. This distinction at the time of frozen section is not absolutely essential, since the treatment of choice for both neoplasms is resection. Many patients with thymic carcinoid have an associated Cushing's syndrome (16), and thus the clinical history may be helpful in distinguishing between the two. Tissue for diagnostic electron microscopy should be procured in such a situation.

A specific type of reactive lymphoid hyperplasia termed giant lymph node hyperplasia, Castleman's disease (17), or angiofollicular hyperplasia (18) is often mistaken for thymoma or lymphoma. Giant lymph node hyperplasia has a predilection for the anterior mediastinum, and typically involves lymph nodes rather than the thymus. Grossly, it is usually encapsulated, often attached to the carina or a main stem bronchus. Intraoperative resection often causes excessive bleeding. The hyaline-vascular type of giant lymph node hyperplasia causes confusion, both on frozen and permanent sections. Randomly scattered atretic lymphoid follicles with concentrically arranged hyaline strands bear resemblance to Hassall's corpuscles and constitute the main detour from a correct diagnosis of giant lymph node hyperplasia. The viewer mistakes the pattern for thymoma. Hassall's corpuscles are rare in thymoma and are not a feature of giant lymph node hyperplasia. Furthermore, the fibrous trabeculae, perivascular spaces, and epithelial cell population common to thymoma are absent in giant lymph node hyperplasia.

Carcinoma metastatic to the thymus is rare and is almost always from a primary lung tumor. A frozen section diagnosis of thymic metastasis is often difficult to establish, since some thymic carcinomas are histologically indistinguishable from primary lung carcinomas, such as small cell or epidermoid carcinoma (19, 20). In the event that a bonafide thymic carcinoma is suspected at the time of frozen section, the pathologist should inform the surgeon that the thymic neoplasm could be either primary or metastatic. In this situation, the surgeon will probably explore the mediastinum further and may submit one or more mediastinal lymph nodes for frozen section. If lymph nodes are positive, a debulking procedure may be performed, or the surgeon may terminate the procedure.

Cystic Thymoma

Large thymomas tend to undergo cystic degeneration. The main differential diagnosis includes thymic cyst. If only one section taken from a cystic area is examined by frozen section, this distinction may be difficult or impossible. Solid portions of the mass should be sampled in an effort to find residual neoplasm. The epithelial lining of a cystic thymoma may have squamous metaplasia and may resemble other mediastinal cysts, or even cystic teratoma. Usually, the location and cyst wall components help to make the distinction (see Mediastinal Cysts, this Chapter).

Rarely, the cystic pattern of thymoma forms a microcystic arrangement and simulates the reticulated pattern of endodermal sinus tumor (yolk sac tumor) (Figs. 10.6 and 10.7) (21, 22). Pure endodermal sinus tumor usually presents in young males, in contrast to thymoma, which is a neoplasm of

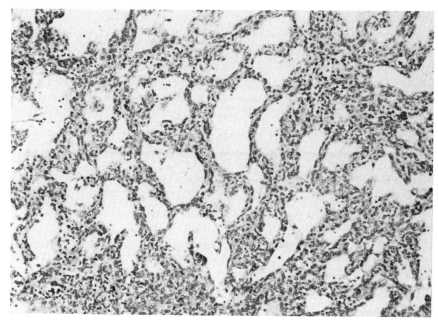

Figure 10.6. Microcystic thymoma.

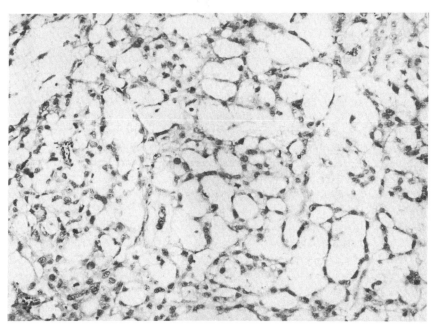

Figure 10.7. Endodermal sinus tumor with reticulated pattern. Compare with Fig. 10.6.

elderly patients. Moreover, endodermal sinus tumor is usually combined with other germ cell components, typically embryonal carcinoma and/or germinoma. The presence of papillary formations with Schiller-Duval bodies, atypical mitoses, zones of necrosis, and hyaline globules (α-fetoprotein) are features of endodermal sinus tumor that serve to distinguish it from a thymoma having microcystic features. For a more detailed discussion of the histologic features of germ cell neoplams, the reader is referred to a comprehensive discussion of the topic (23).

Spindled Thymoma

One of the most frequent histologic variations of thymoma is a spindled pattern, in which the architecture may resemble carcinoid, fibrous mesothelioma, fibrous histiocytoma, hemangiopericytoma, or paraganglioma. The frozen section interpretation in such a situation may be extremely difficult. In reality, a precise histologic distinction is not essential, since the treatment for all the above neoplams is resection. In this setting, it is probably best to classify such lesions as "spindle cell neoplasm," notifying the surgeon of the diagnostic problem. Tissue for diagnostic electron microscopy should be obtained.

Fibrous mesothelioma rarely presents in the mediastinum (24) and should be considered in the differential diagnosis of spindled thymoma. Grossly, it is usually encapsulated, similar to thymoma, and attached by a pleural pedicle. An intact layer of mesothelial cells overlying the neoplasm is a helpful histologic feature on frozen section.

Other primary spindled cell neoplasms are rare in the anterior mediastinum and include nerve sheath neoplasms, vascular neoplasms, and fibrosarcoma. Accurate frozen section of such neoplasms can be exceedingly difficult, and usually requires electron microscopy.

Thymoma: Benign or Malignant?

Once a diagnosis of thymoma has been established by frozen section, the question of "benign" versus "malignant" thymoma arises. The pathological assessment of "benign" or "malignant" thymoma is of little or no importance at the time of frozen section. The most important factor is resectability of the mass, which is a surgical decision. The pathologist will not assist the surgeon by informing him that the thymoma in question is probably malignant. A detailed assessment of mitotic rate or cellular pleomorphism only wastes valuable patient anesthesia time and does not change the operative management once a diagnosis of thymoma is established. Even for the rare thymic carcinomas, treatment of choice is total resection. The histologic distinction between thymoma and thymic carcinoma is often exceedingly difficult even on permanent section, and this distinction at the time of resection is irrelevant to the intraoperative management.

The following enumerates the criteria for determining resectability. In fact, these are often the most reliable indicators of malignant behavior: 1) encasement of great vessels; 2) invasion of hilum; 3) invasion of epicardium and/or myocardium; 4) pulmonary metastases; 5) extensive pleural seeding; 6) pleural effusion.

Thymoma has a peculiar tendency to spread along the pleural surfaces by so-called droplet formation, in which the metastases appear as grossly discrete nodules (10). Some surgeons will resect pleural metastases along with the primary mass. If there is extensive pleural seeding, or if a pleural effusion is encountered, the surgeon will probably not perform a definitive resection. Frozen sections of the pleura may be required to confirm the diagnostic impression.

Germ Cell Neoplasms

The most common primary germ cell neoplasms of the anterior mediastinum are mature cystic teratoma and germinoma. The latter are more common in males, whereas the former present in an equal sex ratio.

The differential diagnostic considerations in the frozen section evaluation of germ cell neoplasms of the mediastinum are listed in Table 10.3.

Germinoma

Since germinoma often has an accompanying lymphocytic component, diagnostic confusion with malignant lymphoma or thymoma is not uncommon. Similarly, germinoma may have a granulomatous response as part of the neoplasm (25). If this is an extensive process, diagnostic confusion with granulomatous inflammation, such as that seen in sarcoidosis, can occur.

The distinction between germinoma and thymoma has already been discussed. Distinction between lymphoma and germinoma can be exceedingly difficult. If the preoperative clinical workup has failed to prove the germ cell origin of the neoplasm (26), the diagnosis is best deferred.

Mature Cystic Teratoma

Mature cystic teratoma represents one of the most common type of mediastinal germ cell neoplasms, and may be confused with a bronchial hamartoma or mediastinal cyst. Teratomas may erode into the tracheo-

Table 10.3.
Frozen Section Evaluation of Germ Cell Neoplasms of the Mediastinum

Histologic Type	Differential Diagnosis
Germinoma	Malignant lymphoma Thymoma Carcinoma Granulomatous inflammation
Mature cystic teratoma	Hamartoma Mediastinal cyst
Embryonal carcinoma	Poorly differentiated carcinoma
Endodermal sinus tumor	Poorly differentiated carcinoma Thymoma Carcinoid
Choriocarcinoma	Poorly differentiated carcinoma

bronchial tree, and be surrounded by extensive necrosis. The presence of teratomatous elements in nonseminomatous germ cell tumors (27–29) should not be confused with the aforementioned entities. Bronchial hamartomas are usually identified grossly by the surgeon as a cartilagenous mass which is incidentally shelled out from the lung during an operative procedure. The distinction between bronchial hamartoma and teratoma is also discussed in detail in Chapter 6, **Lung**.

Mediastinal Cysts

Mediastinal cysts are developmental anomalies and are typically located in the anterior or middle compartment. The usual management for all mediastinal cysts is resection. Precise location of the cyst is very helpful in characterizing it as to specific type. Pericardial cysts are usually located at the right cardiophrenic angle and are lined by mesothelial cells. Bronchogenic cysts are typically found in the subcarinal area. They are often attached to the anterior esophageal wall and are lined by respiratory type mucosa, with or without squamous metaplasia. True esophageal cysts may be lined by epithelium similar to that of bronchogenic cysts and may be difficult to distinguish from bronchogenic cysts. The presence of a double layer of smooth muscle within the cyst wall is helpful in identifying a cyst of esophageal origin. Ideally, the frozen section should include a full thickness section of the cyst wall. The rare gastroenteric cyst, typically found in the posterior mediastinum, is the only cystic maldevelopment associated with other anomalies, specifically vertebral malformations (30). Technically, gastroenteric cysts are duplications of the gut and may be lined by gastric and/or intestinal type epithelium. Mediastinal cysts having an epithelial lining of respiratory epithelium without cartilage or smooth muscle within the cyst wall are probably best classified as undifferentiated cysts of foregut origin.

In contrast to mediastinal cysts, mature cystic teratoma is usually lined by stratified squamous epithelium and contains both ectodermal and endodermal derivatives within its cyst wall. The procedure of choice for mature cystic teratoma, as for mediastinal cysts, is complete resection.

Nonseminomatous Germ Cell Tumors

The differential diagnosis of nonseminomatous germ cell tumors, specifically endodermal sinus tumor is discussed under a separate section (p. 242).

Neurogenic Neoplasms

Neurogenic (sympathetic nerve and nerve sheath) neoplasms are the most common neoplasms of the mediastinum, and typically arise in the posterior mediastinum. They are one of the most common mediastinal neoplasms of childhood (23, 31-34). The frozen section diagnosis of sympathetic neurogenic neoplasms is usually straightforward, with the exception of neuroblastoma. The main frozen section differential diagnosis for neuroblastoma includes malignant lymphoma, Ewing's sarcoma, and embryonal rhabdomyosarcoma. The patient's age, location of the mass, and presence of elevated urinary catecholamines usually establishes the diagnosis in the majority of instances (31). Tissue for electron microscopy should always be submitted in cases where there is uncertainty about the frozen section diagnosis. Although patients with clinical stage I neuroblastoma usually undergo surgery (31), approximately 65% of these patients harbor metastases at the time of diagnosis. After adjuvant therapy, complete resection may be undertaken (34).

SPECIAL PROBLEMS IN FROZEN SECTION DIAGNOSIS OF MEDIASTINAL TISSUES

Involuted Thymus

With aging, the lymphoid component of the thymus decreases in absolute volume. Fat replaces much of the cortex. Within the medulla, Hassall's corpuscles become prominent, and medullary epithelial cells assume a spindled configuration. During mediastinal exploration, the surgeon may not recognize the thymus as such, and may submit it or a part of it for frozen section.

The frozen section appearance of involuted thymic tissue may mislead the pathologist into believing that he is dealing with a mediastinal lymph node containing foci of metastatic squamous carcinoma. Rendering such a frozen section diagnosis is a common diagnostic pitfall. The surgeon may terminate the procedure because the frozen section diagnosis has lead him to believe that the patient has inoperable bronchogenic carcinoma. The pathologist should be certain that the tissue in question is actually a lymph node before rendering such a diagnosis.

The problem of involuted thymus is also discussed in Chapter 6, **Lung.**

Aberrant Thyroid and Parathyroid

Mediastinal thyroid tissue usually represents retrosternal extension of a goiter. Rarely, there is no anatomic connection with the cervical thyroid. The inferior parathyroid glands and the thymus share a common embryonic lineage from the third and fourth branchial pouches. During embryogenesis, parathyroid tissue may descend into the mediastinum. Large parathyroid adenomas primary in the neck may descend via fascial planes into the anterior or posterior mediastinum. Rarely, parathyroid tissue may be encountered in frozen section evaluation of mediastinal masses and must be differentiated from a carcinoid tumor, lymphoid proliferation, or even germinoma. During parathyroid exploration (see Chapter 11, **Parathyroid**) mediastinal tissue, especially thymus, may be submitted in an attempt to identify parathyroid tissue if exploration of the neck is unsatisfactory.

Granulomatous Inflammation

Granulomatous inflammation involving the mediastinum may be encountered in neoplastic or infectious processes. The differential diagnosis of granulomatous processes involving the mediastinum is listed in Table 10.4.

Table 10.4.
Granulomatous Processes of the Mediastinum[a]

Diagnosis	Type Granuloma	Tissue
Granulomatous mediastinitis (tuberculosis, histoplasmosis)	Necrotizing caseating, noncaseating	Lymph node, lung, soft tissue
Sarcoidosis	Necrotizing or nonnecrotizing	Lymph node
Germinoma	Epithelioid with lymphocytic component	Thymus, lymph node, soft tissue
Hodgkin's Disease	Epithelioid	Thymus, lymph node

[a]Adapted from Goodwin RA, Nickell JA, Des Prez RM: Mediastinal fibrosis complicating healed primary histoplasmosis and tuberculosis. *Medicine* 51:227–246, 1972; Schrowengerdt CG, Suyemoto R, Main FB: Granulomatous fibrous mediastinitis. A review and analysis of 180 cases. *J Thorac Cardiovasc Surg* 57:365–379, 1969; and Strimlan CV, Dines DE, Payne WS: Mediastinal granuloma. *Mayo Clin Proc* 50:702–705, 1975. (Refs. 35–37).
If the frozen section displays granulomatous inflammation, tissue culture for microbiological studies, especially Mycobacteria and fungi, should be obtained.

WHEN TO DEFER A FROZEN SECTION

Possible Malignant Lymphoma

Lymphoma and reactive lymphoid hyperplasia (specifically angiofollicular hyperplasia) (17) can present as a primary mediastinal mass. If the frozen section of a mediastinal mass is suspicious for a lymphoproliferative process, the diagnosis should be deferred after notifying the surgeon that the tissue in question could possibly contain a malignant lymphoma. Representative tissue should be biopsied as atraumatically as possible and submitted for special studies, including electron microscopy when necesssary.

The frozen section problem posed in distinguishing lymphocytic thymoma from malignant lymphoma is discussed in detail in a separate part of this chapter (p. 237).

The role of surgical management in malignant lymphoma is controversial (38-40). Some surgeons proceed with partial or complete resection even after the diagnosis has been deferred, mainly on the justification that the mediastinum has already been entered and that postoperative therapy will be facilitated by less tumor burden. Most surgeons will also attempt to resect as much tissue as possible when there is compression of vital structures and/or if the thymus is involved.

Sclerosis

Approximately 50% of all malignant lymphomas arising in the mediastinum are Hodgkin's disease, nodular sclerosing type (Figs. 10.8–10.10). The surgeon may biopsy the periphery of an involved lymph node and submit it for frozen section. Since the capsule and fibrous septae of lymph nodes affected by nodular sclerosing Hodgkin's disease are characteristically

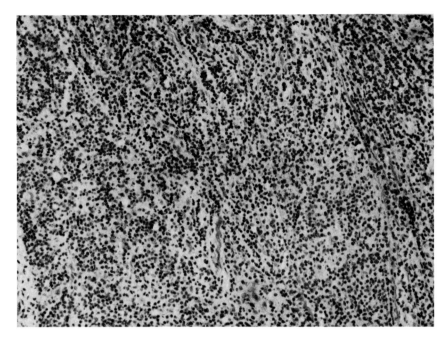

Figure 10.8. Frozen section of Hodgkin's disease, nodular sclerosing type.

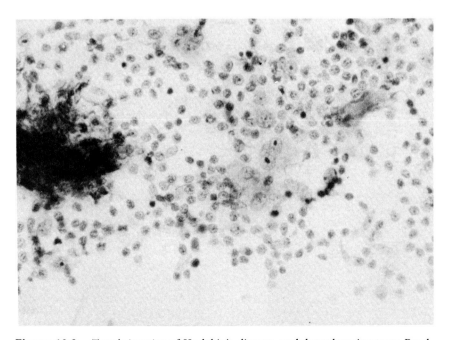

Figure 10.9. Touch imprint of Hodgkin's disease, nodular sclerosing type. Reed-Sternberg cells are present. Hematoxylin and eosin.

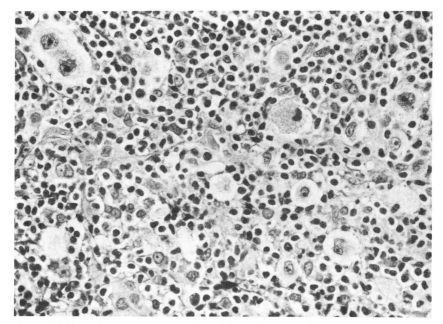

Figure 10.10. Permanent section. Hodgkin's disease, nodular sclerosing type.

sclerotic, the pathologist may encounter a frozen section having only sclerotic tissue admixed with a few lymphocytes, eosinophils, and plasma cells. The differential diagnosis includes idiopathic sclerosing mediastinitis (often secondary to histoplasmosis or tuberculosis) and radiation effect. The pathologist should defer the diagnosis and urge the surgeon to retrieve additional tissue for permanent section and special studies. Fungal cultures may be helpful in confirming an infectious etiology.

Germinoma Versus Lymphoma

Frozen section distinction between germinoma and malignant lymphoma may be exceedingly difficult. The clinical history may be helpful in ruling out lymphoma if the patient is a young male with an elevated human gonadotropin level (26). The general recommended treatment for primary mediastinal germinoma is radiotherapy and/or surgery (27-29, 41-43). Complete resection may be possible in some instances but it is not crucial to patient management, since postoperative radiotherapy is usually highly effective.

If there is doubt about the diagnosis, it should be deferred. Tissue for electron microscopy should be obtained.

REFERENCES

1. Tyers GFO, Larrieu AJ, Nelems JMB: Mediastinal Tumors. In Copeland EM III (ed): *Surgical Oncology.* New York, Wiley & Sons, 1983, p 245–256.
2. Akwari OE, Payne WS, Onofrio BM: Dumbbell neurogenic tumors of the mediastinum: Diagnosis and management. *Mayo Clin Proc* 53:353–358, 1978.

3. Wang KP, Nelson S, Scatarige J, Siegelman S: Transbronchial needle aspiration of a m̮ diastinal mass: Therapeutic implications. *Thorax* 38:556–557, 1983.

4. Jereb M, Us-Krasovec M: Transthoracic needle biopsy of mediastinal and hilar lesions. *Cancer* 40:1354–1357, 1977.

5. Rosenberger A, Adler O: Fine needle aspiration biopsy in the diagnosis of mediastinal lesions. *Am J Roentgenol* 131:239–242, 1978.

6. McNeill TM, Chamberlain JM: Diagnostic anterior mediastinotomy. *Ann Thorac Surg* 2:532–539, 1966.

7. LeGolvan DP, Abell, MR: Thymomas. *Cancer* 39:2142–2157, 1977.

8. Wilkins EW, Castleman B: Thymoma: A continuing survey at the MGH. *Ann Thorac Surg* 28:252–256, 1979.

9. Batata MA, Martini N, Huvos AG, Aguilar RI, Beattie EJ: Thymomas: Clinicopathologic features, therapy, and prognosis. *Cancer* 34:389–396, 1974.

10. Wilkins EW: Thymic tumors: Management of the thymoma. *Surgical Rounds* 7:84–96, 1984.

11. Rosai J, Levine GF. In: *Tumors of the Thymus. Atlas of Tumor Pathology,* series 2, Fasc. 13, Washington, DC, Armed Forces Institute of Pathology, 1976, p. 62.

12. Phloxine preparation. In Luna LG (ed): *Manual of Histologic Staining Methods of the Armed Forces Institute of Pathology,* ed 3. American Registry of Pathology, 1968, p 35–40.

13. Rosai J, Levine GF: In: *Tumors of the Thymus. Atlas of Tumor Pathology,* series 2, fasc. 13. Washington, DC, Armed Forces Institute of Pathology, 1976, p 75.

14. Bernatz PE, Khonsari S, Harrison EG, Taylor W: Thymoma: Factors influencing prognosis. *Surg Clin N Am* 53:885–892, 1973.

15. Slater G, Papatestas AE, Genkins G, Kornfield P, Horowitz SH, Bender A: Thymomas in patients with myasthenia gravis. *Ann Surg* 188:171–174, 1978.

16. Salyer WR, Salyer DC, Eggleston JC: Carcinoid tumors of the thymus. *Cancer* 37:958–973, 1976.

17. Castleman B, Iverson L, Menendez VP: Localized mediastinal lymph node hyperplasia resembling thymoma. *Cancer* 9:822–830, 1956.

18. Keller AR, Hochholzer L, Castleman B: Hyaline-vascular and plasma cell types of giant lymph node hyperplasia of the mediastinum and other locations. *Cancer* 29:670–683,1972.

19. Shimosato Y, Kameya T, Nagai K, Suemasu K: Squamous cell carcinoma of the thymus. An analysis of eight cases. *Am J Surg Pathol* 1:109–121, 1977.

20. Wick MR, Scheithauer BW, Weiland LH, Bernatz PE: Primary thymic carcinomas. *Am J Surg Pathol* 6:613–630, 1982.

21. Mukai K, Adams WR: Yolk sac tumor of the anterior mediastinum. Case report with light and electron microscopic examination and immunohistochemical study of alpha-fetopro-tein. *Am J Surg Pathol* 3:77–83, 1979.

22. DeSmet AA, Silver TM, Hart WR: Endodermal sinus tumor of the anterior mediastinum. *South Med J* 70:757–758, 1977.

23. Salyer WR, Salyer DC: The Mediastinum and Thymus. In Silverberg SG (ed): *Principles and Practices of Surgical Pathology.* New York, Wiley & Sons, 1983, p 727–762.

24. Scharifker D, Kaneko M: Localized fibrous "mesothelioma" of pleura (submesothelial fibroma). A clinicopathologic study of 18 cases. *Cancer* 43:627–635, 1979.

25. Rosai J, Levine G: *Tumors of the Thymus. Atlas of Tumor Pathology.* series 2, fasc. 13. Washington, DC, Armed Forces Institute of Pathology, 1976, p. 186.

26. Javadpour N, McIntire KR, Waldmann TA: Human chorionic gonadotropin (HCG) and alpha-fetoprotein (AFP) in sera and tumor cells of patients with testicular seminoma. *Cancer* 42:2768–2772, 1978.

27. Martini N, Golbey RB, Hajdu SI, Whitmore WF, Beattie EJ: Primary mediastinal germ cell tumors. *Cancer* 33:763–769, 1974.

28. Beattie EJ: Mediastinal germ cell tumors (Surgery). *Semin Oncol* 6:109–112, 1979.

29. Economou JS, Trump DL, Holmes EC: Management of primary germ cell tumors of the mediastinum. *J Thorac Cardiovasc Surg* 83:643–649, 1982.

30. Fallon M, Gordon ARG, Lendrum AC: Mediastinal cysts of foregut origin associated with vertebral anomalies. *Br J Surg* 41:520–533, 1954.

31. Tyers GFO, Larrieu AJ, Nelems JMB: Mediastinal Tumors, In Copeland EM III (ed): *Surgical Oncology.* New York, Wiley & Sons, 1983, p 253.

32. Reed JR, Hallet KK, Feigm DS: Neural tumors of the thorax. Subject review from the AFIP. *Radiology* 126:9–17, 1978.

33. Gale AW, Jelihovsky T, Grant AF, Nicks R: Neurogenic tumors of the mediastinum. *Ann Thorac Surg* 17:434–443, 1974.

34. Bower RJ, Kiesewetter WB: Mediastinal masses in infants and children. *Arch Surg* 112:1003–1009, 1977.

35. Goodwin RA, Nickell JA, Des Prez RM: Mediastinal fibrosis complicating healed primary histoplasmosis and tuberculosis. *Medicine* 51:227–246, 1972.

36. Schrowengerdt CG, Suyemoto R, Main FB: Granulomatous fibrous mediastinitis. A review and analysis of 180 cases. *J Thorac Cardiovasc Surg* 57:365–379, 1969.

37. Strimlan CV, Dines DE, Payne WS: Mediastinal granuloma. *Mayo Clin Proc* 50:702–705, 1975.

38. Bergh NP, Gatzinsky P, Larsson S, Lundin P, Ridell B: Tumors of the thymus and thymic region. II. Clinicopathologic studies on Hodgkin's disease of the thymus. *Ann Thorac Surg* 25:99–106, 1978.

39. Benjamin SP, McCormack LJ, Effler DR, Groves LK: Primary lymphatic tumors of the mediastinum. *Cancer* 30:708–712, 1972.

40. VanHeerden JA, Harrison EG, Berriati PE: Mediastinal malignant lymphoma. *Chest* 57:518–529, 1970.

41. Clamon GH: Management of primary mediastinal seminoma. *Chest* 83:263–266, 1983.

42. Medini E, Levitt SH, Jones TK, Rao Y: The management of extratesticular seminoma without gonadal involvement. *Cancer* 44:2032–2038, 1979.

43. Hurt RD, Bruckman JE, Farrow GM, Bernatz PE, Hahn RJ, Earle JD: Primary anterior mediastinal seminoma. *Cancer* 49:1650–1653, 1982.

11

Parathyroid

B. Balfour Kraemer, M.D.

Successful parathyroid exploration requires close intraoperative interaction between surgeon and pathologist. The surgeon's reliance on frozen section interpretation is judicious, since, in most instances, it is the surgeon's clinical assessment rather than the pathologist's frozen section diagnosis that will determine the intraoperative course of events. The experienced surgeon utilizes frozen section primarily for tissue identification.

THE INTRAOPERATIVE SETTING

During a formal parathyroid exploration, the surgeon will attempt to identify as many parathyroid glands as possible. He plays a game of statistical odds with anatomy, realizing that although the majority of patients have four parathyroid glands, a small percentage of patients will have three or five or more glands, one of which may be outside the neck (1–3). A meticulous exploration of each side of the neck is first carried out. If four glands are not positively identified, depending on which gland(s) are missing, the exploration is extended to include inspection of structures high in the neck, the thyroid bed, tracheoesophageal groove, and superior mediastinum (4,5). A median sternotomy with exploration of the mediastinum is usually not performed during the same anesthesia, unless the patient is in hypercalcemic crisis (5). The thymus may be removed by a transcervical approach. Thyroid lobectomy on the side of the missing gland may be performed in an effort to identify an intrathyroidal parathyroid gland.

INDICATIONS FOR FROZEN SECTION

Tissue Identification

The main indication for frozen section diagnosis in parathyroid surgery is tissue identification. For the surgeon, in situ recognition of parathyroid glands may be obscured by disorted anatomic landmarks or poorly controlled hemostasis. In the case of a hyperfunctioning adenoma, uninvolved parathyroid glands may be smaller than usual and difficult for the surgeon to locate (6). Sometimes, the surgeon may not be able to distinguish parathyroid from thyroid, fat, lymph node, or thymus. Biopsy confirmation of presumed parathyroid tissue facilitates the exploration and helps the surgeon preserve the vascular supply of the gland(s) so identified.

Parathyroid tissue may be removed and then cryopreserved (7). Tissue handled in such a manner is usually from a subtotal or total parathyroidectomy. Cryopreserved parathyroid tissue gives the surgeon a margin of safety and can be heterotopically autotransplanted at some future date if the patient develops persistent hypoparathyroidism following subtotal resection. Cryopreservation is also utilized when the patient has all parathyroid tissue removed during the course of another procedure, such as an extended laryngectomy or total thyroidectomy, where sacrifice of the glands is unavoidable.

Adenoma Versus Hyperplasia

The frozen section distinction between solitary parathyroid adenoma and nodular hyperplasia is often difficult and sometimes impossible. The surgeon who places such a burden on the pathologist places himself in a precarious position in the operating suite, and the pathologist who believes that he can always confidently make this distinction on frozen section overestimates his diagnostic capabilities. This diagnostic problem is discussed in further detail in other sections (see FROZEN SECTION DIAGNOSIS and DEFERRED DIAGNOSIS, this Chapter).

TYPES OF SPECIMENS

Parathyroid Biopsy

Biopsy of a grossly normal parathyroid is usually not performed unless the clinical diagnosis is in doubt or there is some question as to the status of the glands (5). If the surgeon is uncertain as to whether the tissue is parathyroid, biopsy for tissue confirmation is performed. If a hyperfunctioning adenoma is suspected, multiple glands may be biopsied for tissue confirmation.

During the course of biopsy, the surgeon takes great care not to traumatize or devascularize the glands, and so is very conservative in the removal of viable tissue. Biopsy size is usually less than 2 mm. The surgeon may perform multiple parathyroid biopsies and submit them simultaneously to the pathologist on a "parathyroid map" (8). Due to the minute size of these biopsies, special handling is required (see SPECIAL TECHNIQUES, this Chapter).

Single Parathyroid Gland

The removal of a single enlarged parathyroid is performed when the clinical diagnosis of parathyroid adenoma is established. Such a specimen is accompanied by parathyroid biopsy of one or more grossly normal parathyroid glands.

Subtotal Parathyroidectomy

This procedure is the treatment of choice for patients with hyperparathyroidism due to familial MEN syndromes or chronic renal insufficiency (9,10). After all four glands are identified and found to be enlarged, three are removed completely, and 35-50 mg of the fourth gland is left in situ. A variation of this procedure includes the removal of two entire glands, leaving two well vascularized remnants behind (11). This latter procedure is not performed on patients with familial syndromes. Tissues may be cryopreserved for future autotransplantation (see Total Parathyroidectomy).

Total Parathyroidectomy

Selected patients with primary hyperparathyroidism or renal osteodystrophy with reactive (secondary, tertiary) hyperplasia are rendered aparathyroid, and tissue is reserved for autotransplantion. This second procedure is either performed during the same anesthesia or at some future date (7,12,13). A portion of the resected parathyroid tissue is cryopreserved if not immediately transplanted (see SPECIAL TECHNIQUES, this Chapter).

Regional Neck Lymph Nodes

The surgeon may biopsy lymph nodes in the case of suspected parathyroid carcinoma, or in a re-exploration for persistent hypercalcemia, where a diagnosis of sarcoidosis is being considered (14).

Thyroid Lobectomy

Intrathyroidal parathyroid glands are present in 2-8% of the population (15). If the surgeon is unable to identify all four parathyroid glands, he may remove the thyroid lobe on the ipsilateral side of the missing gland in an effort to locate an intrathyroidal parathyroid gland (16–18). This type of resection is more likely to be performed if one of the superior parathyroids has not been identified.

Thymus

Thymic tissue may be removed during parathyroid exploration, since in approximately 10% of the adult population, one or both inferior parathyroid glands are found within the rostral end of the thymic capsule (17). Those parathyroids situated in the lower neck (associated with a cervical tongue of thymus) are easily accessible by a transcervical approach, whereas those embedded within the thoracic thymus may only be retrievable via mediastinotomy or median sternotomy.

Mediastinal Tissue

Mediastinotomy or median sternotomy with exploration is performed on patients who have persistent hyperparathyroidism following an initial unsuccessful neck exploration or when the patient is in hypercalcemic crisis (5,18,19). Parathyroid will be most likely found in association with thymic tissue, but may also be embedded within mediastinal fat or pericardium (6,19).

SPECIAL TECHNIQUES

Cryopreservation

Cryopreservation of parathyroid tissue is usually performed in large medical centers having a surgeon who is active in parathyroid surgical procedures, or in centers having a renal transplant facility. This technique requires a controlled rate freezer that lowers tissue temperature at a rate of $-1°C$, reaching a maximum of $-100°C$. Tissue is preserved in a 10% dimethylsulfoxide, 10% human serum, and 80% tissue culture medium (7,13), and stored in a liquid nitrogen freezer for as long as 18 months.

FROZEN SECTION DIAGNOSIS

Adenoma Versus Hyperplasia

The distinction between adenoma and hyperplasia has been purported to be one of the most difficult tasks that the pathologist must perform in frozen section (20). In reality, the experienced surgeon will usually not force the pathologist to make such a distinction, since his clinical diagnosis, in the majority of instances, is correct. The pathologist may or may not corroborate the clinical impression by frozen section. When he does not, the surgeon has two options. He either heeds the frozen section diagnosis, perhaps changing his operative strategy, or he dismisses the diagnosis and proceeds with his intended operation (8). One situation in which the surgeon will listen closely to the pathologist's interpretation is when two enlarged and two normal appearing glands are identified. The percentage cellularity based on the frozen section of the grossly normal glands will often decide the extent of the resection. Even so, the significance of microscopic hyperplasia in grossly normal or equivocally enlarged parathyroids remains controversial (21).

The gross, histologic, and cytologic features which have been reported to be helpful in distinguishing parathyroid adenoma from hyperplasia (Figs. 11.1–11.3) are listed in Table 11.1. Even when the pathologist has an intact gland for evaluation, distinction between these two entities may be exceedingly difficult. A descriptive frozen section diagnosis is often preferable to attempts at a specific diagnosis. The surgeon appreciates the pathologist's dilemma. Likewise, the pathologist appreciates that the surgeon must act as a pathologist in the operating suite (10).

Parathyroid or Thyroid

Accurate tissue identification is the pathologist's main function in a parathyroid exploration and is usually a straightforward exercise. Occasionally, parathyroid tissue can be mistaken for thyroid, and vice versa. Parathyroid tissue can be intrathyroidal, and thyroid tissue can sequester itself into perithyroidal tissue, mimicking parathyroid or lymph node. Histologically, normal and adenomatous parathyroid may form microfollicles, trabeculae, or acini, and simulate the follicles of normal or adenomatous thyroid (22). A parathyroid adenoma may be composed of a pure oxyphilic cell population, superficially resembling a Hürthle cell lesion of the thyroid.

Table 11.1.
Parathyroid Hyperplasia Versus Adenoma

	Hyperplasia	Adenoma
Pattern	Nodular or diffuse	Expansile mass
Lobularity	Exaggerated	Destroyed
Capsule	None	+ or −
Residual parathyroid	+ or −	+ or −
Cell type	Single or multiple	Usually single
Acini, microfollicles	− or +	Usually +
Stromal fat	0 − ++	0 − +
Intracytoplasmic fat	0 − +	0 − +
Nuclear atypia	Usually none	0 − ++++
Mitoses	+	+
Other glands	Enlarged, normal, or variable	Atrophic or normal

The distinction between parathyroid and thyroid tissue in these instances is often impossible when given only a small biopsy for frozen section.

If the surgeon has performed a thyroid lobectomy during the course of parathyroid exploration, he is usually searching for an intrathyroidal parathyroid adenoma. Most such adenomas are subcapsular, but may rarely be embedded entirely within the substance of the thyroid. Often, the histologic features of the adenoma are sufficiently distinctive from surrounding thyroid to make the diagnosis. Rarely, the parathyroid adenoma may have a microfollicular pattern indistinguishable from a thyroid follicular adenoma.

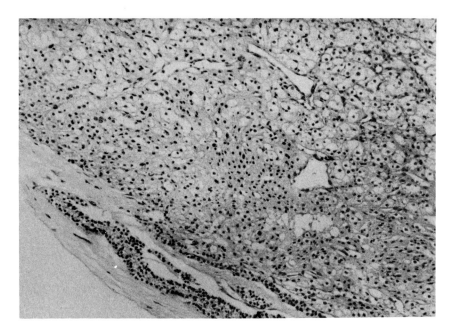

Figure 11.1. Frozen section of hypercellular parathyroid, most consistent with adenoma. Rim of residual parathyroid is present.

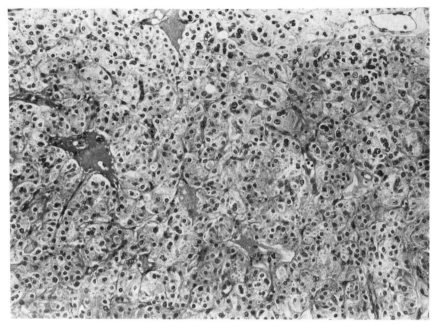

Figure 11.2. Permanent section. Parathyroid adenoma. Note nuclear pleomorphism.

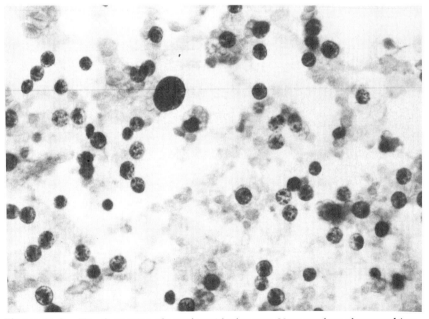

Figure 11.3. Touch imprint of parathyroid adenoma. Note nuclear pleomorphism. Hematoxylin and eosin.

Special stains for fat and glycogen may be helpful if residual normal parathyroid is present. Final diagnosis often rests on permanent sections and immunocytochemistry.

Aberrant Parathyroid

Parathyromatosis

Parathyromatosis, first described by Erdheim in 1904 (23) is defined as nonencapsulated clusters of parathyroid tissue outside the anatomic confines of the parathyroid glands (24). These minute foci of parathyroid are derived from aberrant migration of parathyroid cells during embryogenesis and may be found scattered within the neck or superior mediastinum. Hyperfunctioning foci of parathyromatosis may be responsible for hyperparathyroidism, and may represent some of the reported cases of supernumerary mediastinal parathyroid adenomas or recurrent parathyroid adenomas which "seeded" the area from which they were removed (6,16,25). Parathyromatosis should not be interpreted as foci of metastases.

Supernumerary Parathyroid Adenoma

The most common sites for hyperfunctioning parathyroid in an aberrant location are listed in Table 11.2.

Most supernumerary parathyroid adenomas are found during re-exploration procedures. The search for a supernumerary adenoma is intensified if the surgeon identifies a bilobated or multilobated parathyroid gland in the neck (3). Accurate tissue identification by the pathologist is crucial, since the surgeon's strategy is an aggressive one, and he is determined to find an elusive adenoma which lurks in one of the aforementioned sites (Table 11.2). Multiple frozen section requests are to be anticipated. The patient will undergo a meticulous dissection of both sides of the neck from the angle of the jaw to the inferior limits of the neck and may have the entire mediastinum explored. Tissues resected from such an exploration should be very carefully examined by the pathologist, and any suspicious nodules should be submitted for frozen section.

Parathyroid Carcinoma

The actual incidence of parathyroid carcinoma is very low. Most such neoplasms are functioning (26,27). Nonfunctioning parathyroid carcinomas have been reported to have a poorer prognosis (27). In most instances, the

Table 11.2.
Supernumerary Parathyroid Adenomas: Common Locations

Neck	Mediastinum
Carotid sheath	Thymus
Thyroid	Pericardium
Tracheoesophageal groove	Aorticopulmonary window
Cervical thymus	Mediastinal fat
Retroesophageal space	Deep retroesophageal space

diagnosis is made on clinical grounds. Parathyroid carcinoma is usually invasive and becomes fixed to adjacent structures. Microscopically, chief or oxyphil cells (28) are traversed by broad, haphazardly arranged fibrous bands (Figs. 11.4 and 11.5). Vascular/capsular invasion may be present. As with other endocrine neoplasms, the best criterion for malignancy is identification of metastasis.

Parathyroid carcinoma may secondarily invade the thyroid. In such a situation, the main differential diagnosis is medullary carcinoma of the thyroid. The presence of stromal amyloid, a carcinoid or spindle pattern, and multicentric foci favor medullary carcinoma.

Intraoperative Cytology

The majority of parathyroid specimens are biopsies. These specimens are minute and easily subject to distortion, making tissue identification difficult. Cytologic evaluation circumvents this problem (8,29). Some pathologists have learned to rely only on the cytologic evaluation of such biopsies at the time of frozen section and submit the tissue biopsy only for permanent section (30). Distinguishing parathyroid from thyroid, fat, and lymphoid tissue (thymus or lymph node) is usually possible on the basis of cytology alone. Touch imprints or smear preparations are satisfactory methods which have been described (8). In the situation where a biopsy specimen yields an inadequate cytologic specimen, the biopsy is probably fat. If the biopsy floats in saline, this further supports the probability that it is fat and not parathyroid (8).

Rapid Stains

Fat Stain

A variety of neutral lipid stains have been reported to be of practical value in distinguishing normal from hyperfunctioning parathyroid (31–35). Studies have shown that chief cell intracytoplasmic lipid content, rather than extracellular or stromal fat, more accurately differentiates normal from hyperfunctioning parathyroid (36). Unfortunately, the amount of intracytoplasmic lipid in hyperfunctioning states may vary from one area to the next, and in a small biopsy may not be representative. To complicate matters further, disorders other than hyperparathyroidism may be responsible for decreased lipid stores in parathyroid glands (20).

In a situation where the surgeon finds multiple slightly enlarged glands, use of a fat stain on more than one biopsy may help to establish a frozen section diagnosis of hyperfunctioning parathyroid (37). If both biopsies display little or no intracytoplasmic lipid, it is likely that the parathyroids are hyperplastic.

Fat stains may also be used on frozen section tissue to rapidly distinguish parathyroid from thyroid. This stain is of limited use when trying to distinguish hyperfunctioning parathyroid from thyroid, since lipid stores may be minimal or absent in the former.

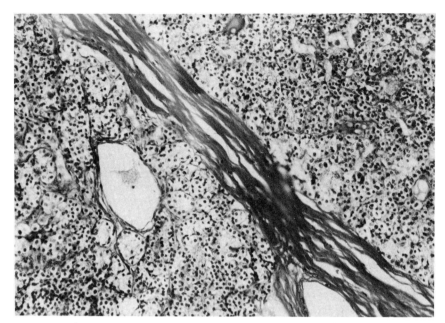

Figure 11.4. Parathyroid carcinoma. Note broad fibrous bands.

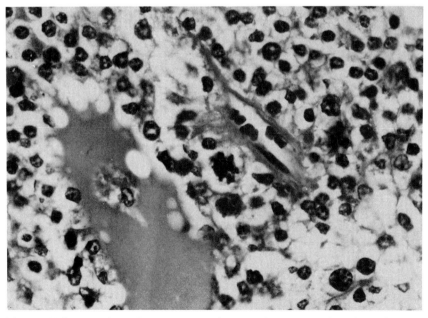

Figure 11.5. Parathyroid carcinoma with atypical mitoses and nuclear pleomorphism.

PAS Stain

Like the fat stain, a PAS stain can help to distinguish thyroid from parathyroid. Resting chief cells contain glycogen in variable quantities. Also like the fat stain, use of a PAS stain is limited when dealing with hyperfunctioning parathyroid, since glycogen supplies are usually diminished or absent.

Weight of the Gland

Total parathyroid gland weight includes actual weight of both the parenchymal and stromal components. The mean glandular weight has been reported to be 32 mg (3). Normal gland weights vary according to age, sex, nutritional status, and anatomic site. Due to the variability of stromal fat in normal and hyperfunctioning states, other techniques have been developed in an effort to more accurately reflect true parenchymal cell weight. The density gradient technique (38) is based on specific gravity differences between normal and hyperplastic glands. Tissue that remains bouyant in a mannitol solution is interpreted as normal, whereas tissue having a density between 1.049-1.069 is interpreted as hyperplastic. Since the original technique was described, false negative results have been reported (39). We have no experience with this method.

DEFERRED DIAGNOSIS

Adenoma Versus Hyperplasia

The frozen section distinction between a solitary parathyroid adenoma and nodular hyperplasia is sometimes impossible. The surgeon who identifies one enlarged parathyroid gland and three other grossly normal glands has already made a tentative diagnosis of parathyroid adenoma before a frozen section is even requested. The pathologist serves a function in confirming that the excised tissue is parathyroid, that it is hypercellular (Fig. 11.1), and that the morphology is consistent with an adenoma. Tissue confirmation and an estimation of percentage cellularity is less confusing and just as helpful to the surgeon. In the instance when multiple parathyroids are identified and appear only slightly enlarged, biopsies should be evaluated as described above. Fat stains may be helpful adjuncts in supporting a diagnosis of hyperfunctioning parathyroid.

Oxyphilic Lesion

Pure oxyphilic adenomas of the parathyroid have been described (40). Biopsy of such an adenoma may be impossible to distinguish from a Hürthle cell lesion of thyroid origin. Functioning parathyroid adenomas may have little or no glycogen or fat, and thus rapid special stains are of limited use. Final diagnosis usually rests on permanent section with immunocytochemistry for thyroglobulin and parathormone.

REFERENCES

1. Alveryd A: Parathyroid glands in thyroid surgery. *Acta Chir Scand (Suppl)* 389:5–42, 1968.
2. Gilmour JR: The gross anatomy of the parathyroid glands. *J Pathol* 46:133–149, 1938.
3. Grimelius L, Akerstrom G, Johannson H, Bergstrom R: Anatomy and histopathology of human parathyroid glands. *Pathol Annu* 16:1–24, 1981.
4. Van Heerden JA, Beahrs OH, Woolner LB: The pathology and surgical management of primary hyperparathyroidism. *Surg Clin N Am* 57:557–563, 1977.
5. Edis AJ: Surgical anatomy and technique of neck exploration for primary hyperparathyroidism. *Surg Clin N Am* 57:495–504, 1977.
6. Wang CA, Mahaffey JE, Axelrod L, Perlman JA: Hyperfunctioning supernumerary parathyroid glands. *Surg Gynecol Obstet* 148:711–714, 1979.
7. Wells SA, Ross AJ, Dale JK, Gray RS: Transplantation of the parathyroid glands: Current status. *Surg Clin N Am* 59:167–177, 1979.
8. Geelhoed GW, Silverberg SG: Intraoperative imprints for the identification of parathyroid tissue. *Surgery* 96: 1124–1141, 1984.
9. Prinz RA, Gamvros OI, Sellu D, Lynn JA: Subtotal parathyroidectomy for primary chief cell hyperplasia of the multiple endocrine neoplasia Type I syndrome. *Ann Surg* 193:26–29, 1981.
10. Block MA: Exploration of parathyroid glands and subtotal resection for hyperplasia. In Nyhus LM and Baker RJ (eds): *Mastery of Surgery*, vol 1. Boston, Little, Brown, & Co. 1984, p 205–212.
11. Kaplan EL, Bartlett S, Sugimoto J, Fredland A: Relation of postoperative hypocalcemia to operative techniques: Deleterious effect of excessive use of parathyroid biopsy. *Surgery* 92:827–834, 1982.
12. Niederle B, Roka R, Brennan MF: The transplantation of parathyroid tissue in man: Development, indications, and results. *Endocrine Rev* 3:245–277, 1982.
13. Mallette LE, Eisenberg KL, Schwaitzberg SD, Suki WN, Noon GP: Total parathyroidectomy and autogenous parathyroid graft placement for treatment of hyperparathyroidism due to chronic renal failure. *Am J Surg* 146:727–733, 1983.
14. Billings PJ, Milroy, EJG: Reoperative parathyroid surgery. *Br J Surg* 70:542–546, 1983.
15. Davis O, Scanlon EF, Pollack ER, Casey JJ, Victor TA: Bilateral intrathyroidal hyperplastic parathyroid glands. *J Surg Oncol* 27:271–274, 1984.
16. Cohn, KH, Silen W: Lessons of parathyroid reoperations. *Am J Surg* 144:511–515, 1982.
17. Paloyan E, Lawrence, AM: Anatomy of the parathyroid glands. In Nyhus LM and Baker RJ (eds): *Mastery of Surgery*, vol. 1. Boston, Little, Brown, & Co. 1984, p 191–196.
18. Paloyan E, Lawrence AM: Parathyroidectomy for primary hyperparathyroidism. In Nyhus LM and Baker RJ (eds): *Mastery of Surgery*, vol 1. Boston, Little, Brown, & Co., 1984, p 197–204.
19. Russell CF, Edis AJ, Scholz DA, Sheedy PF, Van Heerden JA: Mediastinal parathyroid tumors. Experience with 38 tumors requiring mediastinotomy for removal. *Ann Surg* 193:805–809, 1981.
20. Dufour R, Durkowski, C: Sudan IV stain. *Arch Pathol Lab Med* 106:224–227, 1982.
21. Edis AJ, Beahrs OH, van Heerden JA, Akwari OE: "Conservative" versus "liberal" approach to parathyroid neck exploration. *Surgery* 82:466–471, 1977.
22. Boquist, L: Follicles in human parathyroid glands. *Lab Invest* 28:313–320, 1973.
23. Erdheim JEI: Ueber Suhilddrusenaplasie. II. Geschwulste des ductus thyreoglossus. III. Ueber einige Menschliche Keimenderivate. *Beitr Pathol Anat* 35:366, 1904.
24. Reddick RL, Costa JC, Marx SJ: Parathyroid hyperplasia and parathyromatosis. *Lancet* 1:549, 1977.
25. Palmer JA, Brown WA, Kerr WH, Rosen IB, Walters NA: The surgical aspects of hyperparathyroidism *Arch Surg* 110:1004–1007, 1975.
26. Holmes EC, Morton DL, Ketcham AS: Parathyroid carcinoma: A collective review. *Ann Surg* 169:631–640, 1969.
27. Aldinger KA, Hickey RC, Ibanez ML, Samaan NA: Parathyroid carcinoma: A clinical study of seven cases of functioning and two cases of nonfunctioning parathyroid cancer. *Cancer* 49:388–397, 1982.
28. Obara T, Fujimoto Y, Yamaguchi K, Takanashi R, Kino I, Sasaki Y: Parathyroid carcinoma of the oxyphil cell type. *Cancer* 55:1482–1489, 1985.

29. Silverberg SG: Imprints in the operative evaluation of parathyroid disease. *Arch Pathol Lab Med* 99:375–378, 1975.

30. Bloustein PA, Silverberg SG: Rapid cytologic examination of surgical specimens. *Pathol Annu* 12:251–278, 1977.

31. Farnebo LO, Von Unge H: Peroperative evaluation of parathyroid glands using fat stains on frozen sections. Advantages and limitations. *Acta Chir Scand* 520:17–24, 1984.

32. Monchik JM, Farrugia R, Teplitz C, Teplitz C, Brown S: Parathyroid surgery: The role of chief cell intracellular fat staining with osmium carmine in the intraoperative management of patients with primary hyperparathyroidism. *Surgery* 94:877–886, 1983.

33. Ljungberg O, Tibblin S: Peroperative fat staining of frozen sections in primary hyperparathyroidism. *Am J Pathol* 95:633–641, 1979.

34. Kasdon EJ, Cohen RB, Rosen S, Silen W: Surgical pathology of fat stain and problems in interpretation. *Am J Surg Pathol* 5:381–384, 1981.

35. King DT, Hirose FM: Chief cell intracytoplasmic fat used to evaluate parathyroid disease by frozen section. *Arch Pathol Lab Med* 103:609–612, 1979.

36. Roth SI, Gallagher MJ: The rapid identification of "normal" parathyroid glands by the presence of intracellular fat. *Am J Pathol* 84:521–528, 1976.

37. Saffos RO, Rhatigan RM, Urgulu S: The normal parathyroid and the borderline with early hyperplasia: A light microscopic study. *Histopathology* 8:407–422, 1984.

38. Wang CA, Reider SV: A density test for the intraoperative differentiation of parathyroid hyperplasia from neoplasia. *Ann Surg* 187:63–67, 1978.

39. Lockett LJ: A source of false results in the intraoperative parathyroid density test. *Am J Clin Pathol* 78:781–783, 1982.

40. Ordonez NG, Ibanez ML, Mackay B, Samaan NA, Hickey RC: Functioning oxyphil cell adenomas of parathyroid gland: Immunoperoxidase evidence of hormonal activity in oxyphil cells. *Am J Clin Pathol* 78:681–689, 1982.

12

Lymph Nodes

B. Balfour Kraemer, M. D.

The pathologist is often called upon to evaluate a lymph node by frozen section. Before doing so, the patient's clinical history, nature of the operative procedure, and exact anatomic location of the excised lymph node(s) should be known.

INDICATIONS FOR FROZEN SECTION

Intraoperative Staging

For some one stage major operative procedures, the surgeon relies upon frozen section guidance to first determine the status of the regional lymph nodes before undertaking the procedure. Depending upon the nature of the operation, the location and extent of lymph node metastases identified by frozen section is the single most important factor in determining whether or not the intended procedure will be completed or abandoned. The most common operations which routinely utilize intraoperative lymph node staging are radical hysterectomy (1), radical prostatectomy (2,3), radical cystectomy (4,5), lobectomy or pneumonectomy (6), and regional lymph node dissection for metastatic malignant melanoma (7).

Possible Lymphoproliferative Disease

Frozen section diagnosis of lymph node biopsies from patients with known or suspected lymphoproliferative disorders is routinely deferred. A frozen section should be performed to assess the representativity of the biopsy. If facilities permit, frozen section slides for cell surface markers can be prepared (see SPECIAL TECHNIQUES, this Chapter).

Hormone Receptor Assay

A clinically positive lymph node in a patient with a history of a malignancy, typically breast carcinoma, may be biopsied for the express purpose of obtaining receptor analysis data (8). Frozen section evaluation histologically confirms that metastatic disease is present, and ensures that representative tissue is submitted. If the biopsy is small, the frozen section block can be surrendered for receptor assay. The frozen section slide becomes the permanent histologic record.

The Surgeon's Prerogative

The surgeon reserves the right to submit any suspicious lymph node for frozen section diagnosis. His curiosity should be satisfied, and the pathologist should honor such requests, within reason.

TYPES OF SPECIMENS

Peripheral Lymph Node Biopsy

In the ideal situation, the surgeon provides the pathologist with the largest accessible lymph node and gives an exact description of the anatomic site from where the lymph node was excised. This last piece of information is particularly helpful when evaluating a lymph node excised from the neck. The surgeon who designates biopsies with such generic descriptions as "neck node" deserves an immediate phone call or personal visit for more detailed information. The burden is on the pathologist to interpret the clinical history with the histologic findings and to provide a clinicopathologic correlation. The pathologist should know the level of a lymph node metastasis, since this information is important in the management of the patient. For example, metastatic squamous carcinoma involving a supraclavicular lymph node has vastly different clinical implications than metastatic squamous carcinoma involving a high cervical lymph node (9). For the latter, the surgeon will proceed with a neck dissection. For the former, he will direct his attention to a possible infraclavicular primary, such as lung. The site of the lymph node should be correlated with the histology of the metastasis, and a possible primary site should be suggested (see Table 12.1).

Lymphadenectomy Specimens

To the pathologist, lymphadenectomy specimens are grossly unimpressive, nondescript fatty lymph nodes. To the surgeon, they are pieces of tissue which should be examined with great care. Such specimens deserve the undivided attention of the pathologist, for within them is held the immediate future of the operation and, often, the ultimate future of the patient.

Lymphadenectomy specimens may be received en bloc or in multiple segments. The latter is commonly encountered in bilateral retroperitoneal lymph node dissection for testicular nonseminomatous germ cell tumor staging. In such cases, the surgeon should designate the various portions of the dissection and provide orientation if necessary. If frozen sections are requested, the pathologist should be aware of any previous therapy or procedures which might possibly influence the histology of the lymph nodes (i.e., lymphangiography, chemotherapy/radiotherapy).

Lymph nodes submitted for frozen section are done so under the sur-

Table 12.1.
Location of Lymph Node Metastasis in the Neck: Correlation With Posssible Primary Site(s)

Site of Metastasis	Possible Primary Site
Preauricular	Skin upper face and temple
Subdigastric	Lateral and posterior tongue, tonsil, palate
Submaxillary	Skin lateral face, anterior tongue, floor of mouth
Submental	Lip, anterior floor of mouth
Midjugular	Larynx, pharynx
Low jugular	Thyroid, cervical esophagus
Scalene, supraclavicular	Subclavicular
High posterior cervical	Nasopharynx
Low posterior cervical	Thyroid, nasopharynx

geon's presumption that if a favorable frozen section diagnosis is rendered, the planned procedure will be carried out. Since lymphadenectomy specimens may contain from 10 to 30 or more lymph nodes, handling these specimens as frozen section material is problematic. In general, the manner in which these specimens are handled depends to a great degree on the surgeon's demands and the ability of the pathologist to provide rapid frozen section service. If a frozen section suite is equipped to handle a large number of frozen sections simultaneously, the surgeon may take advantage of this and request that all lymph nodes be submitted for frozen section diagnosis. He may even ask that two separate levels be examined, a request that is honored at M.D. Anderson Hospital, typically for lymph node dissections for metastatic prostatic carcinoma. Alternatively, the surgeon may take it upon himself to choose which lymph nodes should be frozen, or may rely on the pathologist's judgement to select suspicious lymph nodes (3). In such a setting, the pathologist should take the time to very carefully dissect out all lymph nodes and examine them grossly at multiple levels in order to select which lymph nodes should be frozen.

The most common lymphadenectomy specimens are listed in Table 12.2. In lymph node dissections for possible metastatic prostatic carcinoma, negative lymph nodes identify patients who are potentially curable by prostatectomy. In contemplated radical cystectomy, location and number of lymph node metastases helps to determine the feasibility of a radical cystectomy (4). For radical hysterectomy, para-aortic and/or obturator lymph nodes may be submitted first to assess extent of disease outside the pelvis and feasibility of curative resection (1,10). Regional lymph node dissections for metastatic malignant melanoma may be submitted for frozen section diagnosis in two situations. If frozen section of inguinal lymph nodes is positive, concominant iliac dissection may be performed (7). One-stage chemotherapy isolation limb perfusion may be preceded by frozen section evaluation of regional nodes. In patients with nonseminomatous germ cell tumors, retroperitoneal dissection of lymph nodes is performed for pathologic staging. These specimens are not routinely submitted for frozen section diagnosis. If postradiation/chemotherapy lymph nodes appear to grossly contain viable tumor at the time of resection, the surgeon may ask for a frozen section to confirm his clinical impression.

Table 12.2.
Lymph Nodes Groups Contained in Lymphadenectomy Specimens

Procedure	Lymph nodes
Radical prostatectomy	Common and external iliac, presacral, hypogastric, obturator
Radical cystectomy	Common and external iliac, hypogastric, obturator, perivesical
Ilioinguinal dissection	Inguinofemoral, common, external, and internal iliac, obturator
Radical hysterectomy	Paraaortic, common and external iliac, obturator, hypogastric
Retroperitoneal dissection for nonseminomatous germ cell tumors	Common and external iliac, paraaortic, preaortic, paracaval

SPECIAL TECHNIQUES

Intraoperative Cytology

Touch imprints are useful adjuncts in frozen section evaluation of lymph nodes and have a high diagnostic specificity and sensitivity (11). Imprint cytology can be utilized as a rapid screening device when multiple lymph nodes are submitted for frozen section. Imprint evaluation for staging breast and gastric carcinoma is used in some institutions in Europe (12,13) and has been reported to have a high predictive value. False negatives or false positives are likely to occur when the cytology is evaluated without tissue correlation.

If lymph node imprint cytology is to be heavily relied upon as a frozen section diagnostic tool, the pathologist must always take into account the anatomic site from where the lymph node was excised before he renders a diagnosis solely on the basis of cytologic findings. Anatomic peculiarities of regional lymph nodes are often easily overinterpreted on cytologic evaluation alone. For example, abdominal lymph nodes from the celiac axis may contain exuberant lipophagic granulomas (lipogranulomas), which form secondary to ingested mineral oil products. Touch imprints taken from such lymph nodes contain numerous epithelioid histiocytes which cytologically can be mistaken for cells of epithelial malignancies (11). Touch imprints taken from postlymphangiogram lymph nodes may display multinucleate giant cells, eosinophils, and histiocytes. Such an imprint might be confused as representing an infectious process. Intrathoracic and low jugular lymph nodes often have large numbers of anthracotic laden histiocytes that may obscure other cell populations in the imprint. Finally, Mullerian gland inclusions in abdominopelvic lymph nodes may be represented on an imprint as clusters of cytologically atypical epithelial cells, and may be overinterpreted as cells of metastatic adenocarcinoma.

Lymph Node Biopsy for Known or Suspected Lymphoproliferative Disease

Hopefully, the surgeon provides the pathologist with the largest accessible lymph node which contains representative neoplasm. Special handling of such lymph nodes is required, and is outlined below:

For processing, the pathologist should have a sterile lymph note at least 1.5 cm in diameter:

1.) Thin slice for frozen section, which will *a*) determine representativity of biopsy, and *b*) provide tissue for cell surface markers (slides remain frozen after preparation).

2.) Aliquot for electron microscopy (glutaraldehyde fixative).

3.) Aliquot for microbiology (as needed) for *a*) routine, *b*) fungal, *c*) Mycobacteria.

4.) Aliquot for special studies (if available) of *a*) surface/cytoplasmic immunoglubulins, *b*) cytogenetics, *c*) flow cytometry.

5.) Touch imprints: *a*) 95% ethanol fixed, *b*) air dried.

6.) Routinely processed tissue: *a*) formaldehyde solution, *b*) B5 fixative (for immunoperoxidase cytoplasmic immunoglobulins).

Lymph Node Biopsy in Patients at Risk for Acquired Immunodeficiency Syndrome (AIDS)

Such a lymph node biopsy should be handled as outlined for known or suspected lymphoproliferative disease, with the additional guidelines (14–18):

1.) The biopsy should be kept sterile and handled with precautions. After frozen section has been performed, contaminated disposables should be double-bagged and discarded as biohazards. The work area and instruments should be immediately disinfected.

2.) Frozen section material for T lymphocyte subsets (Th/Ts) should be prepared.

3.) A small piece of tissue should be submitted for viral culture (Epstein-Barr, Cytomegalovirus).

FROZEN SECTION DIAGNOSIS

Metastatic Signet-Ring Cell Carcinoma

Identification of lymph node metastases from a signet-ring cell primary becomes important in the intraoperative evaluation of gastric carcinomas which are potentially resectable (19,20). The decision to proceed with total gastrectomy may be decided on the basis of negative supra- and infrapyloric or paracardiac lymph nodes (20).

Malignant signet-ring cells are often frustratingly elusive on frozen section. This problem is related to the type of cytoplasmic mucin within the cells, poor visualization of the cell membrane, and location of the malignant cells (Figs. 12.1 and 12.2). When the pattern of metastatic lymph node involvement in signet ring cell carcinoma is sinusoidal, the architecture of the lymph node may remain intact and the sinuses may remain patent. On

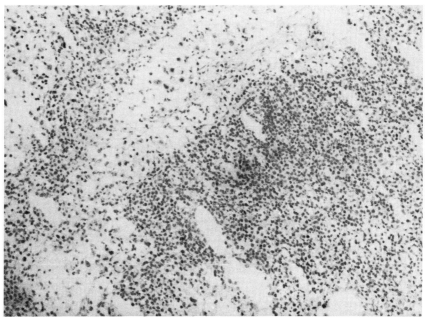

Figure 12.1. Frozen section of lymph node containing metastatic signet-ring cell carcinoma. There is extensive sinusoidal involvement, however, the signet-ring cells are poorly visualized.

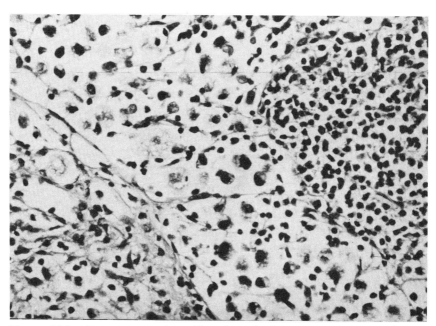

Figure 12.2. Permanent section of lymph node. Same case as Fig. 12.1. Signet-ring cells can be easily visualized within sinusoids.

low power examination, the lymph node may appear histologically unremarkable. Signet-ring cells intermingled with sinus histiocytes become so well camouflaged that frozen section identification of these malignant cells on hematoxylin and eosin sections becomes exceedingly difficult or impossible.

Touch imprints may be helpful in visualizing signet ring cells. Rapid mucin stains are also valuable adjuncts (see Chapter 1). Fixation of the frozen section slide in formaldehyde solution for 1 minute prior to staining may help to improve cellular detail.

Lymph Node Inclusions

The most frequently encountered types of inclusions that can give diagnostic difficulty on frozen section are listed in Table 12.3.

Salivary Gland Inclusions

These inclusions are heterotopic rests within intra- or paraparotid lymph nodes (21). Serous type acini and ductular elements become intimately associated with lymphoid tissue and may be distributed anywhere in the substance of the lymph node. If the ducts undergo squamous or oncocytic metaplasia, they may superficially resemble metastatic carcinoma, or even a salivary gland neoplasm (the evolution of Wharthin's tumor is probably explained by this phenomenon). Salivary gland inclusions may extensively replace the nodal architecture. By themselves, they have no prognostic significance and should not be interpreted as metastasis.

"Thyroid" Inclusions

So called "thyroid inclusions" in cervical lymph nodes have been considered to represent either benign thyroid follicles that have migrated into regional lymphatics (22–26), or metastasis from well differentiated thyroid carcinoma (Fig. 12.3) (27,28). The frozen section identification of thyroid follicles in a cervical lymph node may be an incidental finding in a lymph node that has been removed for another type of head and neck cancer. It is our policy to interpret such lymph nodes as containing metastatic well differentiated thyroid carcinoma. The lymph node metastasis is occult, and the corresponding primary may or may not be grossly detectable. This is particularly true of occult sclerosing papillary thyroid carcinomas (29). The surgeon may inspect the thyroid if it is easily visualized within the operative field. If a suspicious nodule is palpated on the side ipsilateral to the nodal metastasis, thyroid lobectomy will probably be performed. In reality, the significance of the pathologist's frozen section diagnosis and the therapeutic

Table 12.3.
Lymph Node Inclusions, According to Site

Region	Type Inclusion
Head and neck	Salivary gland, "thyroid"
Axillary, inguinal	Nevus cell aggregates
Abdominopelvic	Mullerian, decidua

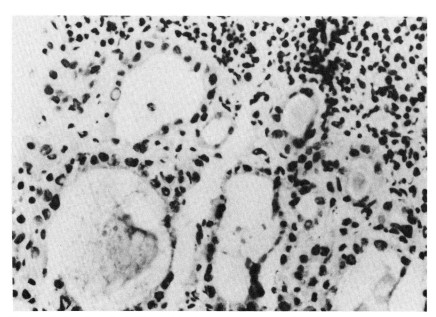

Figure 12.3. So-called "thyroid inclusion" in cervical lymph node. We interpret such lymph nodes as containing metastatic well differentiated thyroid carcinoma.

efficacy of the thyroid resection is limited, since the overall survival for most patients will not be affected by the removal of an occult thyroid primary and/or its metastases. For long term survival of patients, resection seems justified in view of the remote incidence of anaplastic transformation of papillary carcinoma.

Nevus Cells

Microscopic aggregates of nevus cells have been identified in isolated axillary and inguinal lymph nodes (30–32). They pose a problem to the pathologist when they are found in an axillary lymph node of a patient with breast carcinoma. Nevus cells are easily distinguished from metastatic carcinoma on the basis of their location and cytologic features. Nevus cells are typically associated with the lymph node capsule, not the subcapsular sinus (Fig. 12.4). They may rarely be scattered in perinodal fat immediately adjacent to the capsule (Fig. 12.5). Cytologically, they are histologically bland oval or spindled cells which are devoid of nuclear pleomorphism, mitoses, or necrosis. They may rarely contain melanin pigment (33).

Mullerian Type Glandular Inclusions

Mullerian inclusions can be found in surgically excised pelvic and/or para-aortic lymph nodes in approximately 14% of the adult female population (34–37). They represent intranodal metaplastic proliferations of pelvic (coelomic) peritoneum, with Mullerian features.

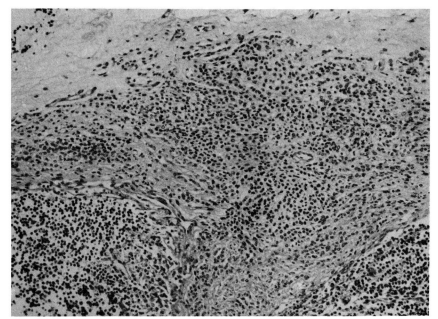

Figure 12.4. Nevus cell aggregates in capsule of axillary lymph node.

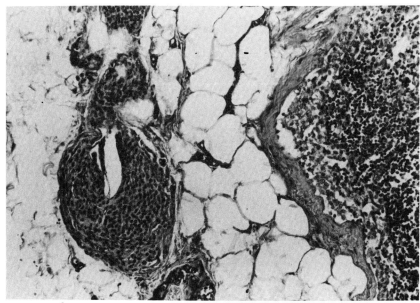

Figure 12.5. Nevus cell aggregate in perinodal fat.

These types of inclusions are usually incidental findings in lymph nodes removed for staging purposes. If coexistent salpingitis is present, Mullerian inclusions may be exuberant, with architectural and cytologic atypia (38).

The location and extent of Mullerian grandular inclusions is variable. They may be found within the lymph node medulla, scattered in the interfollicular zone, or within the sinusoids (Fig. 12.6). One or multiple lymph nodes may contain inclusions.

Histologically, the epithelial lining of Mullerian inclusions is reminiscent of other Mullerian-derived structures, and thus may resemble endosalpingeum, ovarian surface epithelium, endocervix, or endometrium. Proliferating glandular inclusions may display pseudostratification with a cribriform-like arrangement (35). Psammoma bodies may be present.

Frozen section evaluation of Mullerian inclusions can be exceedingly difficult, especially when the inclusions are proliferative or when the area of the lymph node containing the inclusion(s) has been partially crushed. The intraoperative setting usually complicates matters further, since the patient is typically a woman undergoing a staging procedure for a gynecologic malignancy. The question arises: Does this lymph node contain Mullerian inclusions or metastatic carcinoma?

The most important features that help to distinguish benign glandular inclusions from metastatic carcinoma are outlined in Table 12.4.

Decidua

Decidua in extra-Mullerian sites is unusual. Decidual change in an abdominopelvic lymph node is associated with pregnancy (39,40), intranodal endometriosis (41), or progestogen therapy. Frozen section identification

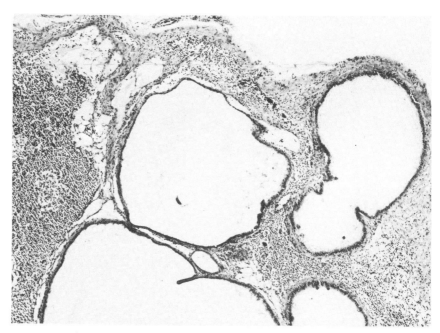

Figure 12.6. Mullerian inclusions in pelvic lymph node.

Table 12.4.
Benign Mullerian Gland Inclusions Versus Metastatic Carcinoma

Lymph Node	Inclusions	Metastasis
Location in lymph node	Interfollicular, medullary, sinus, capsule	Sinus, parenchyma
Histology		
Cilia	$+ - + +$	$-/+$
Epithelial tufting	None	$+$
Necrosis	None	$-/+$
Papillae	None	$-/+$
Pseudostratification	$-/+$	$+$
Desmoplasia	None	$+$
Psammoma bodies	$-/+$	$-/+$
Nuclear pleomorphism	$-/+$	$+ - + +$
Nucleoli	$-$	$+$
Mitoses	$+$[a]	$+$
Cribriform pattern	$-/+$[a]	$-/+$
Squamous metaplasia	$-/+$[b]	$-/+$ (endometrioid primary)

[a]When present, often associated with coexistent salpingitis (38).
[b]May possibly be a postradiation feature (39).

of decidua is easily missed, since it is usually not considered in the differential diagnosis and is misinterpreted as metastatic squamous carcinoma.

Several features help to identify decidua. Decidual cells have a low nucleocytoplasmic ratio, lightly eosinophilic cytoplasm, no nuclear pleomorphism, and no keratinization.

The Fatty Lymph Node

Fat is technically difficult to freeze and cut. Best results are obtained by using some simple variations in routine frozen section. First, a thick slice of lymph node is preferable, since a thicker tissue block is somewhat easier to cut with a microtome. Next, the tissue should be frozen to the lowest temperature possible by the cryostat. Optimal cutting temperature for fat is lower than for most other tissues (optimum temperature is -20 to $-40°C$). Alcohol fixatives are to be avoided, since the tissue may float off the slide.

Granulomatous Inflammation

A granulomatous lesion in a lymph node may be related to foreign body, infection, neoplasia, or immune reaction. Characterization of the granuloma is helpful in establishing its etiology (42). Frozen section identification of granulomatous inflammation, unless obviously of the foreign body type (suture, silicone, lymphangiogram, etc.), should be followed with cultures, including those for routine bacteria, fungi, and Mycobacteria. Some Mycobacterial infections cannot be proven by tissue biopsy alone; culture is often the only means of diagnosing such infections (43).

Radiation Effect

Pelvic lymph nodes removed from patients with invasive carcinoma of the bladder, endometrium, or cervix are often radiated preoperatively. The usual histologic features associated with radiation injury include lymphoid depletion and atrophy (44). Successfully ablated metastases usually form dense fibrocollagenous scarlike accumulations. If metastases remain, they may be viable or extensively necrotic. Bizarre cytologic features induced by radiation may obscure any histologic resemblance of the metastasis to the primary.

Preoperative radiation is also routinely administered to bulky neck lymph node metastases of squamous carcinoma. Radiation shrinks metastatic deposits, facilitating resection. Histologically, metastases may be completely "melted," leaving behind a foreign body granulomatous response to the disintegrating keratinocytes (44).

DEFERRED DIAGNOSIS

Possible Malignant Lymphoma

Frozen section diagnosis of lymph nodes biopsies from patients with known or suspected lymphoproliferative disease should be deferred. A frozen section should be prepared to assess representativity of the biopsy and to have frozen tissue available for special studies (see SPECIAL TECHNIQUES, this Chapter).

Pseudomalignant Crush Artifact

Lymph nodes biopsied via rigid scope methods, such as mediastinoscopy, are subject to significant biopsy trauma (see Chapter 6, **Lung**). Although the pathologist has little control over biopsy procedures, he should urge the surgeon to refrain from handling the biopsy once it has been removed from the patient. Surgeons are naturally curious about the tissues they excise, but in the case of lymph node biopsies, it is the pathologist who should be the first to examine the specimen. The surgeon who squeezes the lymph node to assess its texture will collapse part or all of the delicate nodal framework. Such traumatized biopsies are difficult or impossible to evaluate by frozen section. In the case of metastatic undifferentiated small (oat) cell carcinoma, histologic distinction between this and pseudomalignant crush artifact of lymphoid tissue is often impossible (see Chapter 6, **Lung**).

Necrosis, Infarction, or Sclerosis

An excised lymph node that is entirely sclerotic, infarcted, or necrotic may be a clue that the patient has, or will develop a malignant lymphoma (45,46). Infarcted lymph nodes may herald the presentation of a non-Hodgkin's lymphoma, or less commonly, Hodgkin's disease. Extensive necrosis and/or sclerosis is common in Hodgkin's disease, nodular sclerosing type, and may replace the entire lymph node architecture. In such situations, the diagnosis should be deferred, and the pathologist should ask the surgeon to obtain another biopsy.

Irradiated lymph nodes that display extensive fibrous scarring most likely contained radiosensitive metastases. Frozen section diagnosis should be deferred, but a brief histologic description for the benefit of the surgeon can be added.

REFERENCES

1. Piver MS, Barlow JJ: Para-aortic lymphadenectomy in staging patients with advanced local cervical cancer. *Obstet Gynecol* 43:544–548, 1974.
2. McLaughlin AP, Saltzstein SL, McCullough DL, Gittes RF: Prostatic carcinoma: Incidence and location of unsuspected lymphatic metastases. *J Urol* 115:89–94, 1976.
3. Kramolowsky EV, Narayana AS, Platz CE, Loening SA: The frozen section in lymphadenectomy for carcinoma of the prostate. *J Urol* 131:899–900, 1984.
4. Smith JA, Whitmore WF: Regional lymph node metastasis from bladder cancer. *J Urol* 126:591–593, 1981.
5. Dretler SP, Ragsdale BD, Leadbetter WF: The value of pelvic lymphadenectomy in the surgical treatment of bladder cancer. *J Urol* 109:414–416, 1973.
6. Naruke T, Suemasu K, Ishikawa S: Lymph node mapping and curability at various levels of metastasis in resected lung cancer. *J Thorac Cardiovasc Surg* 76:832–839, 1978.
7. Finck SJ, Giuliano AE, Mann BD, Morton DL: Results of ilioinguinal dissection for stage II melanoma. *Ann Surg* 196:180–186, 1982.
8. Lee Y-TN, Markland FS: Steroid receptors study in breast carcinoma. *Med Pediatr Oncol* 5:153–166, 1978.
9. Molinari R, Cantu G, Chiesa F, Podreca S, Milani F, Del Vecchio M: A statistical approach to detection of the primary cancer based on the site of neck node metastases. *Tumori* 63:267–282, 1977.
10. Wharton JT, Edwards CL: Carcinoma of the cervix and endometrium. In Copeland EM (ed): *Surgical Oncology.* New York, Wiley & Sons, 1983, p 559.
11. Bloustein PA, Silverberg SG: Rapid cytologic examination of surgical specimens. *Pathol Annu* 12:251–278, 1977.
12. Quill DS, Leahy AL, Lawler RG, Finney RD: Lymph node imprint cytology for the rapid assessment of axillary node metastases in breast cancer. *Br J Surg* 71:454–455, 1984.
13. Morris DL, Moore J, Thompson H, Keighley MRB: Peroperative lymph node imprint cytology for staging gastric carcinoma. *Br J Surg* 69:282, 1982.
14. Raphael M, Pouletty P, Cavaille-Coll M, Rozenbaum W, Homond A, Nonnenmacher L, Delcourt A, Gluckman JC, Debre P: Lymphadenopathy in patients at risk for acquired immunodeficiency syndrome. Histopathology and histochemistry. *Arch Pathol Lab Med* 109:128–132, 1985.
15. Brynes RK, Chan WC, Spira TJ, Ewing EP, Chandler FW: Value of lymph node biopsy in unexplained lymphadenopathy in homosexual men. *JAMA* 250:1313–1317, 1983.
16. Stahl RE, Friedman-Kien A, Dubin R, Marmor M, Zolla-Pazner S: Immunologic abnormalities in homosexual men: Relationship to Kaposi's sarcoma. *Am J Med* 73:171–178, 1982.
17. David JM, Mouradian J, Fernandez RD, Cunningham-Rundles S, Metroka CE: Acquired immune deficiency syndrome. A surgical perspective. *Arch Surg* 119:90–95, 1984.
18. Chan WC, Byrnes RK, Spira TJ, Banks PM, Thurmond CC, Ewing EP, Chandler FW: Lymphocyte subsets in lymph nodes of homosexual men with generalized unexplained lymphadenopathy. Correlation with morphology and blood changes. *Arch Pathol Lab Med* 109:133–137, 1985.
19. Cassell P, Robinson JO: Cancer of the stomach: a review of 854 patients. *Br J Surg* 63:603–607, 1976.
20. Fujimaki M, Soga J, Wada K, Tani H, Aizawa O, Kawaguchi M, Ishibashi K, Maeda M, Kanai T, Omori Y, Muto T: Total gastrectomy for gastric cancer. Clinical considerations on 431 cases. *Cancer* 30:660–664, 1972.

21. Brown RB, Gaillard RA, Turner JA: The significance of aberrant or heterotopic parotid gland tissue in lymph nodes. *Ann Surg* 138:850–856, 1953.

22. Meyer JS, Sternberg LS: Microscopically benign thyroid follicles in cervical lymph nodes: Serial section study of lymph node inclusions and entire thyroid gland in five cases. *Cancer* 24:302–311, 1969.

23. Roth LM: Inclusions of nonneoplastic thyroid tissue within cervical lymph nodes. *Cancer* 18:105–111, 1965.

24. Gricouroff G: Epithelial inclusions in the lymph nodes. Diagnostic, histogenetic, and prognostic problems. *Diag Gynecol Obstet* 4:285–294, 1982.

25. Nicastri AD, Foote AW, Frazell EL: Benign thyroid inclusions in cervical lymph nodes. *JAMA* 194:1–4, 1965.

26. Fechner RE: Pathology Quiz (Resident's page). *Arch Otolaryngol* 110:698–700, 1984.

27. Clark RL, Hickey RC, Butler JJ, Ibanez ML, Ballantyne AJ: Thyroid cancer discovered incidentally during treatment for unrelated head and neck cancer: Review of 16 cases. *Ann Surg* 163:665–671, 1966.

28. Butler JJ, Tulinius H, Ibanez ML, Ballantyne AJ, Clark RL: Significance of thyroid tissue in lymph nodes associated with carcinoma of the head, neck, and lung. *Cancer* 20:103–112, 1967.

29. Klinck GH, Winship T: Occult sclerosing carcinoma of the thyroid. *Cancer* 8:701–706, 1955.

30. Johnson WT, Helwig EB: Benign nevus cells in the capsule of the lymph nodes. *Cancer* 23:747–753, 1969.

31. McCarthy SW, Palmer AA, Bale PM, Hirst E: Nevus cells in lymph nodes. *Pathology* 6:351–358, 1974.

32. Azzopardi JG: Problems in breast pathology. In Bennington JL (ed): *Major Problems in Pathology,* vol 11. London, W. B. Saunders, 1979, p 316–317.

33. Lamovec J: Blue nevus of the lymph node capsule. Report of a new case with review of the literature. *Am J Clin Pathol* 86:367–372, 1984.

34. Kempson RL: Benign glandular inclusions in iliac lymph nodes (consultation case). *Am J Surg Pathol* 2:321–325, 1978.

35. Schnurr RC, Delgado G, Chun B: Benign glandular inclusions in para-aortic lymph nodes in women undergoing lymphadenectomies. *Am J Obstet Gynecol* 130:813–816, 1978.

36. Hsu YK, Parmley TH, Rosenhein NB, Bhagava BS, Woodruff JD: Neoplastic and non-neoplastic mesothelial proliferations in pelvic lymph nodes. *Obstet Gynecol* 55:83–88, 1980.

37. Farhi DC, Silverberg SG: Pseudometastases in female genital cancer. *Pathol Annu* 17(Pt.1):47–76, 1982.

38. Kheir SM, Mann WJ, Wilerson JA: Glandular inclusions in lymph nodes. The problem of extensive involvement and relationship to salpingitis. *Am J Surg Pathol* 5:353–359, 1981.

39. Mills SE: Decidua and squamous metaplasia in abdominopelvic lymph nodes. *Int J Gynecol Pathol* 2:209–215, 1983.

40. Covell LM, Discuillo AJ, Knapp RC: Decidual change in pelvic lymph nodes in the presence of cervical squamous cell carcinoma during pregnancy. *Am J Obstet Gynecol* 27:674–676, 1977.

41. Russell HB: Decidual reaction of endometrium ectopic in an abdominal lymph node. *Surg Gynecol Obstet* 81:218–220, 1945.

42. Ioachim HL: Granulomatous lesions of lymph nodes. In *Pathology of Granulomas.* New York, Raven Press, 1983, p 151–187.

43. Roberts FJ, Linsey S: The value of microbial cultures in diagnostic lymph node biopsy. *J Infec Dis* 149:162–165, 1984.

44. Fajardo LF, Berthrong M: Radiation in surgical pathology (Part 1). *Am J Surg Pathol* 2:159–199, 1978.

45. Cleary KR, Osborne BM, Butler JJ: Lymph node infarction foreshadowing malignant lymphoma. *Am J Surg Pathol* 6:435–442, 1982.

46. Maurer R, Schmid U, Davies JD, Mahy NJ, Stansfeld AG, Lukes RJ: Lymph node infarction and malignant lymphoma: a multicentre survey of European, English and American cases. *Histopathology* 10:571–588, 1986.

13

Neuroendocrine Tumors

Elvio G. Silva, M.D.

All neuroendocrine tumors share similar histologic features that make them easy to identify. With minor variations in pattern or cytology, these features persist among tumors in different organs. Identification of neuroendocrine tumors in frozen section is important because their immediate treatment could be significantly different from that of non-neuroendocrine tumors in a similar location. When a tumor is recognized as a neuroendocrine neoplasm, special handling, such as submitting tissue for electron microscopic and hormonal identification, is required.

TERMINOLOGY AND CLASSIFICATION

We classify tumors of the diffuse endocrine system according to their cell size into two groups (1): *1.)* small cell type carcinoma, and *2.)* medium cell type—*a*) carcinoid, and *b*) endocrine carcinoma. The carcinoid and endocrine carcinoma subcategories are based on the absence or presence of abundant mitoses, significant atypia, and necrosis.

Small Cell Carcinomas

The question of whether or not a tumor is neuroendocrine is not of paramount importance in diagnosing small cell carcinomas because all small cell carcinomas are likely to be equally aggressive.

Pathologists are not often asked to render a frozen section diagnosis of small cell carcinoma. The more usual request is to verify by frozen section analysis the representativity for permanent section examination. When a patient has undergone an operation without previous microscopic diagnosis and the pathologist receives tissue for frozen section analysis, the foremost differential diagnosis is lymphoma, especially in the adult patient population. Recognizing lymphoma is particularly important because surgical excision, the most effective treatment for small cell carcinoma at various locations in the body, is not generally indicated in lymphoma. Features seen by light microscopy are useful in differentiating small cell carcinoma from lymphoma. The presence of epithelial differentiation, squamous islands or glands, rosettes, and well demarcated groups of cells help to distinguish carcinoma from lymphoma. Molding between tumor cells is diagnostic of small cell carcinoma, but, because of freezing artifacts, this feature is difficult to observe in frozen section (Fig. 13.1). For differential diagnosis, therefore, it is extremely important to obtain cytologic preparations from the biopsy specimen (Figs. 13.2 and 13.3). When all of these features are not identified in frozen section, the diagnosis should be deferred until the permanent sections have been examined.

Neuroendocrine Tumors of Medium Cell Size

Terminology for endocrine carcinomas varies mainly according to the location of the tumor, although cytologic features and histologic patterns are the same at all sites. The cytologic features and patterns of the carcinoid, or less aggressive type of neuroendocrine tumors, are discussed below.

Cytologic Features

The carcinoid tumors are composed of polygonal cells with a moderate amount of cytoplasm, a round nucleus, finely dispersed chromatin, and an inconspicuous nucleolus. Mitotic figures are rarely seen. A monotonously uniform histologic appearance is characteristic. Since these diagnostic features are not usually observed in frozen section, cytologic preparations from these tumors are essential.

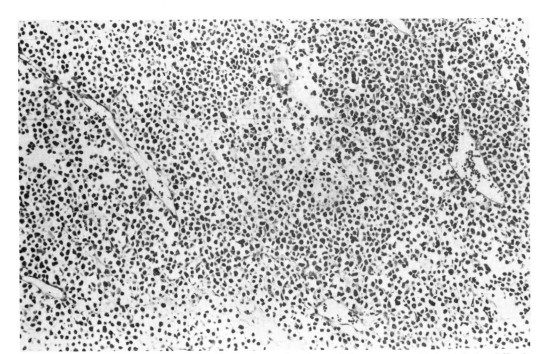

Figure 13.1. Frozen section of small cell carcinoma showing a diffuse pattern which might be difficult to differentiate from lymphoma.

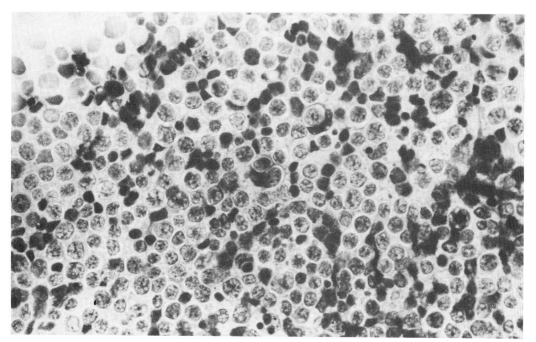

Figure 13.2. Cytologic preparation from same case as Fig 13.1. Small cell carcinoma. Nuclear molding between tumor cells is present.

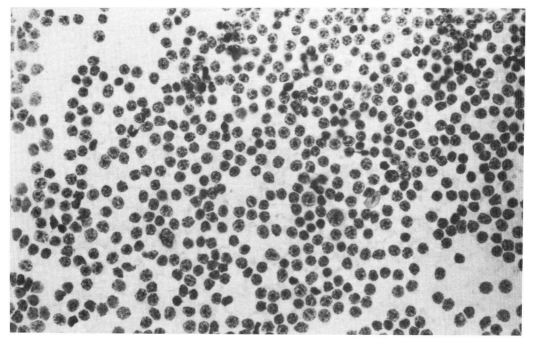

Figure 13.3. Cytologic preparation of small lymphocytic lymphoma. There is lack of cohesion between tumor cells.

Patterns

According to their pattern, neuroendocrine tumors resemble a variety of non-neuroendocrine neoplasms, so that familiarity with the different patterns is important is making the diagnosis. Table 13.1 contains a summary of neuroendocrine tumor patterns and the most common differential diagnoses (Figs. 13.4 and 13.5). In addition to these characteristic patterns and cytologic features, neuroendocrine tumors may occasionally have hypocellular stroma and amyloid between groups of tumor cells.

SPECIAL PROBLEMS ENCOUNTERED DURING FROZEN SECTION OF NEUROENDOCRINE TUMORS

Thyroid

In the thyroid gland, recognition of a neuroendocrine tumor or medullary carcinoma is of paramount significance, because this tumor is treated with total thyroidectomy and lymph node dissection (2). Follicular carcinoma having a microfollicular pattern and Hürthle cell tumor can be mistaken for medullary carcinoma. Follicular neoplasms might be treated with lobectomy only and no lymph node dissection. The differential diagnosis between medullary carcinoma and follicular lesions is based mainly on the identification of small lumina at the center of tumor cell groups; in addition, the features described as typical of neuroendocrine tumors are important diagnostic clues.

See Chapter 3, **Thyroid,** for additional information regarding medullary carcinoma.

Table 13.1.
Neuroendocrine Tumors[a]

Pattern	Differential Diagnosis	Comments
Trabecular	Sex cord tumor in ovary	Tubular (Sertoli cell) and microfollicular (GCT)[b] areas might be identified in sex cord tumors
Insular	Breast carcinoma	Atypical nuclei and variation in cellular characteristics suggest breast carcinoma
	Acinic cell carcinoma	Lattice and cystic patterns and clear cells might be observed in this carcinoma
Glandular	Prostatic carcinoma Breast carcinoma	High mitotic rate, prominent nucleoli, and variation in cell size and shape suggest a nonendocrine carcinoma
Spindle	Sarcoma and spindle carcinoma Adenocarcinoma	Cellularity, atypia, and lack of cellular uniformity suggest sarcoma and sarcomatoid carcinoma

[a]In addition to characteristic pattern and cytologic features of these tumors, sometimes the stroma is hypocellular and amyloid material can be identified between groups of tumors cells.
[b]GCT, granulosa cell tumor.

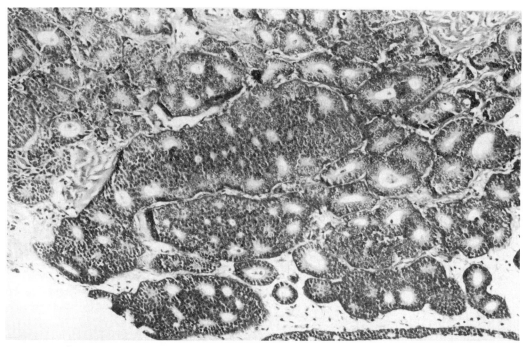

Figure 13.4. Carcinoid displaying insular and glandular pattern.

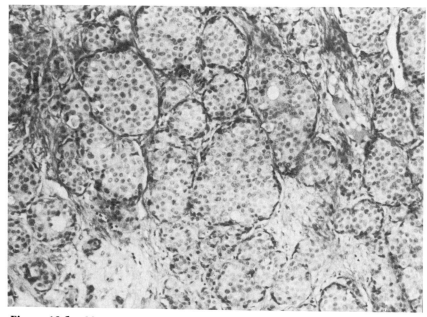

Figure 13.5. Metastatic carcinoma of breast, easily confused with insular carcinoid. Variation in cell size, and nuclear atypia suggest a poorly differentiated carcinoma.

Lung

Differentiating between carcinoid tumors in lung tissue and metastases (e.g., from breast or prostatic carcinoma) by frozen section is not crucial because both tumors are treated in the same manner—surgical excision. The differences in these types of tumors are important in the handling of tissue for further studies, for example, submitting tissue for estrogen receptor analysis in cases of metastatic breast carcinoma. The presence of cellular atypia, mitotic figures, and necrosis suggests metastatic adenocarcinoma over carcinoid. It is not unusual, however, to see foci of breast carcinoma without mitotic figures or necrosis. Therefore the main histologic feature useful in this differential diagnosis is cellular atypia. Since this feature does not show up well in frozen sections, cytologic preparations are essential. See Chapter 6, **Lung,** for additional information regarding carcinoid.

Pancreas and Midportion of Duodenum

Determining the neuroendocrine nature of a pancreatic or duodenal neoplasm is crucial to immediate patient management. The diagnosis of resectable adenocarcinoma in the head of the pancreas or the second portion of duodenum is followed by a radical duodenopancreatectomy (Whipple's operation), a procedure carrying a high mortality rate (3,4). If the pathologic findings point to the diagnosis of neuroendocrine tumor (namely islet cell tumor) the surgeon usually performs only a local resection of the neoplasm; this operation is less complicated and has better postoperative results. Obtaining cytologic preparations in addition to the frozen section is indispensable to the differential diagnosis of these pancreatic neoplasms (Figs. 13.6 and 13.7). One special type of neuroendocrine tumor, the somatostatinoma, which often occurs in the duodenum, is characterized by a predominantly glandular pattern, and is easily confused with adenocarcinoma (5,6). Frequently this type of neuroendocrine neoplasm also contains psammoma bodies, which, in addition to the cytologic features, are helpful in identifying this lesion (Fig. 13.8). Psammoma bodies are not usually found in a nonpapillary adenocarcinoma.

Ovary

Neuroendocrine Versus Non-neuroendocrine Tumors

Different kinds of primary ovarian tumors including nonendocrine neoplasms, sex cord tumors, and dysgerminomas may be mistaken for neuroendocrine neoplasms, but they are treated in similar fashion. Differentiating between neuroendocrine and non-neuroendocrine tumors of the ovary is important only in cases in which the latter may represent a metastasis. The differential diagnosis implies different treatments; when a carcinoma is recognized as metastatic, a search for its possible origin in the gastrointestinal tract is mandatory during the exploratory laparotomy.

See Chapter 5, **Gynecologic Specimens,** for additional information regarding the ovary.

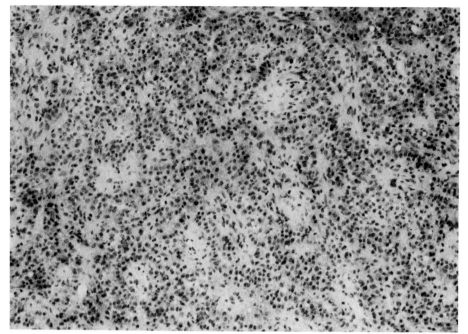

Figure 13.6. Frozen section. Islet cell tumor showing an organoid pattern is difficult to differentiate from a poorly differentiated adenocarcinoma.

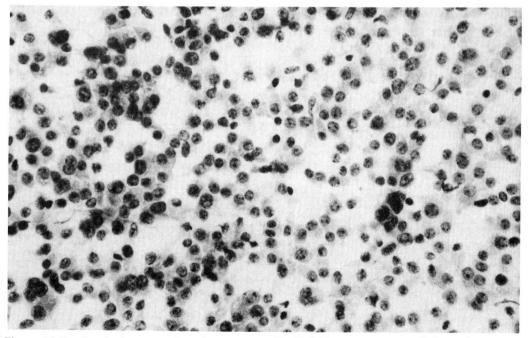

Figure 13.7. Cytologic preparation of same case as Fig 13.6. The monotonous cellular uniformity and lack of significant atypia or mitoses favor an endocrine neoplasm over poorly differentiated carcinoma.

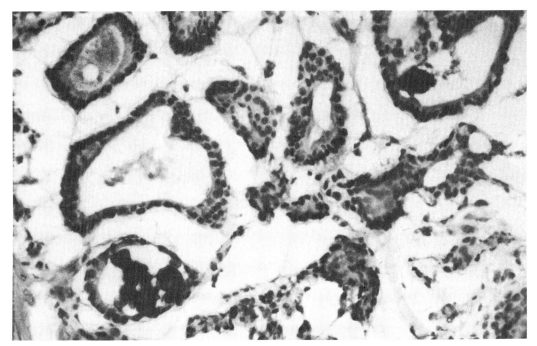

Figure 13.8. Psammomatous carcinoid of duodenum. The presence of psammoma bodies and the absence of atypical cells are useful features in identifying this neoplasm.

Carcinoid: Primary Versus Metastatic Tumors

Primary versus metastatic carcinoid involvement in the ovary should be differentiated if possible. Since both types are neuroendocrine tumors, the only means of distinguishing them is to identify another component such as teratoma, Sertoli-Leydig cell tumor, or mucinous tumor. If any of these components is found, the carcinoid is primary in the ovary. Bilaterality of a carcinoid tumor in the ovary is diagnostic of metastatic disease. When a carcinoid in the ovary is identified as metastatic, a search for and resection of the primary is mandatory.

REFERENCES

1. Silva EG: Tumors of the diffuse endocrine system, histochemical and electron-optic aids, and pitfalls in diagnosis. *CRC Crit Rev Clin Lab Sci* 21:19–49, 1984.
2. Guillamondegui OM, Goepfert H: Thyroid cancer. In: Gates G (ed): *Current Therapy in Otolaryngol Head and Neck Surgery.* Philadelphia, Becker, 1984–1985, p 270–275.
3. Bradley EL, Zeppa R: The pancreas. In Sabiston DC, Jr (ed): *Davis-Christopher Testbook of Surgery: The Biological Basis of Modern Surgical Practice.* Philadelphia, W. B. Saunders, 1981, p 1281.
4. Tepper J, Nardi G, Suit H: Carcinoma of the pancreas: Review of MGH experience from 1963 to 1973: Analysis of surgical failure and implications for radiation therapy. *Cancer* 37:1519–1524, 1976.
5. Chen R, Tang C-K, Lee JY-Y, Kurland CL: Duodenal somatostatin-containing tumor with psammoma bodies. *Hum Pathol* 16:517–519, 1985.
6. Dayal Y, Doos WG, O'Brien MJ, Nunnemacher G. DeLellis RA, Wolfe HJ: Psammomatous somatostatinomas of the duodenum. *Am J Surg Pathol* 7:563–665, 1983.

14

Bone Radiation-Injured Tissue, Skin and Soft Tissue

Elvio G. Silva, M.D.

BONE

The only reason for examining a frozen section from a lesion in bone is to determine whether the tissue sample is adequate for diagnosis. If the tissue is not ossified/calcified, some of its fragments may be examined by frozen section. It is very important to recognize lymphomas in order to prepare the tissue for proper studies; for this we rely on cytologic preparations. If the lesions are calcified, cytologic preparations can be made from the soft tissues component in and around the calcified portion of the specimen.

Frozen section might also be requested for patients undergoing arthroplasty or other orthopaedic procedures to be certain that no inflammation or infection is present in the area to be operated upon. The tissue submitted for frozen section in such cases is usually synovium or intramedullary contents.

In cases of tumor-containing cartilage, frozen section slides should be stained with hematoxylin and eosin because metachromatic stains (i.e., toluidine blue) often do not stain cartilage.

RADIATION-INJURED TISSUE

Frozen section evaluation of tissues that have received radiotherapy usually entails problems because of the presence of atypical cells. The morphologic manifestations of radiation injury may be seen as soon as 10 days after treatment and may persist for as long as 5 years or longer (1).

The atypical cells associated with radiotherapy may be seen in stroma and epithelium. Irradiated cells often demonstrate atypical features relative to surrounding noninjured cells. In a group of 10 to 15 epithelial cells, for example, only a minority will be atypical (Fig. 14.1). The nuclei affected by radiation are enlarged, hyperchromatic, and irregular in shape.

Clues to detecting atypical changes caused by radiotherapy are the

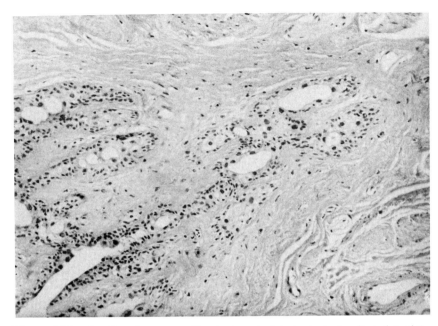

Figure 14.1. Irradiated prostate. Glands show isolated, atypical enlarged nuclei.

presence of nuclear and cytoplasmic vesicles and angulated cytoplasmic projections. In addition, the stroma shows edema with fibrin and eosinophils, telangiectatic blood vessels with prominent endothelial cells, dilated lymphatics, and foam cells in vessel walls (1-3).

SKIN

Frozen section of biopsied skin is done most commonly to evaluate the margins of basal cell carcinoma. Although this is usually an easy task, differentiating a basal cell carcinoma that involves the dermis from tangentially sectioned hair follicles is sometimes a problem. The presence, in one area, of more than two nests of basaloid cells with irregular distribution, many mitotic figures, and no surrounding or overlying pilosebaceous structures is diagnostic of basal cell carcinoma (Fig. 14.2 and 14.3).

Although some writers have suggested the use of frozen section to diagnose malignant melanoma (4,5), our policy is not to freeze pigmented lesions. If a malignant melanoma is frozen for histologic examination, the pathologist must be aware that any lesion, and tissue in general, will be thicker in frozen than in permanent sections. Shafir and associates (6) studied frozen and permanent sections of 29 skin melanomas and found that the melanomas in frozen section were 0.1 to 0.4 mm thicker than those in permanent section (6). Our results were similar when we compared the thickness of several tumors in frozen section with their thickness in the permanent section (Silva, unpublished data).

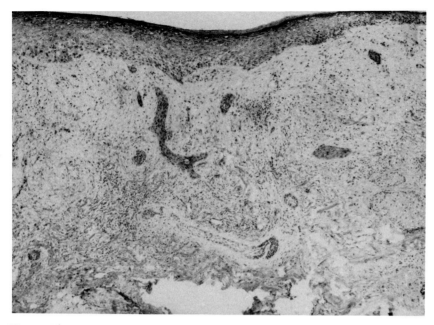

Figure 14.2. Frozen section of basal cell carcinoma. Groups of basaloid cells show a disorganized distribution in the dermis.

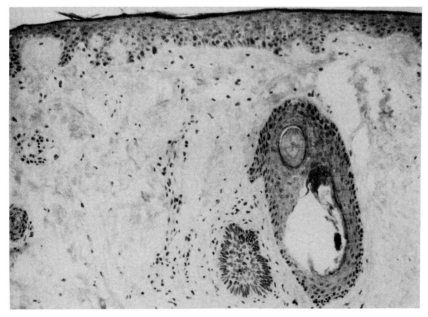

Figure 14.3. Single groups of basal cells which are part of the hair follicle are present.

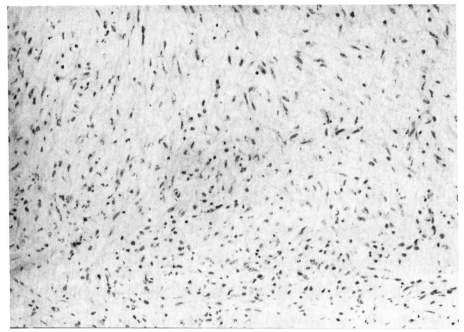

Figure 14.4. Frozen section showing reactive fibrous tissue at the margin of resection of a spindle cell sarcoma.

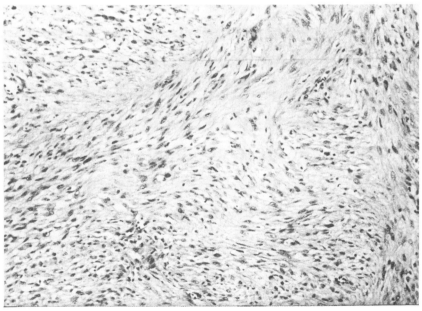

Figure 14.5. Spindle cell sarcoma. It is necessary to obtain a section from the primary tumor to compare it with the histologic features displayed at the margin (see Fig. 14.4.).

SOFT TISSUE

In the case of soft tissue lesions, the frozen section technique is used primarily for histologic evaluation of margins of resection. These margins need to be studied when a generous excision is not possible, or when lesions are surrounded by fibrotic tissue which obscures the advancing margin. A frozen section from the tumor must be obtained before the margins of resection are evaluated, even in cases where the diagnosis of the tumor is known. Variations on morphology may result from additional treatment. A frozen section from the lesion will determine the exact character of the tumor and differentiate it from surrounding tissue (Figs. 14.4 and 14.5).

Margins of resection are difficult to evaluate in three types of soft tissue tumors: those that are status-post radiotherapy having a major fibroblastic component, angiosarcoma, and desmoid tumors. Radiotherapy may result in a markedly atypical cellular population in connective tissue. Such a proliferation might be difficult to differentiate from sarcomatous cells (see RADIATION-INJURED TISSUE, this Chapter). For margins of resection of angiosarcoma sections from both the central and peripheral portions of the neoplasm must be compared with the margins of resection. The reason for submitting sections from these two different areas is because the peripheral areas are usually better differentiated than the central areas. The differential diagnosis between proliferating vessels in the soft tissue and a neovascular lesion should be based on the absence or presence of atypical endothelial cells. For evaluation of the margins of resection of desmoid tumors, the connective tisue must be devoid of fibrosis.

Soft tissue lesions are rarely diagnosed exclusively by frozen section. This is done only when lesions are too deep to be diagnosed from biopsy, as is often the case with retroperitoneal and mediastinal masses. For these patients, frozen section is done to confirm that the lesion is of soft tissue origin; such a tumor needs no further classification, because it must be completely excised. There are very few sarcomas that might be confused with other types of tumors. In our experience, we have encountered such a problem when a malignant schwannoma with glandular elements was interpreted as carcinoma. Tissue for frozen section examination is needed, however, because other processes may be occurring at these sites that are not best treated with resection, such as infections, lymphomas, and germ cell tumors (7). Fortunately, these three processes are easily differentiated from soft tissue neoplasms. Biopsies are necessary to determine definitive treatment regimens. Tissue for culture is also required for diagnosis of infectious processes. Tissue for cell markers in lymphoma may be taken as needed.

Frozen section examination has been proposed in cases of necrotizing fasciitis to facilitate early treatment of this rapidly progressive, potentially fatal soft tissue infection (8).

REFERENCES

1. Fajardo LF, Berthrong M: Radiation injury in surgical pathology. Part I. *Am J Surg Pathol* 2:159–199, 1978.
2. Berthrong M, Fajardo LF: Radiation injury in surgical pathology. Part II. Alimentary tract. *Am J Surg Pathol* 5:153–178, 1981.

3. Fechner RE: The surgical pathology of iatrogenic lesions. In Silverberg SG (ed): *Principles and Practice of Surgical Pathology.* New York, John Wiley & Sons, 1983, p. 77.

4. Little JH, Davis NC: Frozen section diagnosis of suspected malignant melanoma of the skin. *Cancer* 34:1163–1172, 1974.

5. Milton GW: Aetiology of melanoma. In Milton GW (ed): *Malignant Melanoma of the Skin and Mucous Membrane.* New York, Churchill Livingstone, 1977, p 21.

6. Shafir R. Hiss J, Tsur H, Bubis JJ: Pitfalls in frozen section diagnosis of malignant melanoma. *Cancer* 51:1168–1170, 1983.

7. Logothetis CJ, Samuels ML, Selig DE, Dexeus FH, Johnson DE, Swanson DA, von Eschenbach AC: Chemotherapy of extragonadal germ cell tumors. *J Clin Oncol* 3:316–325, 1985.

8. Stamenkovic I, Lew PD: Early recognition of potentially fatal necrotizing fasciitis: The use of frozen-section biopsy. *N Engl J Med* 310:1689–1693, 1984.

Index

Page numbers in *italics* denote figures; those followed by "t" denote tables.

293